Clinical Oral Medicine

Clinical Oral Medicine

Editor: Theresa Martino

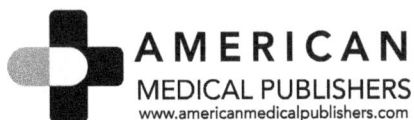

AMERICAN
MEDICAL PUBLISHERS
www.americanmedicalpublishers.com

AMERICAN
MEDICAL PUBLISHERS
www.americanmedicalpublishers.com

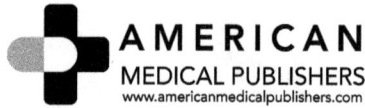

Cataloging-in-Publication Data

Clinical oral medicine / edited by Theresa Martino.
    p. cm.
Includes bibliographical references and index.
ISBN 978-1-63927-639-4
1. Oral medicine. 2. Dentistry. 3. Mouth--Diseases.
4. Mouth--Diseases--Treatment. I. Martino, Theresa.
RC815 .C55 2023
617.522--dc23

American Medical Publishers,
41 Flatbush Avenue,
1st Floor, New York,
NY 11217, USA

ISBN 978-1-63927-639-4 (Hardback)

Contents

Permissions

List of Contributors

Index

Preface

Oral medicine is referred to as a discipline of dentistry which is focused on the care of oral health. It is concerned with the diagnosis and management of various medical problems that affect the orofacial region. It is focused on the treatment of oral mucosal abnormalities, including temporomandibular disorders, salivary gland disorders and oral cancer. It is also concerned with the diagnosis and management of facial pain occurring due to neurologic or musculoskeletal conditions, and smell and taste disorders, along with the identification of various infectious and systematic diseases. Oral medicine is a non-surgical specialty, which includes procedures like therapeutic injections, small excisions, diagnostic biopsies, along with other minor surgical interventions. It also manages the oral and dental problems of cancer patients who have oral mucositis, oral pathology associated with radiation therapy, and bisphosphonate-related osteonecrosis of the jaws. Various conditions that are managed by oral medicine include pemphigus vulgaris, Behçet's disease and lichen planus. This book provides comprehensive insights on clinical oral medicine. It will prove to be immensely beneficial to students and researchers in this field.

The information contained in this book is the result of intensive hard work done by researchers in this field. All due efforts have been made to make this book serve as a complete guiding source for students and researchers. The topics in this book have been comprehensively explained to help readers understand the growing trends in the field.

I would like to thank the entire group of writers who made sincere efforts in this book and my family who supported me in my efforts of working on this book. I take this opportunity to thank all those who have been a guiding force throughout my life.

Editor

Isolation and Identification of Potentially Pathogenic Microorganisms Associated with Dental Caries in Human Teeth Biofilms

Xiuqin Chen, Eric Banan-Mwine Daliri[iD], Ramachandran Chelliah and Deog-Hwan Oh *

Department of Food Science and Biotechnology, College of Agriculture and Life Sciences, Kangwon National University, Chuncheon 200-701, Korea; cxq20135331@gmail.com (X.C.); ericdaliri@kangwon.ac.kr (E.B.-M.D.); ramachandran865@gmail.com (R.C.)
* Correspondence: deoghwa@kangwon.ac.kr

Abstract: Dental caries is attributed to the predominance of cariogenic microorganisms. Cariogenic microorganisms are pathological factors leading to acidification of the oral microenvironment, which is related to the initiation and progression of caries. The accepted cariogenic microorganism is *Streptococcus mutans* (*S. mutans*). However, studies have found that caries could occur in the absence of *S. mutans*. This study aimed to assess the presence of potentially cariogenic microorganisms in human teeth biofilm. The microorganisms were isolated from human mouth and freshly extracted human maxillary incisors extracted for reasons of caries. The isolates were sorted based on their acidogenic and aciduric properties, and the *S. mutans* was used as the reference strain. Four potentially cariogenic strains were selected. The selected strains were identified as *Streptococcus salivarius* (*S. salivarius*), *Streptococcus anginosus* (*S. anginosus*), *Leuconostoc mesenteroides* (*L. mesenteroides*), and *Lactobacillus sakei* (*L. sakei*) through morphological analysis followed by 16S rRNA gene sequence analysis. The cariogenicity of isolates was analyzed. We show, for the first time, an association between *L. sakei* (present in fermented food) and dental caries. The data provide useful information on the role of lactic acid bacteria from fermented foods and oral commensal streptococci in dental caries.

Keywords: cariogenic microorganisms; isolation; cariogenic potential; dental caries

1. Introduction

Dental caries is a biofilm-mediated disease in which the cariogenic bacterial group is a limited subset of the many species found in biofilms on the surface of the tooth [1]. Caries results in the damage of the calcified structure of the dental apatite (tooth enamel). Despite the numerous efforts made by scientists to simulate the biomineralized crystallization–amorphous boundary of hard tissue in nature and to induce the epitaxial growth of enamel with current technology, damage of tooth enamel is irreversible [2,3]. Dental caries is a preventable disease that places a considerable burden on the economy and quality-of-life [1]. The data from the Global Burden of Disease (GBD) confirmed that untreated permanent dental caries remains the most common health condition globally in 2015 (34.1 percent) [4]. The GBD latest study in 2017 estimates that 3.5 billion people worldwide are affected by oral diseases, with untreated dental caries is one of the commonest non-communicable diseases worldwide [5]. Besides, increasing evidence suggests that dental caries may has adverse effects on cardiovascular diseases [6], such as coronary heart disease [7], hypertension [8], and arteriosclerosis [9]. Furthermore, an association between dental caries and pregnancy outcomes has been identified [10]. Therefore, tooth-preserving preventive care must be taken seriously.

At present, the accepted etiology of caries is a four-factor theory that includes oral microorganisms, oral environment, host, and time. Long-term changes in the availability of microbial metabolic substrates may change the ecological balance of the microbiome [11]. Frequent intake of sugars results in saccharification (acid production) by oral microbes. There is evidence to suggest that sugar supplementation can disrupt the homeostasis between acid-producing and none-acid-producing microorganisms [12]. *S. mutans* has been a major focus in the etiology of dental caries, it has long been considered as a pathogenic bacteria of dental caries, because it not only produces lactic acid but also grows at low pH. However, *S. mutans* was not detected in 10 to 20 percent of dental caries patients, so it is now clear that *S. mutans* is not the only pathogenic bacterium related to the etiology of dental caries [13]. A meta genetic analysis data have shown that caries is caused by an overall change in the composition of the oral microbiome [14]. In the absence of *S. mutans*, other acid-producing species could perform the cariogenic function [15,16]. Therefore, to prevent dental caries, it is necessary to control cariogenic microorganisms (including but not limited to *S. mutans*). Evidence is emerging that acid-producing bacterial species other than *S. mutans*, species of the genera *Veillonella* [17], *Scardovia* [18], *Lactobacillus* [19], *Propionibacterium* [20], and low-pH non-*S. mutans streptococci* [21] present in dental biofilm, as colonizers may result in cariogenic conditions in the mouth.

Pathogenic factors of oral microorganisms play key roles in caries development. The coalition of multiple pathogenic microorganisms contributes to initiate and advanced disease. The composing of oral microbiota can easily change by diet and environment [22]. Acidogenic and aciduric microorganisms in the tooth biofilm play an important role in the pathogenesis of dental caries. Studies on the potential cariogenicity of those microorganisms could provide a scientific reference for the prevention and treatment of dental caries. It is still a far way to fully understand due to the complexity of oral bacterial community dynamics. There is no reference demonstrating the specific definition of cariogenic oral microorganisms. In our study, acidogenic and aciduric microorganisms were isolated from the different niche of individuals (the number of the people with caries: 7; the number of caries-free people: 11; the number of infected teeth: 18), and the data showed that potential pathogenic bacteria were presented in all groups of samples (caries, caries-free, and infected tooth). Furthermore, the cariogenicity of isolates was measured.

2. Materials and Methods

2.1. Isolation and Identification of Potentially Cariogenic Microorganisms

The process of isolation and screening of strains is shown in Figure 1.

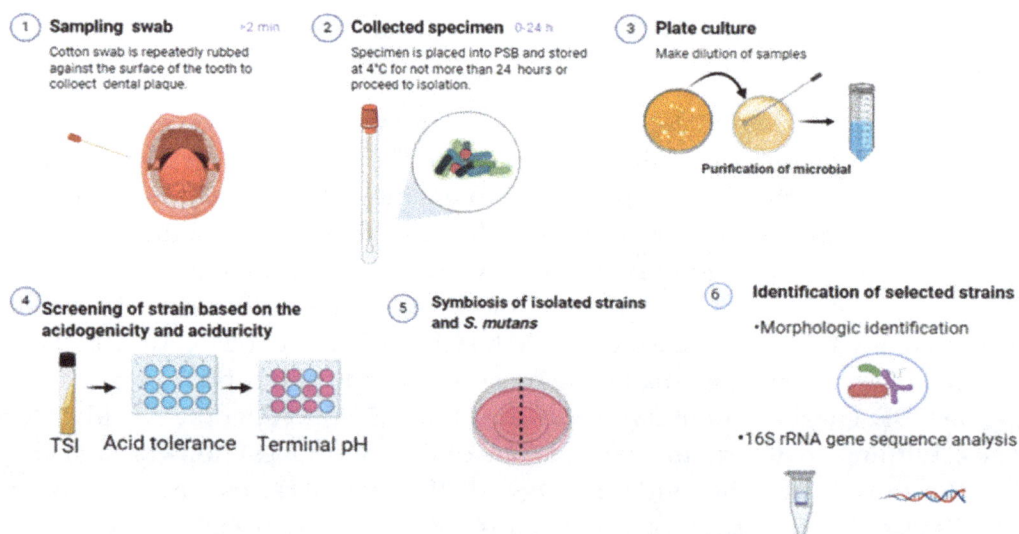

Figure 1. The process of isolation and screening of potentially cariogenic microorganisms in human teeth biofilms. TSI: triple sugar iron agar; PSB: protein solubilization buffer; *S. mutans: Streptococcus mutans.*

2.1.1. Sample Collection and Isolation of Bacterial Strain

A total of 18 volunteers aged 21–56 years provided dental biofilm samples in which 7 of them are previously reported dental caries (DMFT > 0); the subjects were trained to sample and completed the questionnaire. All participants were informed about the aim of this study and signed informed consent before entering the study, the dental condition and diet habits were recorded for each participant. The modified protocol of a previous study was used to collect oral microorganisms [23]. Briefly, supragingival biofilm samples were collected using a sterile cotton swab in the morning before tooth brushing and breakfast. On the other hand, microorganisms also isolated from freshly extracted human maxillary incisors extracted for caries reasons (kindly provided by Limedentistry, Chuncheon, Korea). Infected teeth and the swabs containing biofilm samples were separately placed into 1 mL of 0.1% buffered peptone water (BPW, Difco, New York, NY, USA) and stored at 4 °C to use for not more than 24 h before the experiment. Samples were then sonicated for 30 s, vortexed to disperse, and the suspension dilutions were plated on Lactobacillus MRS agar (MRS, Difco), Tryptone Soy agar (TSA, Difco) with the addition of 5% defibrinated sheep blood, and Eosin methylene blue agar (EMB Difco). Single pure colonies were in a given sector of a plate, well-isolated colonies were selected and subcultured for isolation on a solid medium to ensure purity.

2.1.2. Screening of Strains Based on Cariogenicity

The isolated microorganisms were screened based on their acidogenicity and aciduricity using a method described previously with some modification [23]. Briefly, all isolated microorganisms were inoculated onto slant of the triple sugar iron (TSI) agar to determine the ability of organisms to ferment glucose, lactose, and sucrose, leave the cap on loosely and incubate the tube at 37 °C in ambient air for 18 to 24 h. Changing the color of the TSI to yellow suggesting fermentation of sugar from which strains were selected. Besides, the acid tolerance of selected strains has been measured, prepare Brain Heart Infusion (BHI, Difco) and MRS broth media supplemented with 1% (m/v) sucrose, the pH of media adjusted dropwise with 1 M HCl to get "acid medium" (pH 5.5, enamel demineralization critical pH). Isolated strains overnight culture were inoculated into "acid medium" and conventional medium, respectively, the survival rate of selected microorganisms was measured, immediately after resuspension (Time 0) and after 60 min (Time 60); the isolates with a survival rate more than 90% were selected. Furthermore, the acidogenicity of strains was measured through growing in the broth media supplemented with 1% (m/v) sucrose overnight, and the terminal pH of the suspension was measured by pH meter (Orion Star A211, Thermos Fisher, Beverly, MA, USA). The acidogenicity of strains was classified according to previously published descriptions, low (pH $\geq$ 5.5), moderate (3.5 $\leq$ pH $\leq$ 5.5), and high (pH $\leq$ 3.5); high and moderate acid-producing microorganisms were selected (data not shown). Finally, four strains were selected with high acidogenicity and high acid tolerance.

2.1.3. Symbiosis of Isolated Strains and *S. mutans*

The cariogenic biofilm of human teeth is a unique 3D circular structure made up of multiple species, with *S. mutans* at its core and other acidogenic microorganisms on its periphery, this community is the causative factor [24]. Cariogenic microorganisms are symbiotic in the biofilm. Therefore, we evaluated the symbiosis of isolated strains and *S. mutans* through the disk diffusion test. Wafers were plated on the BHI agar plate where *S. mutans* had been placed; 35 µL suspension and supernatant of isolated strains were added into wafers, respectively, and the plate was left to incubate at 37 °C overnight. In the same way, wafers containing the suspension and supernatant of *S. mutans* were placed on the agar plate where isolated strains had been placed. The results showed that all four selected strains and *S. mutans* are symbiotic (data not shown).

2.1.4. Bacterial Identification—Morphological and Biotyping

After selecting potential cariogenic oral microorganisms, single colonies were inoculated on the BHI broth and incubated at 37 °C in ambient air for 18 to 24 h. Gram staining reactions were performed for each selected strains, and the microbe morphology was observed under the microscope. Besides, the type of hemolysis of individual colonies was evaluated; 16S rRNA sequencing was used to identify the selected cariogenic isolates to the genus level and to determine whether there were clusters of similar organisms [25].

2.2. Evaluation of Cariogenicity of Isolated Oral Microorganisms

The evaluation criterion of pathogenic bacteria associated with dental caries is not well-established. Acidogenicity and aciduricity are generally accepted as characteristics of cariogenic microorganisms [26]. Cariogenic microorganisms must not only produce acids but must also have the ability to grow in a rather hostile acidic milieu. The taxa distinctive of low pH of bacteria represent potential importance in disease progression from initial to more advanced caries. It is reported that enrichment and acid production of acid-tolerant microflora in the oral is the mean cause of the demineralization of tooth enamel [27]. Besides, cariogenicity also depends on the ability of microorganisms to adhere to the tooth surface. Therefore, the ability of biofilm formation is considered to be an essential characteristic. With the sugar intake frequently, over time, the acid-induced adaptation and selection processes of oral microorganisms may shift the demineralization and remineralization balance into a net mineral loss, leading to the progression of dental caries. Therefore, the degree of enamel demineralization can be used to assess the cariogenic characteristics of a bacterium [28].

2.2.1. Measurement of Acidogenicity

Acidogenicity of isolated potentially pathogenic oral bacteria was measured according to the method reported previously [29]. Briefly, bacteria were inoculated in BHI, and growth was monitored by SpectraMax i3 plate reader (Molecular Devices Korea, LLC, Seoul, Korea) until the optical density reached 0.5 (approximately 10^8–10^9 CFU/mL) at 595 nm. An amount of 0.1% BPW (pH 7.0) was used to wash the bacterial cells and incubated at 37 °C for 2 h for starvation. *S. mutans* KCTC 3065 (purchased from Korean Collection for Type Cultures, Daejeon, Korea) and isolates were inoculated into 2 mL of artificial saliva supplemented with 0.5% of sodium chloride and 2% of soy peptone separately. One percent (m/v) extra sucrose was added into the above artificial saliva solution to measure the sucrose dependence of acid production, while a sample without extra sucrose was used as control. Bacteria were grown at 37 °C and determined the pH of suspension using the pH meter.

2.2.2. Measurement of Acid Tolerance

Acid tolerance of isolated potentially pathogenic oral bacteria was measured using a previously reported method with slightly modified [29]. Briefly, 200 µL of an overnight culture of *S. mutans* and isolates were washed by glycine buffer adjust to pH 3.5 (potential killing pH) and then incubated at 37 °C for 2 h. The choice of the pH 3.5 as a detection line of aciduricity was based on the defining killing pH [27]. Bacteria would adapt to acids when exposed to a sublethal pH in the mouth. Therefore, the adapted bacteria and intrinsically acid-tolerant ones will survive in a lethal pH (pH 3.5) environment, while non-acid-tolerant bacteria will not. Acid tolerance was presented as the percentage survival rate, which was calculated with the following formula: (number of cells following incubation at pH 3.5)/(number of cells before incubation at pH 3.5) × 100.

2.2.3. In Vitro Biofilm Formation and Quantification

The biofilm formation and quantification assay were performed using a method described previously with some modification [30]. Briefly, *S. mutans* and isolates grew in BHI medium with the addition of 1% (m/v) sucrose, and we monitored the growth until reaching an optical density of 0.5

at 595 nm. Resin denture (Shefu INC, Jersey, NJ, USA) were purchased online and dipped in the 70% ethanol for 30 min to eliminate the interference of natural microorganism on the surface of the resin denture. Sterile distilled water (DW) was used to rinse the disinfected resin denture and remove the remaining ethanol residue. Furthermore, the materials dried in a laminar flow safety cabinet and kept the ultra-violet lamp on during the period of desiccation to make sure the resin denture would not be contaminated with other bacteria. Identical disinfected resin dentures were individually transferred to the wells of 24-well plates (Spl LifeSciences, Pocheon, Korea) filled with 2 mL of BHI medium with the addition of 1% (m/v) sucrose per well and was inoculated with the bacteria that were growing in the logarithmic phase to achieve a final concentration of 3–4 log CFU/mL. Three separate treatments were performed and a group of wells filled with 2 mL of BHI medium with the addition of 1% (m/v) sucrose without bacterial inoculation was used as the control; static biofilms were grown on the surface of the resin denture for 48 h at 37 °C.

In vitro static biofilm was formed on the surface of resin dentures and quantified through crystal violet (CV) assay and cell enumeration. Resin dentures were washed three times with 0.1% BPW to remove the planktonic bacteria and transferred to a new 24-well plate, and then, 2 mL of 1% CV (m/v) were added into each well for 30 min to stain the biofilm. Subsequently, the stained denture was washed with running water to remove the crystal violet from the surface. The biofilm bound by CV was eluted with 2 mL of 70% ethanol and incubated at room temperature for 30 min. The absorbance of the resulting CV solution was measured at a wavelength of 595 nm using the SpectraMax i3 plate reader (Molecular Devices Korea, LLC, Seoul, Korea).

The number of viable sessile cells was determined using the protocol described previously [31]. In brief, after growing in the medium for 48 h, attached biofilms of each strain were individually washed three times with 0.1% BPW and transferred to the 15 mL plastic tube filled with 5 mL 0.1% BPW and 0.5 g sterile glass beads (<106 μm). Additionally, adhered cells were removed by vortexing on a vortexer at speed of 4000 r/min for 1 min. One hundred microliters of serial dilutions of suspension were spread onto BHI agar plates. The plates were incubated at 37 °C for 24 h, and colonies were expressed as log CFU/tooth. CV assay and cell enumeration were performed in three independent experiments with at least three technical replicates for each.

2.2.4. Dissolution of Tooth Enamel

The main chemical component of tooth enamel is hydroxyapatite (HAP). The ability to dissolve HAP and release Ca^{2+} ions from the tooth is a clinical feature of cariogenic bacteria [32]. The ability of isolated strains to dissolve HAP was determined using protocols described previously with slight modification [28]; the assay was conducted as follows. Freshly extracted human intact teeth extracted for periodontal disease reasons (kindly provided by Limedentistry, Chuncheon, Korea) and were sterilized and dried using the protocol of resin denture sterilization described in Section 2.2.3. The disinfected teeth were placed in each well of 24-well plates filled with 2 mL of BHI medium with the addition of 1% (m/v) sucrose per well and were inoculated with 1% isolated bacteria, respectively. After 96 h of incubation at 37 °C, the Ca^{2+} ions release was measured using o-Cresolphthalein Complexone (OCPC) colorimetric method. An amount of 1 mL aliquot of calcium assay solution was reacted with 10 μL of the test samples. The absorbance of the resulting solution was measured at a wavelength of 575 nm. To eliminate the interference of different human teeth to the experimental results, each tooth was repeatedly disinfected and used alternately after each experiment; the data of Ca^{2+} ions release were expressed as average. The teeth were immersed in the medium without inoculation as the negative control, the pH of the medium adjusted by citric acid to 4.5.

2.3. Statistical Analysis

Each experiment was performed in triplicate, and mean values for all indicators were calculated from the independent triplicate trials. All the numerical data obtained were analyzed by one-way ANOVA using GraphPad software version 5 and Tukey's multiple comparison test at 5% levels.

3. Results and Discussion

3.1. Isolation and Identification of Potentially Cariogenic Microorganisms

A total of 106 strains were isolated from samples using plate cultural method, among which four strains were identified to have similar characteristics of acid-production and acid resistance with the reference strain (*S. mutans* KCTC3065). The identification based on their morphological characteristics and the results of the 16S rRNA sequencing of the isolates are summarized in Table 1. The four selected strains were identified as *S. salivarius*, *S. anginosus*, *L. mesenteroides*, and *L. sakei*. It is worth noting that potential cariogenic bacteria were isolated from all three different sources including the group of no previously reported dental caries (DMFT = 0). Our results are in agreement with Richard et al. (2018), who proposed that interspecies competition of oral microbiota is altered before visible lesions appear on the tooth [33]. Interestingly, *L. mesenteroides* along with *L. sakei* are frequently found on meat [34]. Besides, *L. sakei* is commonly found in Korean Kimchi, which is a traditional Korean fermented vegetable; Kimchi is processed with cabbage and various seasonings that are consumed by every Korean family throughout the year [35]. Soo Youn Lee et al. (2018) have shown that the *L. mesenteroides* and *L. sakei* isolated from Kimchi have the potential to decrease obesity symptoms [36]. It is worth noting that the biofilm samples were collected from Koreans who have diet habits of frequent Kimchi intake. Our results, therefore, lead us to speculate that these bacteria may have come from dietary residues in the mouth. It is reported that *L. sakei* from Kimchi are promising anti-noroviral candidates [37]. Studies have shown that *L. sakei* CRL1862 and *L. mesenteroides* Com75 could be environmentally friendly agents against foodborne pathogens [38,39]. No study or evidence has however demonstrated that the intake of probiotics may have potential cariogenic or cariostatic effects. Ananieva et al. (2017) isolated *L. mesenteroides* from people who were diagnosed with acute profound caries [40]. However, fewer studies investigated their cariogenic associations. Though *S. salivarius* and *S. anginosus* have been considered as oral commensal flora, some findings suggest that *S. salivarius* and *S. anginosus* isolated from deep proximal caries lesion could be considered as indices for caries activity [41,42].

Table 1. Morphological characteristics and biotyping of the bacterial isolates.

No.	Gram	Hemolytic	Isolated Source	NCBI Blast Sequencing Results
C-1	+	γ-hemolysis	Human mouth (caries)	*Streptococcus salivarius*
C-2	+	β-hemolysis	Infected teeth	*Streptococcus anginosus*
C-3	+	γ-hemolysis	Human mouth (caries)	*Leuconostoc mesenteroides*
C-4	+	β-hemolysis	Human mouth(caries-free)	*Lactobacillus sakei*

3.2. Cariogenicity of Isolated Oral Microorganisms

3.2.1. Acidogenic Potential of Isolated Oral Microorganisms and Their Acid Tolerance

Half a percent of sodium chloride and 2% of soy peptone were added into artificial saliva to simulate a real oral environment. The sucrose metabolize ability of isolated bacteria to produce acid was expressed as pH value (Figure 2). When 1% (m/v) sucrose was added into the growth medium, the amount of acid production by both isolates and reference strain increased significantly ($p < 0.05$). The pH of the culture medium of all bacteria were reduced to 4–5 after the 24 h culture and below the enamel demineralization critical pH (pH 5.5). The acid tolerance of the bacteria was defined as the percentage of cell survival obtained after exposition in pH 3.5 for 60 min, the results are shown in Figure 3. The data revealed that the range of percentage of survival of all strains was 45.07–65.36% in which *L. mesenteroides* showed the highest acid tolerance with 65.36% cell survival. Meanwhile, there was no significant difference between *S. salivarius*, *S. anginosus*, *L. sakei*, and *S. mutans*. *L. mesenteroides* displayed the highest acid tolerance and was isolated from a person who has dental caries reported.

Currently, the pathway of acid metabolism of these strains is incompletely explored. Besides, evidence suggests that the link between acid tolerance and acidogenicity of bacteria is inconsistent [23]. This is in agreement with our results in this study (Figures 3 and 4). In our study, when comparisons were made across isolates and reference strain (*S. mutans* KCTC 3065), there were no statistically significant differences for acid production (Figure 2). Likewise, all the isolates showed high acid tolerance, in particular *L. mesenteroides*. Hence, these results, along with the previously reported microbiological pathology of dental caries, lead us to speculate that the isolates in this study may be cariogenicity, although more evidence is needed.

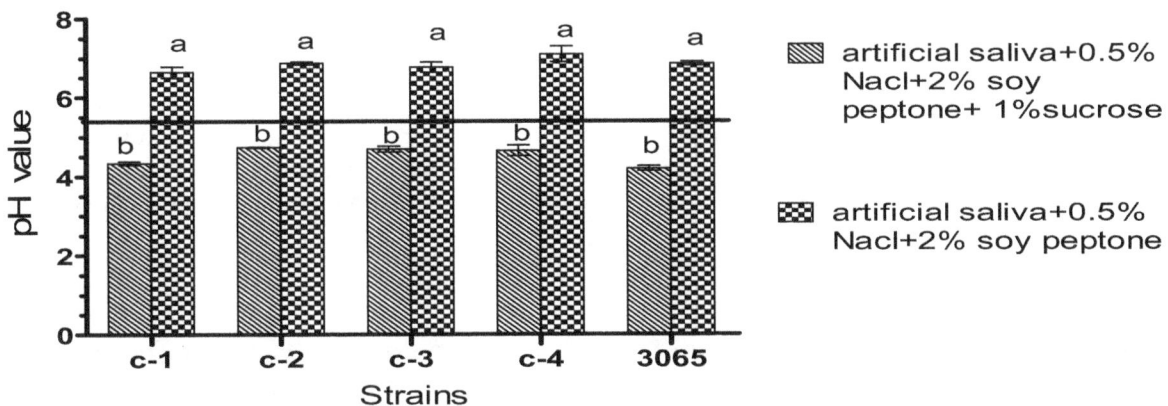

Figure 2. Sucrose-dependent acid production. The change of pH values after 24 h culture: 3065: *S. mutans* KCTC 3065; C-1: *Streptococcus salivarius*; C-2: *Streptococcus anginosus*; C-3: *Leuconostoc mesenteroides*; C-4: *Lactobacillus sakei*. Black solid line: enamel demineralization critical pH. Vertical bars represent standard error of the mean ($n = 3$), different letters in the same group indicate a significant ($p < 0.05$) treatment effect.

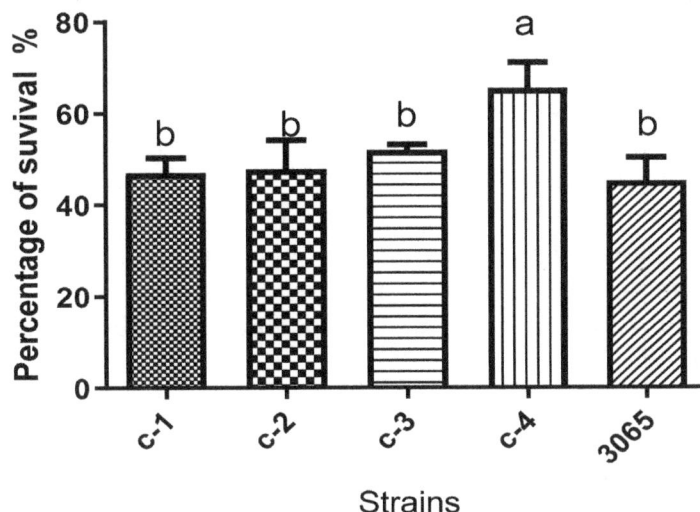

Figure 3. Aciduricity (acid tolerance). Percentage (%) of bacterial survival obtained after exposition to glycine buffer in pH 3.5 for 60 min: 3065: *S. mutans* KCTC 3065 C-1: *Streptococcus salivarius*; C-2: *Streptococcus anginosus*; C-3: *Leuconostoc mesenteroides*; C-4: *Lactobacillus sakei*. Vertical bars represent standard error of the mean ($n = 3$), different letters in the same group indicate a significant ($p < 0.05$) treatment effect.

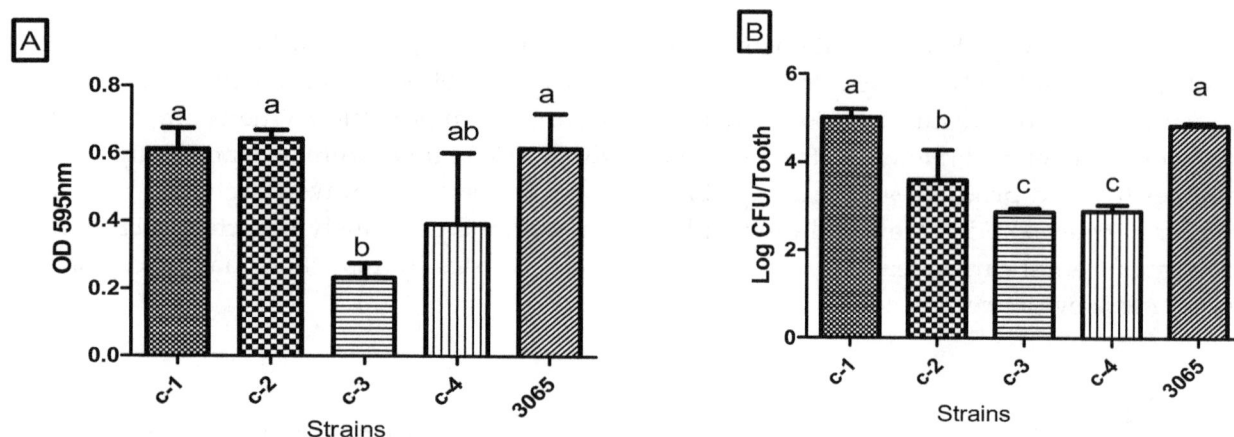

Figure 4. Biofilm formation of four isolated strains and one reference strain. Biofilms were formed on the surface of resin dentures and quantified through crystal violet assay (**A**) and cell enumeration (**B**) 3065: *S. mutans* KCTC 3065 C-1: *Streptococcus salivarius*; C-2: *Streptococcus anginosus*; C-3: *Leuconostoc mesenteroides*; C-4: *Lactobacillus sakei*. Vertical bars represent standard error of the mean ($n = 3$), different letters in the same group indicate a significant ($p < 0.05$) treatment effect.

3.2.2. In Vitro Biofilm Formation and Quantification

Adherence of isolates and reference strain to substrates are shown in Figure 4. The optical density (OD) value reflects the presence of extracellular polymeric substances (EPS) and bacterial cells in the biofilm. The adherent cells of bacteria positively correlated with the OD value of biofilm except for *S. anginosus*. The results showed that the living cells of *S. anginosus* in the biofilm is less than *S. salivarius* and *S. mutans* (Figure 4B), while there is no significant difference in the biofilm biomass among the three strains (Figure 4A). This could be explained by the fact that strains differ in their polymer production and quorum-sensing phenotypes; when cells reach a certain density, some bacteria activate polymer production, while others stop it [43]. The number of adherent *S. salivarius* (5.03 log) and *S. anginosus* (3.59 log) were significantly higher than that of *L. sakei* (2.89 log) and *L. mesenteroides* (2.87 log). There was no significant difference between *S. salivarius*, *S. anginosus*, and *S. mutans* KCTC 3065 on the biofilm biomass. According to a study by Chenbin et al. (2020), *S. salivarius*, along with *S. anginosus* isolated from dental caries samples showed moderate biofilm formation [42]. Interestingly, researchers confirmed that *S. anginosus* could complement the biofilm defect of the *S. mutans* [44]. Our findings suggest that extensive production of extracellular aggregates of *S. salivarius* and *S. anginosus*, along with *S. mutans* KCTC 3065, promotes bacterial attachment and biofilm formation that could be considered as an index for caries activity in caries-active patients. It is confirmed that *S. mutans* is the dominant species in many subjects with dental caries, but not all. Gross et al. (2012) reported that elevated levels *S. salivarius*, *S. sobrinus*, and *S. parasanguinis* are also associated with caries, especially in subjects with no or low levels of *S. mutans* [44]. Similarly, this study suggests species of *S. salivarius*, *S. anginosus*, and *L. sakei* as alternative pathogens, which synthesize large amounts of exopolysaccharides when sucrose is available.

3.2.3. Dissolution of Tooth

As evident from the data in Figure 5A, Ca^{2+} ions released from the tooth was negligible within 24 h incubation in each bacteria. However, after 96 h incubation, Ca^{2+} ions release caused by *S. mutans* was 78.8 μg/mL, and that caused by *S. salivarius* was 76.5 μg/mL. Ca^{2+} ions release of isolates gradually increased except *L. mesenteroides* during the 96 h incubation period. The result showed that *S. anginosus* possesses a significantly higher potential to dissolve tooth with 39.3 μg/mL of Ca^{2+} ions release, when compared to *L. mesenteroides* (16.5 μg/mL). A little amount of Ca^{2+} ions release was detected when the teeth were immersed in a growth medium without inoculation (15.1 µg/mL). This finding suggested that these no-mutans bacteria could also be potential targets for anti-microbial strategies to arrest the progression of caries. The terminal pH of each culture was measured, and the results are shown in Figure 5B. The data revealed that the range of terminal pH of all isolates was 4–5 in which $S. mutans$ groups showed the highest acid production (pH 4.2). The dissolution of hydroxyapatite is reversible, and the release of Ca^{2+} ions has potential buffering effects. It is reported that the Ca^{2+} concentrations in saliva range between 20 and 55 µg/mL [45]. From the data of this study, we could conclude that among all the isolates, $S. salivarius$ showed the strongest cariogenicity. When comparisons were made across $L. mesenteroides$ and other isolates, the lowest Ca^{2+} ions was release by $L. mesenteroides$. The results of high acid production but low tooth demineralization could be explained by the fact that some type of $L. mesenteroides$ strain produce butyric acid instead of lactic acid, since there is lack of evidence to confirm the association between butyric acid and dental caries [46]. These results suggested that acid production and acid resistance alone could not determine the cariogenicity of a bacterium. The highest dissolution of the tooth was caused by the control group ($S. mutans$ KCTC 3065), and this confirmed the accepted theory that $S. mutans$ plays an important role in the etiology of dental caries [46]. Besides, non-mutans Streptococci microbes isolated from special niches have also been proven to contribute to dental caries.

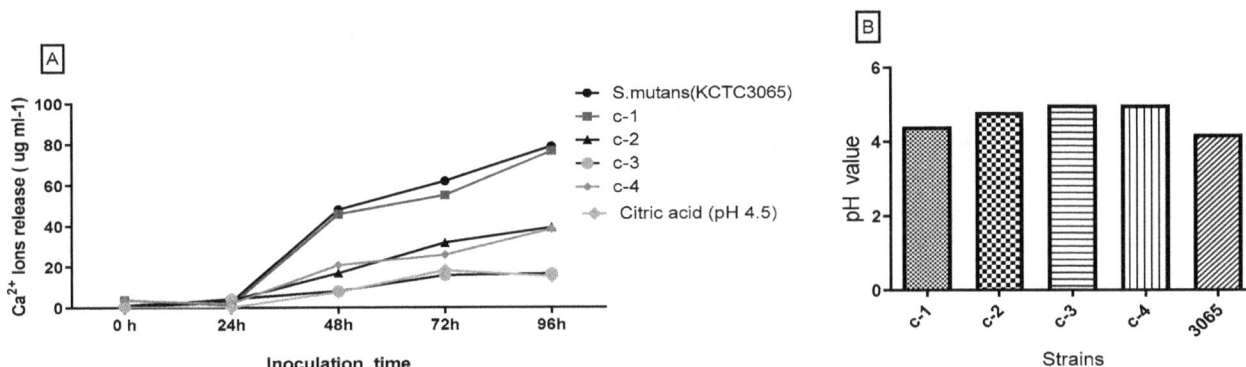

Figure 5. Calcium release from the tooth surface and acidification of cultures caused by isolated bacterial and reference strains. C-1: $Streptococcus salivarius$; C-2: $Streptococcus anginosus$; C-3: $Leuconostoc mesenteroides$; C-4: $Lactobacillus sakei$. Each tooth was repeatedly disinfected and used alternately after each experiment, the data of Ca^{2+} ions release (**A**) and the terminal pH (**B**) of each culture were expressed as average. The teeth were immersed in the medium (pH 4.5) without inoculation as the negative control.

Research on the prevention and treatment of dental caries should be based on a "holistic" instead of focusing purely on a single classical pathogen such as the $S. mutans$ [47]. Results of the in vitro microbiological tests in this study showed that three isolated species ($S. salivarius$, $S. anginosus$, and $L. sakei$) play a subsidiary role in the pathogenesis of caries. However, it is yet premature to classify these strains as cariogens. The communal behavior of non-mutan microorganisms within the oral milieu, and its cariogenicity have been studied by a number of researchers. Pereira et al. analyzed the role of $Candida albicans$ in the etiology of dental caries [48]. In another interesting study, molecular approaches were used to detect all bacterial species associated with dental caries. The data tend to imply that $Propioni bacterium$ may be involved in the procession of caries [49].

4. Conclusions

In this study, the in vitro studies have supported the high acidogenic potential of $S. salivarius$, $S. anginosus$, and $L. sakei$. At present, controversy continues regarding the role of bacteria from fermented food in the microbial etiology of dental caries. For the first time, our data support the associations between dental caries and probiotics present in fermented food ($L. sakei$). This study developed a method of testing a bacterium for its cariogenicity. The results revealed that although mutans streptococci is a major contributor in the etiology of dental caries, some other non-mutans organisms can also contribute to dental caries etiology. *S. salivarius* and *L. sakei* have been reportedly used as probiotics for treating bad breath and regulating intestinal flora. This study highlights the importance of considering the risk of acidogenic and acid-tolerant probiotics on causing dental caries. Isolated pathogens in this study may play a subsidiary role possibly acting in the incidence of dental caries, as residents of the plaque biofilm. Future in vivo trials are needed to confirm the cariogenicity of the isolates in this study.

Author Contributions: Conceptualization, X.C., E.B.-M.D. and D.-H.O.; data curation, X.C.; formal analysis, X.C., E.B.-M.D. and R.C.; funding acquisition, D.-H.O.; investigation, X.C. and R.C.; methodology, X.C.; project administration, D.-H.O.; resources, D.-H.O.; supervision, D.-H.O.; software, X.C.; validation, X.C. and D.-H.O.; visualization X.C. and R.C.; writing—original draft, X.C.; writing—review and editing, X.C. and E.B.-M.D. All authors have read and agreed to the published version of the manuscript.

References

1.   Pitts, N.B.; Zero, D.T.; Marsh, P.D.; Ekstrand, K.; Weintraub, J.A.; Ramos-Gomez, F.; Tagami, J.; Twetman, S.; Tsakos, G.; Ismail, A. Dental caries. *Nat. Rev. Dis. Primers* **2017**, *3*, 1–16. [CrossRef] [PubMed]

2.   Shao, C.; Jin, B.; Mu, Z.; Lu, H.; Zhao, Y.; Wu, Z.; Yan, L.; Zhang, Z.; Zhou, Y.; Pan, H.; et al. Repair of tooth enamel by a biomimetic mineralization frontier ensuring epitaxial growth. *Sci. Adv.* **2019**, *5*, eaaw9569. [CrossRef] [PubMed]

3.   Yang, X.; Yang, B.; He, L.; Li, R.; Liao, Y.; Zhang, S.; Yang, Y.; Xu, X.; Zhang, D.; Tan, H.; et al. Bioinspired peptide-decorated tannic acid for in situ remineralization of tooth enamel: In vitro and in vivo evaluation. *ACS Biomater. Sci. Eng.* **2017**, *3*, 3553–3562. [CrossRef]

4.   Peres, M.A.; Macpherson, L.M.D.; Weyant, R.J.; Daly, B.; Venturelli, R.; Mathur, M.R.; Listl, S.; Celeste, R.K.; Guarnizo-Herreño, C.C.; Kearns, C.; et al. Oral diseases: A global public health challenge. *Lancet* **2019**, *394*, 249–260. [CrossRef]

5.   WHO. Sugars and Dental Caries. 2017. Available online: https://www.who.int/news-room/fact-sheets/detail/sugars-and-dental-caries-90k (accessed on 17 March 2020).

6.   Burcham, Z.M.; Garneau, N.L.; Comstock, S.S.; Tucker, R.M.; Knight, R.; Metcalf, J.L. Patterns of oral microbiota diversity in adults and children: A crowdsourced population study. *Sci. Rep.* **2020**, *10*, 2133. [CrossRef]

7.   Kim, K.; Choi, S.; Chang, J.; Kim, S.M.; Kim, S.J.; Kim, R.Y.; Cho, H.J.; Park, S.M. Severity of dental caries and risk of coronary heart disease in middle-aged men and women: A population-based cohort study of Korean adults, 2002–2013. *Sci. Rep.* **2019**, *9*, 10491. [CrossRef]

8.   Goh, C.E.; Trinh, P.; Colombo, P.C.; Genkinger, J.M.; Mathema, B.; Uhlemann, A.C.; LeDuc, C.; Leibel, R.; Rosenbaum, M.; Paster, B.J. Association between nitrate-reducing oral bacteria and cardiometabolic outcomes: Results from origins. *J. Am. Heart Assoc.* **2019**, *8*, e013324. [CrossRef]

9.   Misaki, T.; Fukunaga, A.; Shimizu, Y.; Ishikawa, A.; Nakano, K. Possible link between dental diseases and arteriosclerosis in patients on hemodialysis. *PLoS ONE* **2019**, *14*, e0225038. [CrossRef]

10.   Cho, G.J.; Kim, S.Y.; Lee, H.C.; Kim, H.Y.; Lee, K.M.; Han, S.W.; Oh, M.J. Association between dental caries and adverse pregnancy outcomes. *Sci. Rep.* **2020**, *10*, 5309. [CrossRef]

11.   Nyvad, B.; Takahashi, N. Integrated hypothesis of dental caries and periodontal diseases. *J. Oral Microbiol.* **2020**, *12*, 1710953. [CrossRef]

12.   Du, Q.; Fu, M.; Zhou, Y.; Cao, Y.; Guo, T.; Zhou, Z.; Li, M.; Peng, X.; Zheng, X.; Li, Y.; et al. Sucrose promotes caries progression by disrupting the microecological balance in oral biofilms: An in vitro study. *Sci. Rep.* **2020**, *10*, 2961. [CrossRef] [PubMed]

13.   Krishnan, K.; Chen, T.; Paster, B.J. A practical guide to the oral microbiome and its relation to health and disease. *Oral Dis.* **2017**, *23*, 276–286. [CrossRef] [PubMed]

14.   Jiang, Q.; Liu, J.; Chen, L.; Gan, N.; Yang, D. The oral microbiome in the elderly with dental caries and health. *Front. Cell. Infect. Microbiol.* **2019**, *8*, 442. [CrossRef] [PubMed]

15. Fechney, J.M.; Browne, G.V.; Prabhu, N.; Irinyi, L.; Meyer, W.; Hughes, T.; Bockmann, M.; Townsend, G.; Salehi, H.; Adler, C.J. Preliminary study of the oral mycobiome of children with and without dental caries. *J. Oral Microbiol.* **2019**, *11*, 1536182. [CrossRef]

16. Ling, Z.; Kong, J.; Jia, P.; Wei, C.; Wang, Y.; Pan, Z.; Huang, W.; Li, L.; Chen, H.; Xiang, C. Analysis of oral microbiota in children with dental caries by PCR-DGGE and barcoded pyrosequencing. *Microb. Ecol.* **2010**, *60*, 677–690. [CrossRef]

17. Widyarman, A.S.; Theodorea, C.F. Effect of reuterin on dual-species biofilm in vitro of streptococcus mutans and veillonella parvula. *J. Int. Dent. Med. Res.* **2019**, *12*, 77–83.

18. Kressirer, C.A.; Smith, D.J.; King, W.F.; Dobeck, J.M.; Starr, J.R.; Tanner, A.C. Scardovia wiggsiae and its potential role as a caries pathogen. *J. Oral Biosci.* **2017**, *59*, 135–141. [CrossRef]

19. Eşian, D.; Man, A.; Burlibasa, L.; Burlibasa, M.; Perieanu, M.V.; Bică, C. Salivary level of Streptococcus mutans and Lactobacillus spp. related to a high a risk of caries disease. *Rom. Biotechnol. Lett.* **2017**, *22*, 12496–12503.

20. Obata, J.; Fujishima, K.; Nagata, E.; Oho, T. Pathogenic mechanisms of cariogenic Propionibacterium acidifaciens. *Arch. Oral Biol.* **2019**, *105*, 46–51. [CrossRef]

21. Zeng, Y.; Youssef, M.; Wang, L.; Alkhars, N.; Thomas, M.; Cacciato, R.; Qing, S.; Ly-Mapes, O.; Xiao, J. Identification of non-streptococcus mutans bacteria from predente infant saliva grown on mitis-salivarius-bacitracin agar. *J. Clin. Pediatr. Dent.* **2020**, *44*, 28–34. [CrossRef]

22. Chen, H.; Jiang, W. Application of high-throughput sequencing in understanding human oral microbiome related with health and disease. *Front. Microbiol.* **2014**, *5*, 508. [CrossRef]

23. Banas, J.A.; Takanami, E.; Hemsley, R.M.; Villhauer, A.; Zhu, M.; Qian, F.; Marolf, A.; Drake, D.R. Evaluating the relationship between acidogenicity and acid tolerance for oral streptococci from children with or without a history of caries. *J. Oral Microbiol.* **2020**, *12*, 1688449. [CrossRef]

24. Kim, D.; Barraza, J.P.; Arthur, R.A.; Hara, A.; Lewis, K.; Liu, Y.; Scisci, E.L.; Hajishengallis, E.; Whiteley, M.; Koo, H. Spatial mapping of polymicrobial communities reveals a precise biogeography associated with human dental caries. *Proc. Natl. Acad. Sci. USA* **2020**, *10*, 1073. [CrossRef] [PubMed]

25. Krzyściak, W.; Papież, M.; Jurczak, A.; Kościelniak, D.; Vyhouskaya, P.; Zagórska-Świeży, K.; Skalniak, A. Relationship between pyruvate kinase activity and cariogenic biofilm formation in streptococcus mutans biotypes in caries patients. *Front. Microbiol.* **2017**, *8*, 856. [CrossRef] [PubMed]

26. Takahashi, N.; Nyvad, B. The role of bacteria in the caries process: Ecological perspectives. *J. Dent. Res.* **2011**, *90*, 294–303. [CrossRef]

27. Senneby, A.; Davies, J.; Svensäter, G.; Neilands, J. Acid tolerance properties of dental biofilms in vivo. *BMC Microbiol.* **2017**, *17*, 165. [CrossRef] [PubMed]

28. Nikawa, H.; Yamashiro, H.; Makihira, S.; Nishimura, M.; Egusa, H.; Furukawa, M.; Setijanto, D.; Hamada, T. In vitro cariogenic potential of Candida albicans. *Mycoses* **2003**, *46*, 471–478. [CrossRef]

29. Lapirattanakul, J.; Takashima, Y.; Tantivitayakul, P.; Maudcheingka, T.; Leelataweewud, P.; Nakano, K.; Matsumoto-Nakano, M. Cariogenic properties of Streptococcus mutans clinical isolates with sortase defects. *Arch. Oral Biol.* **2017**, *81*, 7–14. [CrossRef]

30. Hussain, M.S.; Kwon, M.; Tango, C.N.; Oh, D.H. Effect of electrolyzed water on the disinfection of bacillus cereus biofilms: The mechanism of enhanced resistance of sessile cells in the biofilm matrix. *J. Food Prot.* **2018**, *81*, 860–869. [CrossRef]

31. Park, E.-j.; Hussain, M.S.; Wei, S.; Kwon, M.; Oh, D.H. Genotypic and phenotypic characteristics of biofilm formation of emetic toxin producing Bacillus cereus strains. *Food Control.* **2019**, *96*, 527–534. [CrossRef]

32. Featherstone, J.D. Dental caries: A dynamic disease process. *Aust. Dent. J.* **2008**, *53*, 286–291. [CrossRef] [PubMed]

33. Lamont, R.J.; Koo, H.; Hajishengallis, G. The oral microbiota: Dynamic communities and host interactions. *Nat. Rev. Microbiol.* **2018**, *16*, 745–759. [CrossRef] [PubMed]

34. Papadopoulou, O.S.; Iliopoulos, V.; Mallouchos, A.; Panagou, E.Z.; Chorianopoulos, N.; Tassou, C.C.; Nychas, G.E. Spoilage potential of pseudomonas (p. fragi, p. putida) and lab (leuconostoc mesenteroides, lactobacillus sakei) strains and their volatilome profile during storage of sterile pork meat using gc/ms and data analytics. *Foods* **2020**, *9*, 633. [CrossRef] [PubMed]

35. Rubab, M.; Chellia, R.; Saravanakumar, K.; Mandava, S.; Khan, I.; Tango, C.N.; Wang, M.H.; Oh, D.H. Preservative effect of Chinese cabbage (*Brassica rapa subsp. pekinensis*) extract on their molecular docking, antioxidant and antimicrobial properties. *PLoS ONE* **2018**, *13*, e0203306. [CrossRef]

36. Lee, S.Y.; Sekhon, S.S.; Ko, J.H.; Kim, H.C.; Kim, S.Y.; Won, K.; Ahn, J.Y.; Lee, K.; Kim, Y.H. Lactic acid bacteria isolated from Kimchi to evaluate anti-obesity effect in high fat diet-induced obese mice. *J. Toxicol.* **2018**, *10*, 11–16. [CrossRef]

37. Seo, D.J.; Jung, D.; Jung, S.; Yeo, D.; Choi, C. Inhibitory effect of lactic acid bacteria isolated from kimchi against murine norovirus. *Food Control.* **2020**, *109*, 106881. [CrossRef]

38. Pérez-Ibarreche, M.; Mendoza, L.M.; Vignolo, G.; Fadda, S. Proteomic and genetics insights on the response of the bacteriocinogenic Lactobacillus sakei CRL1862 during biofilm formation on stainless steel surface at 10 °C. *Int. J. Food Microbiol.* **2017**, *258*, 18–27. [CrossRef]

39. Shao, X.; Fang, K.; Medina, D.; Wan, J.; Lee, J.L.; Hong, S.H. The probiotic, Leuconostoc mesenteroides, inhibits Listeria monocytogenes biofilm formation. *J. Food Saf.* **2020**, *40*, e12750. [CrossRef]

40. Ananieva, M.; Faustova, M.; Basarab, Y.O.; Loban, G. Kocuria rosea, kocuria kristinae, leuconostoc mesenteroides as caries-causing representatives of oral microflora. *Wiad. Lek.* **2017**, *70*, 296–298.

41. Kirilova, J.N.; Topalova-Pirinska, S.Z.; Kirov, D.N.; Deliverska, E.G.; Doichinova, L.B. Types of microorganisms in proximal caries lesion and ozone treatment. *Biotechnol. Biotechnol. Equip.* **2019**, *33*, 683–688. [CrossRef]

42. Bin, C.; Al-Dhabi, N.A.; Esmail, G.A.; Arokiyaraj, S.; Arasu, M.V. Potential effect of Allium sativum bulb for the treatment of biofilm forming clinical pathogens recovered from periodontal and dental caries. *Saudi J. Biol. Sci.* **2020**, *27*, 1428–1434. [CrossRef] [PubMed]

43. Nadell, C.D.; Xavier, J.B.; Levin, S.A.; Foster, K.R. The evolution of quorum sensing in bacterial biofilms. *PLoS Biol.* **2008**, *6*, e14. [CrossRef] [PubMed]

44. Gross, E.L.; Beall, C.J.; Kutsch, S.R.; Firestone, N.D.; Leys, E.J.; Griffen, A.L. Beyond streptococcus mutans: Dental caries onset linked to multiple species by 16s rRNA community analysis. *PLoS ONE* **2012**, *7*, 11. [CrossRef] [PubMed]

45. Shaw, L.; Murray, J.; Burchell, C.; Best, J. Calcium and phosphorus content of plaque and saliva in relation to dental caries. *Caries Res.* **1983**, *17*, 543–548. [CrossRef]

46. Traisaeng, S.; Batsukh, A.; Chuang, T.H.; Herr, D.R.; Huang, Y.F.; Chimeddorj, B.; Huang, C.M. Leuconostoc mesenteroides fermentation produces butyric acid and mediates Ffar2 to regulate blood glucose and insulin in type 1 diabetic mice. *Sci. Rep.* **2020**, *10*, 7928. [CrossRef] [PubMed]

47. Banas, J.A.; Drake, D.R. Are the mutans streptococci still considered relevant to understanding the microbial etiology of dental caries? *BMC Oral Health* **2018**, *18*, 129. [CrossRef]

48. Pereira, D.F.A.; Seneviratne, C.J.; Koga-Ito, C.Y.; Samaranayake, L.P. Is the oral fungal pathogen Candida albicans a cariogen? *Oral Dis.* **2018**, *24*, 518–526. [CrossRef]

49. Aas, J.A.; Griffen, A.L.; Dardis, S.R.; Lee, A.M.; Olsen, I.; Dewhirst, F.E.; Leys, E.J.; Paster, B.J. Bacteria of dental caries in primary and permanent teeth in children and young adults. *J. Clin. Microbiol.* **2008**, *46*, 1407–1417. [CrossRef]

2

Oral Primo-Colonizing Bacteria Modulate Inflammation and Gene Expression in Bronchial Epithelial Cells

Elliot Mathieu [1], Chad W. MacPherson [2], Jocelyn Belvis [2], Olivier Mathieu [2], Véronique Robert [1], Vinciane Saint-Criq [1], Philippe Langella [1], Thomas A. Tompkins [2] and Muriel Thomas [1,*]

[1] Micalis Institute, AgroParisTech, INRAE, Université Paris-Saclay, 78350 Jouy-en-Josas, France; elliot.mathieu@inrae.fr (E.M.); veronique.robert@inrae.fr (V.R.); vinciane.saint-criq@inrae.fr (V.S.-C.); philippe.langella@inrae.fr (P.L.)

[2] Rosell Institute for Microbiome and Probiotics, Lallemand Health Solutions Inc., Montreal, QC H4P 2R2, Canada; cmacpherson@lallemand.com (C.W.M.); jbelvis@lallemand.com (J.B.); omathieu@lallemand.com (O.M.); ttompkins@lallemand.com (T.A.T.)

* Correspondence: muriel.thomas@inrae.fr

Abstract: The microbiota of the mouth disperses into the lungs, and both compartments share similar phyla. Considering the importance of the microbiota in the maturation of the immunity and physiology during the first days of life, we hypothesized that primo-colonizing bacteria of the oral cavity may induce immune responses in bronchial epithelial cells. Herein, we have isolated and characterized 57 strains of the buccal cavity of two human newborns. These strains belong to *Streptococcus*, *Staphylococcus*, *Enterococcus*, *Rothia* and *Pantoea* genera, with *Streptococcus* being the most represented. The strains were co-incubated with a bronchial epithelial cell line (BEAS-2B), and we established their impact on a panel of cytokines/chemokines and global changes in gene expression. The *Staphylococcus* strains, which appeared soon after birth, induced a high production of IL-8, suggesting they can trigger inflammation, whereas the *Streptococcus* strains were less associated with inflammation pathways. The genera *Streptococcus*, *Enterococcus* and *Pantoea* induced differential profiles of cytokine/chemokine/growth factor and set of genes associated with maturation of morphology. Altogether, our results demonstrate that the microorganisms, primo-colonizing the oral cavity, impact immunity and morphology of the lung epithelial cells, with specific effects depending on the phylogeny of the strains.

Keywords: oral microbiota; early life; bronchial epithelial cells; immuno-modulation

1. Introduction

The buccal cavity (BC) is the body's entrance for nutriments, air, environmental pollutants and microorganisms. It is a complex ecosystem built by different ecological niches that include the surfaces of hard and soft tissues and saliva [1–3]. In humans, the BC is colonized by more than 500 different microbial species, and most of the bacteria belong to the phyla *Firmicutes*, *Proteobacteria*, *Actinobacteria*, *Bacteroidetes* and *Fusobacteria* [1,4,5]. Numerous descriptions have established an association between buccal microbiota and both local and distal diseases [6–8]. In respiratory diseases such as asthma, differences in the profile of buccal microbiota have been observed in children as soon as 12 months of age [9]. In addition to modulating the buccal microbiota in other chronic respiratory diseases, the BC may also serve as a potential source of respiratory pathogens [8,10]. The installation of the buccal microbiota matches with the maturation of the lung microbiota; therefore, the exchange of microorganisms (and/or metabolites) between both compartments may impact the course of respiratory diseases. The dense and highly diverse buccal ecosystem, which shares similar phyla with the lung microbiota, is easily accessible to study the characteristics of microorganisms that migrate to the lungs.

The human lung microbiota has a low density, about 10^3 bacteria per cm^2 of lung tissue, and a subtle balance is maintained between microbial immigration and elimination [11–15]. Within this constant balance, the two main bacterial phyla represented are *Bacteroidetes* and *Firmicutes* [12,14,16,17]. It has been shown that the lung microbiota forms within the two to three postnatal months in humans and the first weeks in mice [18,19]. The progressive arrival of these microorganisms coincides with the maturation of the immune system [14]. Increasing evidence suggests that the early lung ecosystem impacts future respiratory health. For example, in mice, specific bacterial stimuli during early life are critical for susceptibility to allergic asthma in young adults [20]. Another example of the importance of early life microbial colonization of the mouse airway is the improved long-term tolerance to allergens through the microbial-induction of a transient peak in expression of the programmed death-ligand 1 (PD-L1) by pulmonary dendritic cells [21]. In humans, lower diversity of microbial exposure in urban than in rural areas results in a higher incidence of allergy and asthma [22–24]. These observations, among others, support the hypothesis that exposure to a wide range of diverse microbial signals during the first few months of life has a major impact on the susceptibility to respiratory diseases such as asthma [25–28]. The postnatal period is a pivotal time in respiratory health, making the primo-colonizing bacteria of special interest to screen for new probiotics.

Cells that compose the airway epithelium act as the first line of defense against the external environment and are able to initiate innate and adaptive immune responses [29–31]. Bronchial epithelial cells (BEC) express various innate sensors (e.g., toll-like receptors (TLRs), NOD-like receptors (NLRs) and C-type lectins receptors (CLRs)) that can detect microbes and activate molecular cascades in host cells, triggering the induction of tolerance or inflammation [32,33]. The mediation and regulation of the immune responses are controlled by the secretion of cytokines, chemokines and growth factors. Cytokine secretion, for example, is a major feature of the inflammatory process in allergic reaction. In asthma, changes in the epithelium structure, disruption of epithelial tight junctions and epithelium thickening are observed [30,34]. The physiological characteristics of the bronchial epithelium, which are modulated during disease, influence the homeostasis between the lung and its microbiota [14]. For example, a longer residence time of mucus in the airways may favor the selection of certain bacteria with a high tropism for mucus, leading to the persistence of pathogens [35]. These observations highlight the importance of the BECs in respiratory health and disease, making them a target of importance to study the relationship between external signals and the host.

We hypothesized that early life buccal bacteria induce specific immunomodulatory responses in BECs. The goal of our study was to isolate commensal bacterial strains from the BC of babies and to elucidate their impacts on the immune modulation and global changes in gene expression in BECs. The effect of *Streptococcus*, *Enterococcus* and *Pantoea* strains on BEAS-2B cells was evaluated by using genome-wide human expression microarrays and cytokine and chemokine multiplexing immunoassays. The isolation of buccal commensals and the understanding of their interaction with the BECs is a first step toward understanding the underlying cellular mechanisms at play, the identification of novel beneficial microbes and the possible management of respiratory health.

2. Materials and Methods

2.1. Bacterial Strains, Media and Growth Conditions

Bacterial strains were isolated from the BC of human newborns, using swabs (Portagerm Amies agar and swab—sterile zone, Biomerieux, Marcy-l'Étoile, France). Donors were two males born via vaginal route at term, and the mothers did not receive antibiotic therapy during pregnancy. After written consent was obtained, a pack of 10 swabs was given to the parents. Sampling was performed by the parents as soon as the first day of life, once or twice daily and for 5 to 10 consecutive days. Samples were stored at 4 °C until collection. Swabs were placed in sterile Brain Heart Infusion (BHi) (BD/Difco,

Fisher Scientific, Thermo Fisher Scientific, Waltham, MA, USA) broth medium supplemented with 5 g·L^{-1} of yeast extract (Gibco®, Thermo Fisher Scientific, Waltham, MA, USA). After dilution, bacteria were cultivated on BHi agar medium supplemented with 10 mL·L^{-1} of hemin (H 9039, 50 mL/100 mL) and 5 g·L^{-1} of yeast extract. Plates were incubated for 24–48 h, at 37 °C, under aerobic and anaerobic conditions. Representative bacterial colonies were selected based on the difference in shape, size and color. Isolated strains were subcultured on BHi agar medium, and the purity of the culture was determined before storage in 16% glycerol at −80 °C.

2.2. Bacterial Strain Identification

Strains were identified at the genus level, using sequencing PCR amplicons of 16S rRNA genes. 16S PCR was performed by using the primers 1492R (5′-ACGGCTACCTTGTTACGACTT-3′, position 1517R) and 27F (5′-AGAGTTTGATCCTGGCTCAG-3′, position 008F) [36]. PCR-amplified sequences were run on 1 % agarose gel and then sent for sequencing to Eurofins (Eurofins Scientific, Germany). Nucleotide sequences were analyzed by using Basic Local Alignment Search Tool (BLAST) and compared to the NCBI non-redundant database [37].

2.3. Bacterial Strains Preparation for Challenge Assay

Bacterial strains were thawed and then incubated in BHi. After overnight culture, cultures were passaged once, and on the day of the challenge assay, bacterial cultures were centrifuged, and the pellet was washed with 1 mL of phosphate buffered saline (PBS) (Gibco®, Thermo Fisher Scientific, Waltham, MA, USA). Bacterial cultures were used in post-logarithmic phase, and therefore the time of culture was adapted for each strain. After a second centrifugation, PBS was removed, and bacterial pellet was resuspended in Roswell Park Memorial Institute (RPMI) 1640 Medium (Lonza, Basel, Switzerland). Bacterial cells were enumerated by using the BD Accuri™ C6 (BD Biosciences, Franklin Lakes, NJ, USA) and stored on ice until further used, for 10 min.

2.4. BEAS-2B Human Bronchial Epithelial Cell Challenge

BEAS-2B human bronchial epithelial cell line was obtained from the American Type Culture Collection (ATCC CLR-9609). Cells were maintained in RPMI-1640 medium supplemented with 10% fetal bovine serum (Eurobio, Les Ulis, France), 1% penicillin/streptomycin (Sigma-Aldrich, St. Louis, MO, USA) and 1% L-glutamine (Gibco®, Thermo Fisher Scientific, Waltham, MA, USA) in 75 cm^2 tissue culture flask (Sarstedt, Nümbrecht, Germany) and incubated at 37 °C, in a 5% CO2 atmosphere, in a humidified incubator. Cells were passaged before reaching 80% confluency, using Tripsin-EDTA (Gibco®, Thermo Fisher Scientific, Waltham, MA, USA). To prepare the challenge assay, cells were detached and enumerated, using an automated cell counter (Bio-Rad TC20 (Bio-Rad, Hercules, CA, USA), and seeded at 5 × 10^4 cells/mL, in a 25 cm^2 tissue culture flask (TPP, Trasadingen, Switzerland) (T25) with 5 mL fresh medium, and incubated at 37 °C, 5 % CO2. At 80% confluency, cells were challenged with the bacterial treatments. Prior to the challenge, BEAS-2B cells were enumerated, and appropriate bacterial concentration was calculated in order to get a MOI of 100:1 (100 bacterial cells for each BEAS-2B cell). Medium was removed from the T25, and 5 mL of one of the bacterial conditions, diluted in RPMI-1640 (without supplements), was added to the flask. After a 6 h incubation period at 37 °C, 5 % CO2, supernatants were collected, and Bovine Serum Albumin (BSA) (Sigma-Aldrich, St. Louis, MO, USA), at a final concentration of 0.5 %, was added to each sample, to prevent protein degradation. Supernatants were then stored at −80 °C, and RNA was extracted from the challenged cells.

A similar protocol, in which 24-well plates replaced T25, was used to generate IL-8 secretion data.

2.5. Human Cytokine and Chemokine Profiling

Cytokine and chemokine profiling was done by using the Bio-Plex Pro™ 27-Plex Human Cytokine Panel (Bio-Rad, Hercules, CA, USA), the Bio-Plex Pro™ 40-Plex Human Chemokine Panel (Bio-Rad,

Hercules, CA, USA) and the single-Plex TSLP (Bio-Rad, Hercules, CA, USA). For all plexes, all cytokines and chemokines were multiplexed on the same 96-well plate (1 plate for each plex). Cytokine and chemokine standards were serially diluted, and protein profiling from all challenges were done as per the manufacturer's instructions (Bio-Rad), with 4 biological replicates. Quality controls (from the kit) were also included, only for the 40-plex, to ensure the validity of the results obtained. Protein concentrations were calculated by using the Bio-Plex Manager™ software and expressed in pg/mL.

IL-8 was quantified by using ELISA Max™ Standard Set Human IL-8 (BioLegend, San Diego, CA, USA); manufacturer instructions were followed.

2.6. RNA Extraction and RNA Cleanup

After the challenge assay, supernatant was removed, and 2 mL Trizol Reagent (Invitrogen, Carlsbad, CA, USA) was added to the 25 cm^2 tissue culture flask. After 5 min incubation with gentle agitation at room temperature, cell lysates were transferred to two PhaseLock tubes (Quantabio, Beverly, MA, USA), and 0.2 volumes of chloroform (v/v) was added to each tube. Tubes were shacked vigorously and centrifuged (12,000× g for 10 min at 4 °C). Aqueous phase containing RNA was transferred to a new tube, and RNA was precipitated by adding 0.5 volumes (v/v) of isopropyl alcohol. After centrifugation (12,000× g for 10 min at 4 °C), RNA pellets were washed with 70% ethanol and dried by placing them into a flow hood. Pellets were resuspended in 20 µL RNase-free water, and a step of RNA cleanup was performed, following the manufacturer's instructions (RNeasy mini kit, Qiagen, Hilden, Germany). RNA was quantified by using Nanodrop, and RNA integrity (RIN) was determined with Bioanalyzer (RNA 6000 Nano Kit, Agilent Technologies, Santa Clara, CA, USA). RNA was then stored at −20 °C, until needed. Only RNA samples with a RIN > 8 were used in reverse transcription (RT) of mRNA into cDNA for subsequent gene expression microarrays [38].

2.7. RNA Reverse Transcription and Fluorescent Labeling

First, 10 µg aliquots of RNA were SpeedVac. As previously described by MacPherson et al., 10 µL of freshly prepared oligo dT-master mix (1.5 µL of oligo dT23 primers (3 µg/µL) and 8.5 µL of RNase free water per sample) were added to samples and then incubated at 70 °C for 10 min, in a dry bath [38]. Two cDNA synthesis master mixes were prepared by mixing 4 µL of 5X First Strand Buffer, 2 µL of 0.1 M DTT, 2 µL of dNTP home mix (6.67 mM of GTPs, dATPs, dTTPs and 2 mM of dCTPs), 1 µL of Superscript III (200 U/µL) and 1 µL of a 1 mM mix of Cy3 or Cy5, for each sample. Then, 10 µL of freshly prepared cDNA master mix was added per sample. After gentle flicking, tubes were incubated at 42 °C for 3 h, in a dry bath protected from light. After incubation, 1 µL of RNase mix (0.05 mg/mL RNase A and 0.05 U/µL RNase H) was added to each sample and incubated at 37 °C for 30 min. Labeled cDNA was purified, following the manufacturer's instructions, to remove unincorporated Cy3 or Cy5 dyes (PCR Purification Kit, Qiagen, Hilden, Germany). Labeled and purified cDNA samples were stored with a foil cover at −20 °C, until needed.

2.8. Microarrays Analysis

Genome-wide expression analysis was performed by using Agilent Whole Human 4x44K microarrays (Agilent Technologies, Santa Clara, CA, USA). Microarrays were prepared for pre-hybridization, hybridization and post-hybridization, as previously described MacPherson et al. [38]. Arrays were scanned at 10 µm resolution, using a ScanArray 5000 instrument from Perkin-Elmer (Waltham, MA, USA) and ScanArray software (version 3.0). Images for Cyanine 5 and Cyanine 3 were saved as TIFF format, and a composite image was created and saved as JPEG.

2.9. LDH Cytotoxicity Assay

LDH was quantified by colorimetric method in the supernatant of cell culture by using the Pierce LDH Cytotoxicity Assay Kit (Thermo Fisher Scientific, Waltham, MA, USA). BEAS-2B Bronchial epithelial cells were challenged with bacterial strains, as described in Section 2.4, BEAS-2B Human

Bronchial Epithelial Cell Challenge. After 6 h of incubation, cell supernatants were recovered, and LDH was quantified, following the manufacturer's instructions. Briefly, 50 μL of supernatants was transferred to a 96 wells-plate, and 50 μL of the reaction mixture (containing Substrate mix and Assay buffer) was added to each well. After 30 min incubation at room temperature, 50 μL of Stop solution was added into each well. To determine LDH activity, absorbance at 490 and 680 nm was measured by using a plate-reading spectrophotometer. To obtain the maximum LDH activity control ("Lysis 3 h" in Figure S2), BEAS-2B cells were challenged for 3 h at 37 °C, 5 % CO2 with Lysis buffer (10 % in RPMI). Spontaneous LDH activity control corresponds to RPMI medium only. The percentage of cytotoxicity was calculated as follows:

$$\% \text{ Cytotoxicity} = \frac{\text{Bacteria treated LDH activity} - \text{Spontaneous LDH activity}}{\text{Maximum LDH activity} - \text{Spontaneous LDH activity}} \times 100 \qquad (1)$$

2.10. Data and Statistical Analysis

2.10.1. Human Cytokine and Chemokine Profiling

All data are shown as the mean pg/mL ± standard error of the mean (SEM). Statistical analysis was performed by using GraphPad Prism's Version 8 (GraphPad Software, Inc., San Diego, CA, USA), one-way analysis of variance (ANOVA) or non-parametric Kruskal–Wallis test followed by Dunn's multiple comparison test were used to determine statistical significance. The p-values are as follows: *: $p < 0.03$, **: $p < 0.002$, ***: $p < 0.0002$ and ****: $p < 0.0001$.

For each condition and cytokine/chemokine, ratios were calculated as follows:

$$Ratio = \frac{(bacteria\ stimulated\ average)}{(medium\ average)} \qquad (2)$$

Ratio values were then entered into MeV to create the heat map and hierarchical clustering gene leaf order; Euclidian distance was used as distance metric.

2.10.2. Microarray Data Processing

The signal intensity of all spots was quantified and normalized (Global LOWESS) by using ImaGene version 9.0 (BioDiscovery, El Segundo, CA, USA). Statistical analysis was done with MultiExperiment Viewer (MeV) version 4.8 (TM4 microarray software suite, J. Craig Venter Institute, Rockville, MD, USA). Genes were considered significantly differentially expressed when (a) a t-test p-value of less than 0.05 and (b) a cutoff in transcript abundance of least 1.5-fold change were reached.

Ingenuity Pathway System (IPA) was used to discover relevant biological patterns and genes network modulated by the bacterial challenges. IPA is a web-based bioinformatics application for analyzing and understanding large gene-expression datasets. A p-value < 0.05 (-log(p-value) > 1.3) was considered to be statistically significant for the enrichment of pathways in IPA (p-value calculated by using Fisher's exact test).

Information about the microarray platform and the expression data files can be found on the NCBI Gene Expression Omnibus (GEO; http://www.ncbi.nlm.nih.gov/geo/) under GEO Series record GSE154245.

3. Results

3.1. Strains Isolated from the Swabs

A total of 57 isolates were isolated from the BC of two babies (males, born by vaginal route) and identified by using 16S PCR sequencing. When assessing the abundance in the samples from both donors, the genus *Streptococcus* was the most represented, with 23 members (Figure 1a). *Staphylococcus* and *Enterococcus* strains ($n = 15$ each) were in a close amount. Three sequences were identified as strains belonging to the genus *Rothia* and one to the genus *Pantoea*. We next displayed the distribution of the strains over eight days for one donor (Figure 1b). Note that we were not able to perform such kinetics for the second donor (due to the lack of sampling or the difficulty in purifying strains), making the comparison between the two donors impossible. As shown in Figure 1b, the *Staphylococcus* strains were mainly isolated from the BC samples from the first day of life and were rapidly replaced by the other genera. The *Streptococcus* strains were isolated from day two and were present in all the samples from this day. The three *Rothia* strains of the library were isolated from this donor on days three and four. The *Pantoea* strain was isolated on day five, and, finally, the *Enterococcus* strains were the most isolated in the samples on days seven and eight.

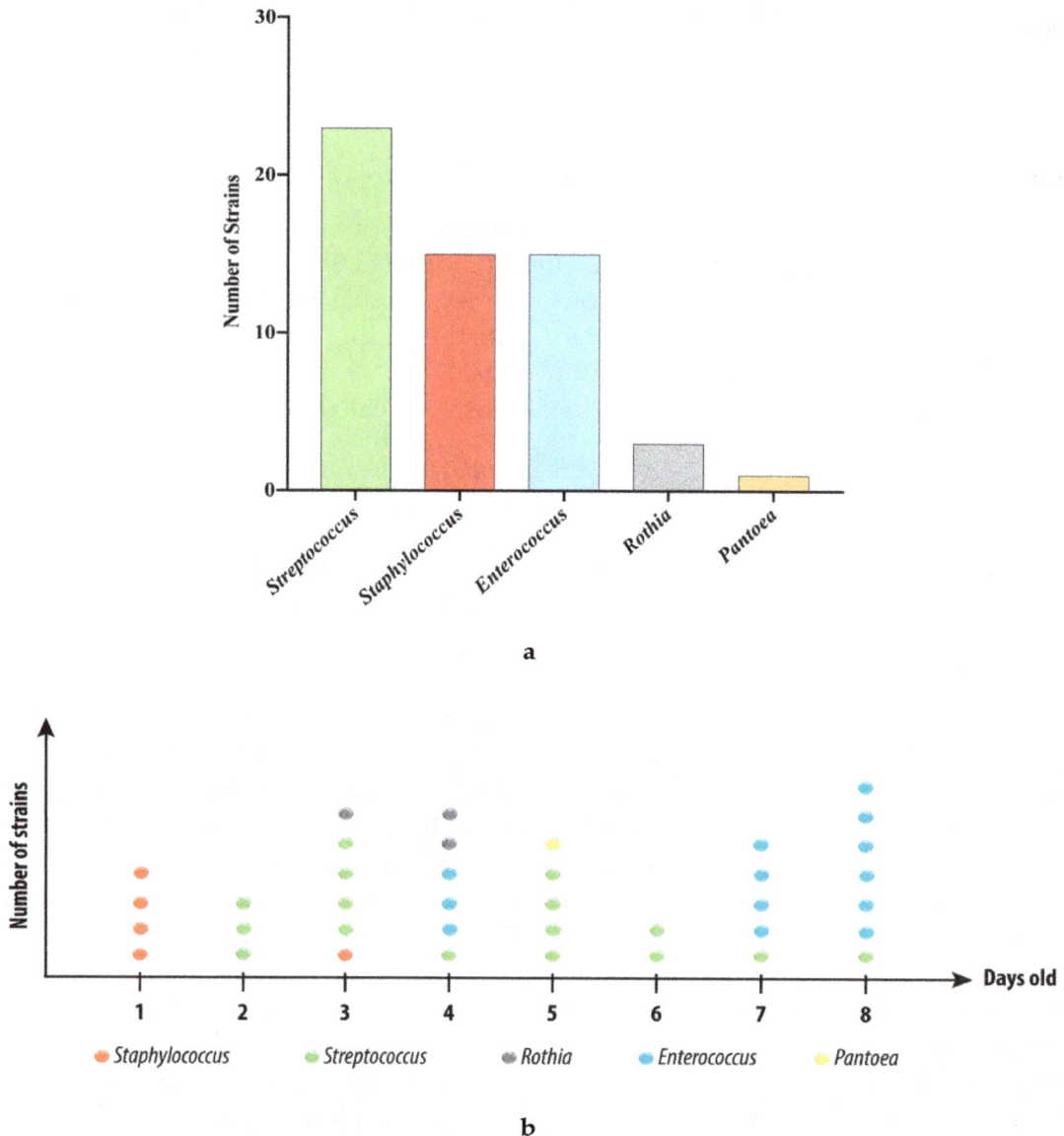

Figure 1. The bacterial library contains members of the early life buccal core microbiota. (**a**) Genera repartition of the 57 strains identified in all the samples (days are mixed) from both donors. (**b**) Bacterial distribution through the days for one donor ($n = 38$). Strains were identified at the genus level, using 16S PCR sequencing. Data are presented as the number of strains per genera. Each dot represents a strain.

3.2. Cytokines and Chemokines Production Profiling in BEAS-2B Cells, Following Bacterial Treatments

From these 57 strains, we selected 11 strains of interest, which comprised *Streptococcus*, *Enterococcus* and *Pantoea*. The other strains (46 strains) mainly displayed a pro-inflammatory profile after a co-incubation with the BEAS-2B cells (data not shown). Particularly, the *Staphylococcus* strains isolated from the first day of life induced Interleukin (IL)-8 secretion (Figure 2). We evaluated the impact of the 11 bacterial strains on the protein levels of cytokine and chemokine secreted by the BEAS-2B cells in the supernatant, following challenge with the bacterial strains. Cytokines and chemokines were quantified by using fluorescent-magnetic-bead-based multiplex immunoassay. Most of our bacterial treatments did not significantly increase of pro-inflammatory markers such as IL-8, IL-6, TNFα (Figure 3a–c) and IL-1β (Figure S1) in comparison to controls. Only the *Pantoea EMP364* strain induced significant production of these pro-inflammatory proteins (Figure 3a–c). Most strains did not induce more than 10.1 % cytotoxicity (measured by LDH release) (Figure S2), although *Streptococcus EMS383* induced up to 60% cytotoxicity. None of the conditions induced Th2-related cytokines IL-2, IL-4, IL-5, IL-7, IL-9, IL-12p70, IL-13 and IL-17A secretion by the BEAS-2B cells following bacterial treatments (data not shown). *Pantoea EM-364* produced an increased production of chemokine markers such as C-C Motif Chemokine Ligand (CCL) 20 and C-X-C Motif Chemokine Ligand (CXCL) 2 (Figure 3e,f). Although not significant, the *Enterococcus* strains increased the production of CCL2 and CXCL2 (Figure 3d,f). Along with *Pantoea EM-364*, they also induced the production of most of the chemokines measured (Figure S1). *Streptococcus* strains only increased CCL25 secretion by the BEAS-2B cells (Figure S1). Most of the *Streptococcus* strains promoted the production of FGF basic (Figure S1), e.g., *EMS353*: 89.80 pg/mL ± 16.19 vs. RPMI: 4.37 pg/mL ± 2.12), while the *Enterococcus* strain had no effect on the production of this growth factor. The opposite pattern was observed for granulocyte colony-stimulating factor (G-CSF) release (Figure S1; e.g., *EME343*: 29.25 pg/mL ± 4.51 vs. RPMI: 0 pg/mL ± 0). The macrophage migration inhibitory factor (MIF) was strongly secreted by BEAS-2B cells in response to *Streptococcus EMS336* (19,847 pg/mL ± 9844), EMS3101 (40,117 pg/mL ± 20,635), *EMS353* (73,039 pg/mL ± 21,501) and *EMS371* (124,956 pg/mL ± 47,693), while all the *Enterococcus* strains had no effect on the production of this cytokine (Figure S1). Figure 4 shows the heat map of the ratios for each cytokine and chemokine detected in each condition and demonstrates that cytokine and chemokine production, by the BEAS-2B cells, was genus-specific. Indeed, similar secretion patterns within the *Streptococcus* genus were seen, as well as within the *Enterococcus* genus.

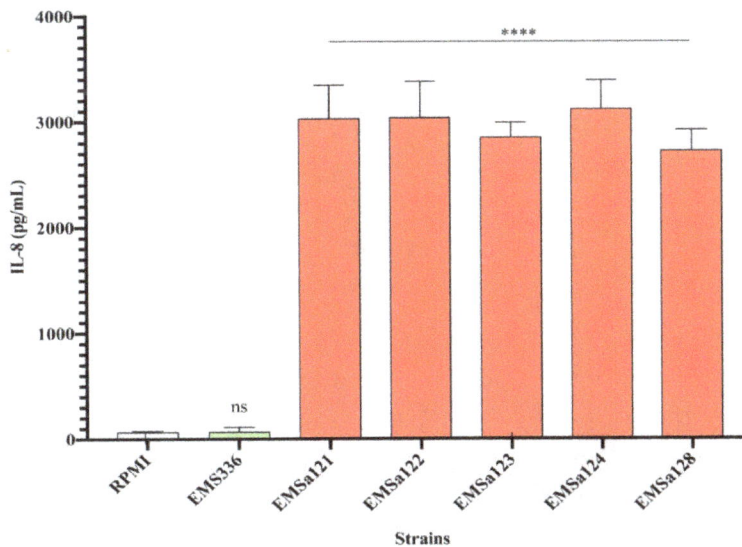

Figure 2. IL-8 produced by the BEAS-2B cells in response to primo-colonizing *Staphylococcus* strains. All strains of *Staphylococcus* (EMSa) and *Streptococcus* (EMS) were isolated from the buccal cavity of human newborns. *Staphylococcus* was isolated on the first day of life. For the challenge assay, BEAS-2B cells were co-incubated with bacterial strains (MOI of 100:1) for 6 h in 24-well plates. IL-8 was quantified by using ELISA immunoassays. Data are the mean of secreted IL-8 (pg/mL) ± SEM of at least two biological replicates (with two technical replicates each). *p*-values: *: $p < 0.03$, **: $p < 0.002$, ***: $p < 0.0002$ and ****: $p < 0.0001$.

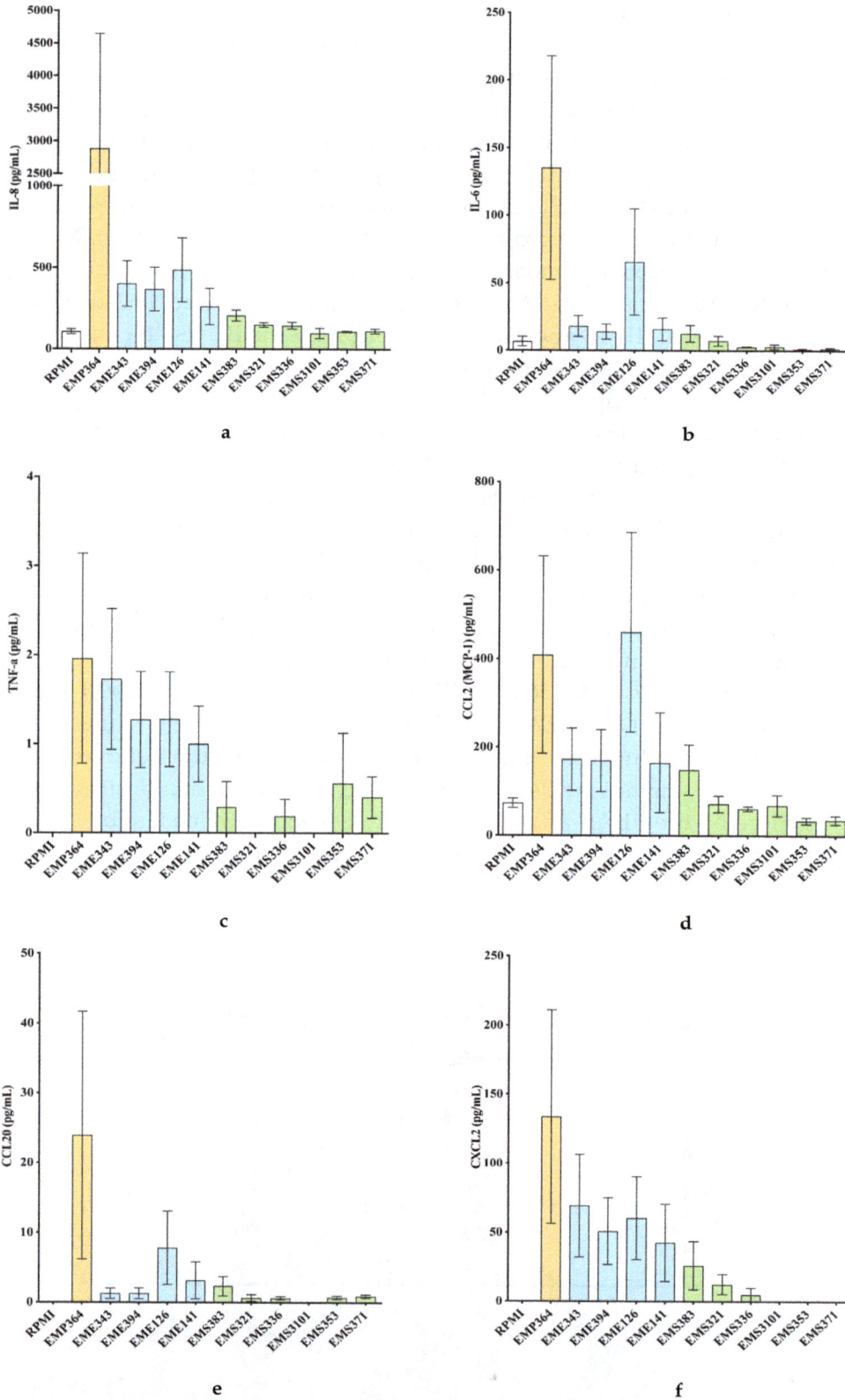

Figure 3. Cytokines and chemokines profiling of the BEAS-2B cells in response to bacterial stimulation: (**a**) IL-8, (**b**) IL-6, (**c**) TNF-α, (**d**) CCL2, (**e**) CCL20 and (**f**) CXCL2. Strains are identified as follows: *EMS, Streptococcus* strains; *EME, Enterococcus* strains; *EMP, Pantoea*. For the challenge assay, BEAS-2B cells were co-incubated with bacterial strains (MOI of 100:1) for 6 h, in 25 cm^2 tissue culture flasks. Cytokines and chemokines were quantified by using multiplex-magnetic-beads-based assay. Data are the mean of secreted proteins (pg/mL) $\pm$ SEM of four biological replicates (with two technical replicates each). *p*-values: *: $p < 0.03$, **: $p < 0.002$, ***: $p < 0.0002$ and ****: $p < 0.0001$.

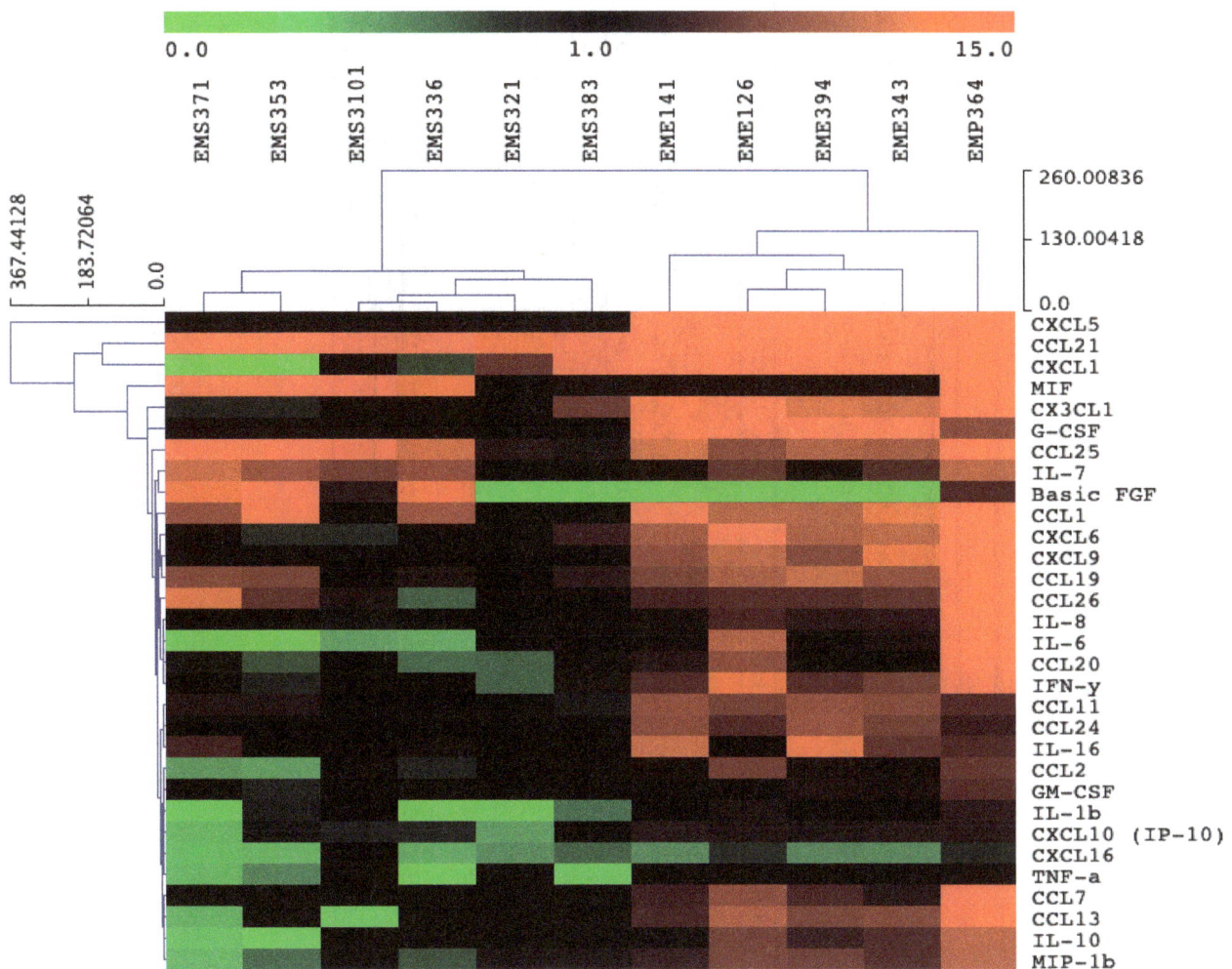

Figure 4. Similar patterns of cytokine, chemokine and growth factor production can be observed depending on the genera. Heatmap showing ratios (treatment/control, values not shown) of secreted proteins after 6 h incubation with bacterial strains. Strains are identified as follows: *EMS*, *Streptococcus* strains; *EME*, *Enterococcus* strains; *EMP*, *Pantoea*. Data are the mean of the ratio of four biological replicates. Heat map produced by using MeV. Hierarchical clustering gene leaf order, and Euclidian distance used as distance metric.

3.3. Analysis of Differential Gene Expression of BEAS-2B Cells, Using Microarray Analysis

To determine if early life buccal commensal bacteria influenced the transcriptional response of BECs, Human bronchial epithelial BEAS-2B cells were challenged with bacterial cultures (MOI = 100) for 6 h. RNA was extracted, and cDNA was prepared for a comparative microarray analysis of BEAS-2B cells stimulated individually with a selection of bacterial strains, or with quiescent cells serving as the control. Note that we were able to recover RNA from the flasks of 7 out of the 11 bacterial co-culture. As shown in Figure 5, the number of genes differentially expressed was strain-dependent. Most of the bacterial conditions differentially regulated between 148 and 303 genes; however, *Streptococcus EMS3101* downregulated up to 617 genes. This last treatment modulated a high number of genes (Figure 5). Among the whole set of genes, *IL-8*, *CCL2* and Activating Transcription Factor 3 (*ATF3*) were strongly upregulated (Table 1), and IL-8 was the most differentially expressed in BEAS-2B co-cultured with three out of four *Enterococcus* strains, with a maximum fold change of 14.5 for *EME343*.

Table 1. Top 10 differentially upregulated genes identified by genome-wide human expression microarrays. * Genes were considered significantly differentially expressed when (a) a t-test *p*-value was less than 0.05 and (b) a cutoff in transcript abundance reached at least 1.5-fold change. The 10 most upregulated genes for each strain are displayed in the table.

EME343		EME394		EME126		EME141		EMS321		EMS383		EMS3101	
Gene	Fold Change	Gene	Fold Change	Gene	Fold Change	Gene	Fold Change	Gene	Fold Change	Gene	Fold Change	Gene	Fold Change
IL8	14.502	IL8	12.219	IL8	8.043	CCL2	4.718	ATF3	5.989	CCL2	6.741	SNORD3B-1	4.091
CCL2	9.667	CCL20	11.190	CCL2	6.391	GADD45A	3.706	IL8	5.036	C1QTNF9	6.711	HIST2H2AA4	3.981
ATF3	7.888	IL1A	9.573	TNFAIP3	4.777	PTX3	3.620	CCL2	3.968	SULT1B1	5.156	CCL2	3.108
TNFAIP3	6.536	CXCL2	7.994	CLDN1	3.609	DDIT3	3.497	EGR1	3.734	CLDN1	4.469	SLC5A7	3.086
PTX3	6.242	CCL2	7.351	IER3	3.527	CLDN1	3.257	STC2	3.732	CHAC1	4.310	HIST1H2BI	3.074
CDKN1A	6.132	PTX3	5.996	NDRG1	3.296	STC2	3.160	PTX3	3.420	ATF3	4.124	HIST1H2AC	2.910
IL1A	6.088	EGR1	4.945	CXCL1	3.220	CXCL2	3.052	DDIT3	3.307	ASNS	4.020	HIST1H2BC	2.848
SLC7A11	5.094	STC2	4.444	PTX3	2.892	MAFF	2.901	CHAC1	3.166	TRIB3	3.930	HIST2H4B	2.759
EGR1	4.936	ATF3	4.391	CSN1S1	2.471	PPP1R15A	2.601	CLDN1	3.116	STC2	3.792	HIST1H4L	2.676
CXCL2	4.823	CHAC1	4.344	CEBPB	2.432	EGR1	2.573	VEGFA	2.963	SLC7A11	3.502	HIST4H4	2.593

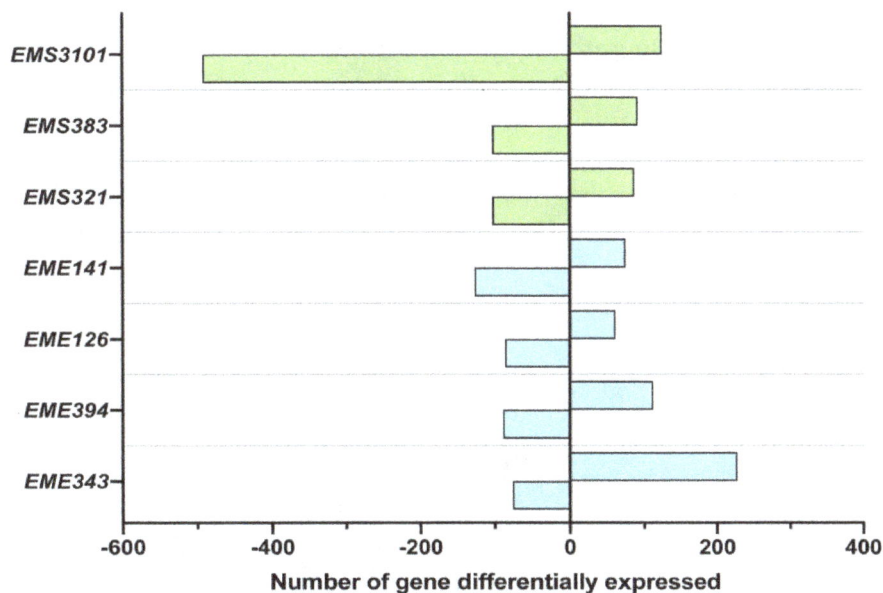

Figure 5. The number of differentially expressed genes is specific to the strain. Following bacterial challenge for 6 h, RNA from the BEAS-2B cells culture was analyzed by genome-wide expression analysis, using Agilent Whole Human 4x44K microarrays. Gene expression changes were expressed as fold of bacteria-treated compared to untreated control (culture medium only). Genes were considered significantly differentially expressed when (i) a t-test p-value of less than 0.05 and (ii) a cutoff in transcript abundance of least 1.5-fold change were observed. Data are expressed as the number of gene differentially expressed. Strains are identified as follows: *EMS*, *Streptococcus* strains; *EME*, *Enterococcus* strains.

3.4. Gene Enrichment Analysis

In order to identify relevant biological patterns from the whole set of genes differentially regulated by the BC strains, enrichment analysis was performed by using Ingenuity Pathway Analysis (IPA) software. The enrichment and pathway analysis was realized on gene sets with a 1.5-fold-change cutoff for each condition. The analysis revealed enrichment in molecular and cellular functions corresponding to the gene sets related to "cell signaling", "cell death and survival", "cellular movement", "cellular development", "cell-to-cell signaling and interactions" and "inflammation". As shown in Figure 6, the different bacteria induced strain-specific gene modulation in these clusters of molecular and cellular functions. Overall, *Streptococcus EMS3101* and *Enterococcus EME343* were the two strains that induced the most gene modulation in the assay conditions used. For example, the *Streptococcus EMS3101* had the greatest impact on genes involved in "cell death and survival", "cellular movement" and "cellular development" related functions. Interestingly, for the *Streptococcus*, only *EMS321* was found to regulate genes enriched in the "inflammation" cluster. All the *Enterococcus* strains displayed a similar pattern of enrichment. Of note, the *EME141* strain had less impact on genes differentially expressed related to "inflammation", "cell-to-cell signaling" and "interactions and cell signaling" functions than the other *Enterococcus* strains.

To get further insight into the pathways impacted by the bacterial treatments, IPA canonical pathway analysis was performed. We mainly focused our attention to pathways related to the "inflammation", "cell-to-cell signaling and interactions" and "cell signaling functions" to assess the immunomodulatory impact of BC strains on airway epithelial cell immunity. Based on IPA, enrichment pathways of differentially expressed genes were observed for glucocorticoid receptor signaling, IL-6 signaling, role of IL-17F in allergic inflammatory airway diseases, IL-17 signaling, tumor necrosis factor receptor (TNFR) 1 and 2 signaling, acute phase response signaling, TLRs signaling, IL-10 signaling, and the Janus kinase/signal transducers and activators of transcription (JAK/STAT) signaling (Figure 7). Overall, this analysis confirmed that *Enterococcus* strains had the strongest impact on the selected pathway of the inflammation and cell signaling. However, the EME141 strain had a significant lower impact on these pathways compared to the other *Enterococcus* strains. Only the glucocorticoid receptor signaling and the acute phase response signaling pathways were significantly enriched from the gene set corresponding to EME141. The *Streptococcus* strains were significantly associated in less than half of the selected pathways, and these associations were more likely to be random than with the *Enterococcus* strains (except for EME141) (Figure 7). Examples of genes that were upregulated in these pathways included *IL-8* (14.5-fold), *CCL2* (9.67-fold), *ATF3* (7.88-fold), *CXCL2* (7.99-fold) and *IL-1A* (up to 9.57-fold).

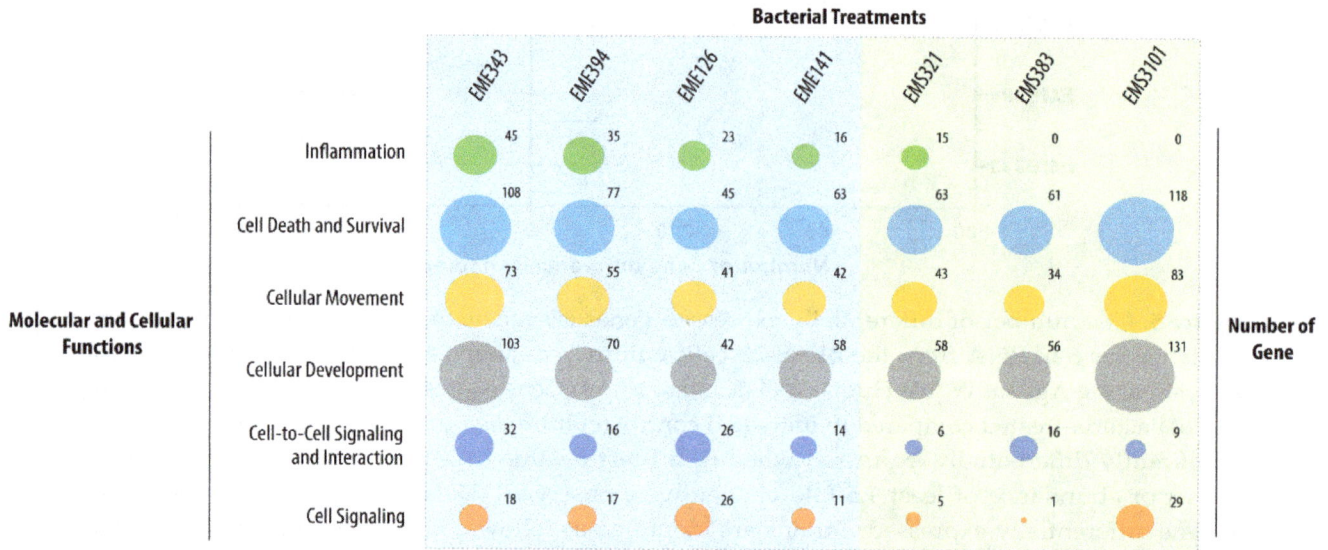

Figure 6. Number of genes significantly enriched in top molecular and cellular functions. Analysis was performed by using IPA. The area of the bubbles is proportional to the number of genes differentially expressed. Enrichment analysis of molecular and cellular functions are statistically significant when a p-value <0.05. The p-values range from 1.15×10^{-2} to 1.29×10^{-13}.

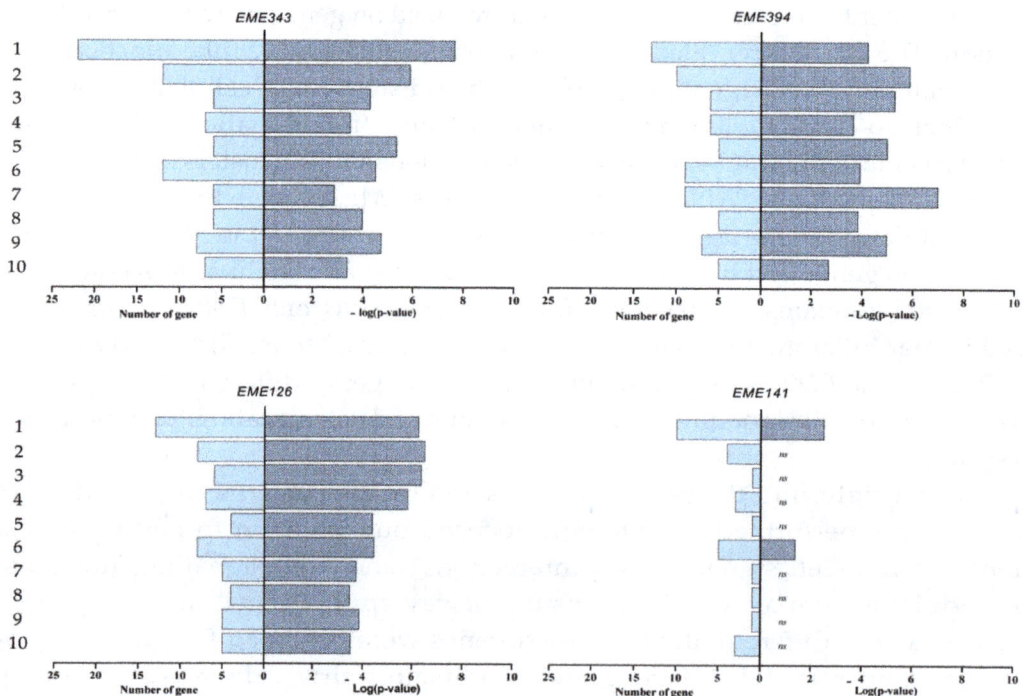

Figure 7. *Cont.*

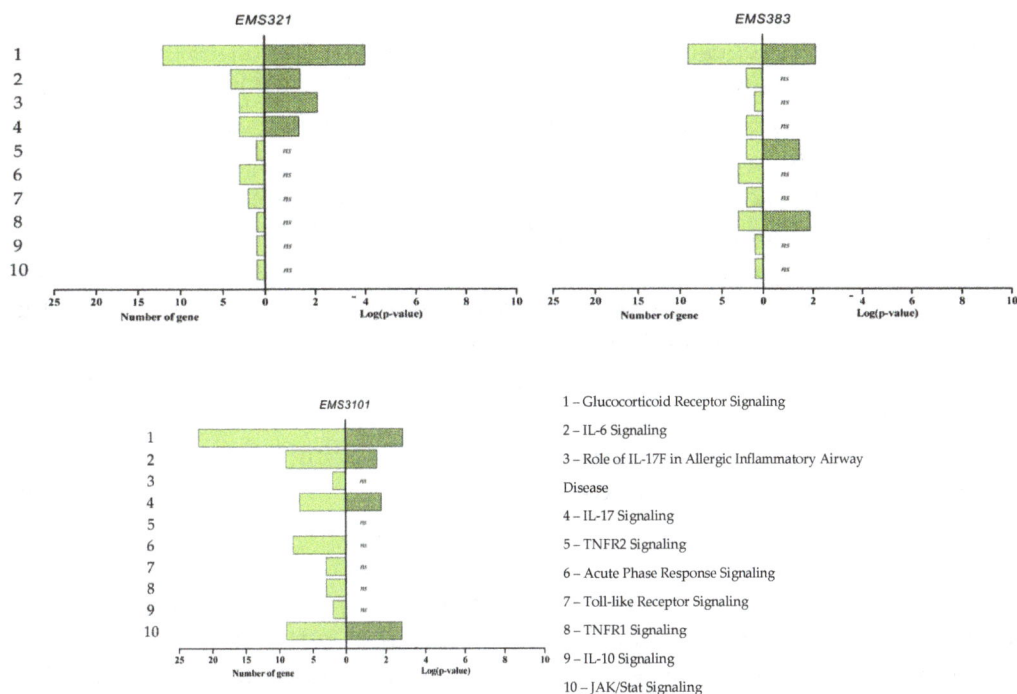

Figure 7. Significant canonical pathways of inflammation and the immune system modulated in BEAS-2B cells by our BC bacteria. Strains are identified as follows: *EMS*, *Streptococcus* strains; *EME*, *Enterococcus* strains. Fold change cutoff = 1.5. The *y*-axis is the $-\log(p\text{-value})$, as produced by IPA, and the *x*-axis is the pathways modulated in BEAS-2B cells. The canonical pathways are predicted pathways that are changing based on gene expression; the higher the $-\log(p\text{-value})$ is, the less likely the association is random.

4. Discussion

This study aimed to isolate cultivable commensal strains from the buccal cavity of human newborns and evaluate their impact on bronchial epithelial cells. We isolated pioneer members of the early life buccal microbiota, and our results provide new insight on the ability of primo-colonizing bacteria to modulate inflammatory pathways in BEAS-2B cells. We also showed that strains from the different genera induced specific differential cytokine/chemokine/growth factor secretion profiles. All together, these data suggest that early life buccal bacterial strains may differentially stimulate and shape the lung immunity.

The isolation process led to the creation of a library made by bacterial strains originating from the oral cavity of human newborns. It is important to note here that the methods of sampling, storage, transport and isolation used in this study may have resulted in the loss of strict anaerobic, sub-dominant and fastidious bacteria. However, the objective of this study was not to identify all the cultivable bacteria of the BC; instead, we sought some representative strains, in order to assess their immunomodulatory effects. Strains that were identified belong to genera that have been shown to be part of the buccal core microbiota during early life. A recent study by Daspher and colleges has shown that members of *Streptococcus*, *Staphylococcus* and *Rothia* genera were early life colonizers of the BC [39]. In our library, *Enterococcus* species were also present. This genus is generally less represented in buccal and lung microbiome [40]. Based on the strains we have identified, the colonization of the BC appears to be sequential. *Staphylococcus* was the only genus detected on the first day of life, while, apart from being the most isolated genus, the *Streptococcus* strains were isolated in every sample from day two onward (Figure 1b), suggesting a persistent colonization of the oral cavity by this genus rather than a transitory passage. Our findings are in accordance with previous studies that have shown that *Streptococcus* is the dominant genus in the oral cavity of newborns [41–44]. Our intention to target the primo-colonizing bacteria was motivated by recent reports describing the early life as a pivotal time for determining the susceptibility to develop chronic respiratory diseases such as asthma. In particular, Arrieta and colleagues have suggested that the first 100 days of life represent an "early-life critical window" where gut dysbiosis influences the risk to develop asthma [45]. The authors demonstrated a causal role of certain bacterial taxa (e.g., *Veillonella* and *Faecalibacterium*) during this period in averting asthma development. Furthermore, increasing evidence suggests that the early lung ecosystem impacts the future respiratory health [20,21]. While no causal role has been established for the microbial communities of the BC in asthma, a recent report has highlighted changes in the composition of the buccal microbiota as soon as three months of age in infants that further developed allergy and asthma later in life [9]. Herein, we had access to precious early life microbial strains of the BC that may be an important stimulator of local and distal immunity. The characterization of their immunomodulatory potential is of major interest in the development of new therapeutic approach for the management of chronic respiratory diseases.

An important observation in this study is that primo-colonizing bacteria clearly induced different response profiles, depending on their phylogeny. Interestingly, the *Staphylococcus* strains isolated in the first days of life displayed strong pro-inflammatory profiles. As shown in Figure 2, some strains were able to induce high production of IL-8. We can presume that there is a mutual benefit for the host and for the *Staphylococcus* strains to this pro-inflammatory response. Thus, it would be interesting to determine the impact of these pro-inflammatory stimuli at birth, which may participate in the acquisition of tolerance by the innate system. We focused our attention on a selection of 11 strains and the measurement of cytokines and chemokines in BEAS-2B cell supernatants. Our results have shown that the *Streptococcus* and *Enterococcus* strains were inducing differential production profiles. Overall, the pattern of cytokines and chemokines production was specific to the genera. We observed distinct clusters of response between the *Enterococcus* and the *Streptococcus*, and the strain *Pantoea EMP-364* induced a significant upregulation of most of the cytokines and chemokines we tested. Interestingly, we observed an significant production of MIF, up to 124,956 pg/mL (Figure S1, *EMS371*), induced by the *Streptococcus* strains. MIF overexpression has been shown to be linked to an increased level of IL-8, TNF-α, IL-6 and IL-1β in BAL fluid and sputum of asthmatic patients [46,47]. This proinflammatory cytokine also mediates the anti-inflammatory effect of glucocorticoids [47]. Herein, the high levels of MIF secreted in response to *Streptococcus* strains were not corelated to a significant production of IL-8, TNF-α, IL-6 and IL-1β by the BEAS-2B cells, under the experimental condition used. Previous observations showed that the secretome of a beneficial probiotic strain, *Lactobacillus rhamnosus* R0011, induced an important production of MIF by the HT-29 intestinal epithelial cells and attenuated proinflammatory mediators [48]. Moreover, MIF has been shown to induce MAPK activation within Type II alveolar epithelial cells, leading to enhanced cellular proliferation, potentially contributing to repair of damaged alveolus in response to infection [49]. Taken together, induction of MIF by the *Streptococcus* strains used in this study highlights a potential novel beneficial outcome of host–microbe interactions within the lung environment and warrants further investigation. We next thought to evaluate the differential gene expression of BEAS-2B, to refine our observations on the specificity of the response induced by the strains. The analysis of differential gene expression of BEAS-2B cells using genome-wide microarray showed that the *Streptococcus* and *Enterococcus* strains induced a differential gene expression profile. It is important to note here that no microarray data are available for one *Pantoea* (EMP364) and three *Streptococcus* (EMS336, EMS353 and EMS371). These three strains of *Streptococcus* were shown to form a dense network in the culture medium during co-culture with epithelial cells. These networks might have stuck to the cell layer when recovering the supernatant, and we were never able to recover RNA following co-culture with these strains. This observation was specific to these three strains of *Streptococcus* only. EMS321, EMS383 and EMS3101 did not form such a network. It has been previously shown that oral *Streptococcus* possesses filamentous capacities that vary among species of the same genus [50]. Herein, we chose not to specify the species, for confidential reasons due to the partnership with an industrial company. Overall, the *Enterococcus* strains induced higher expression fold change for most of the genes involved in pro-inflammatory pathways. Genes such as

IL8 (maximum fold change = 14.50 for *EME343*), *CCL2* (maximum fold change = 9.67 for *EME343*), *ATF3* (maximum fold change = 7.89 for *EME343*), TNF-α Induced Protein 3 (*TNFAIP3*) (maximum fold change = 6.54 for *EME343*), Pentraxin 3 (*PTX3*) (maximum fold change = 6.24 for *EME343*), *CXCL2* (maximum fold change = 7.99 for *EME394*), *IL1A* (maximum fold change = 9.57 for *EME394*) and *CCL20* (maximum fold change = 11.19 for *EME394*) were the common top upregulated genes in cells incubated with the *Enterococcus* strains (Table 1). The enrichment analysis of the expression data showed an increased enrichment of molecular and cellular functions related to "inflammation", "cell signaling", and "cell-to-cell signaling and interactions" for the *Enterococcus* in regards to the *Streptococcus* (Figure 6). The analysis of the canonical pathway related to these clusters of molecular and cellular functions reinforced the differences observed between these two genera but also highlighted differences in regards to the strains. The gene sets were enriched in pathways such as glucocorticoid receptor signaling, IL-6 signaling, role of IL-17F in allergic inflammatory airway diseases, IL-17 signaling, TNFR1 and 2 signaling, IL-10 signaling and JAK/STAT signaling (Figure 7). These pathways are downstream pathways of cytokines signal transduction and play an important role in the immune response of the host [51–53]. Altogether, these differences suggest that, in response to the bacterial stimuli, the epithelial cells might respond specifically by recruiting and stimulating different immune cell populations, depending on their phylogeny.

Newborn lungs, as the immune system, are fully functioning at birth but still developing, and several factors can influence normal morphogenesis. In humans, lung formation starts during the embryonic phase, and the alveolarization finishes at early adult age. Herein, we observed the differential expression of some genes related to the regulation of the postnatal lung morphogenesis such as *EGR1* and *VEGFA* (Table 1). Vascular endothelial growth factor (VEGF) signaling has been shown to play a role in early lung morphogenesis, and BAL VEGF levels may be used to identify preterm infants with a risk of developing BPD [54,55]. The growth factor VEGF was detectable and measurable with the multiplex analysis, but the high variability between replicates did not allow the assessment of the extent of VEGF production (data not shown). We found a high number of genes significantly enriched for the glucocorticoid receptor-signaling pathway. Glucocorticoid receptors, once activated in developing lung, induce a series of morphological alteration in the pulmonary architecture and stimulate lung maturation [56]. Moreover, glucocorticoid treatments were shown to be effective in infant at risk to develop respiratory diseases and are commonly used in women at risk of preterm birth in order to help mature fetal lungs [56–58]. We also noted differential production of basic-FGF, C-GSF, GM-CSF and IL-1b that have all been shown to be involved in lung morphogenesis. Similar to their potential impact on the pulmonary immune maturation, the strains studied in this project may have a differential impact on the morphological and functional maturation of the airways.

To our knowledge, this is the first study to establish the impact of bacterial strains, isolated from the buccal cavity during the first week of life of two babies, on human bronchial epithelial cells in vitro. Although it gives new insight into the impact of different bacterial genera of the oral cavity to modulate lung epithelial cells responses, our study has some limitations. First, the bacteria studied in this project originated from two donors. Even though the strains isolated in our study are in accordance with previous reports on the composition of the BC microbiota, sampling should be performed on a higher number of babies, in order to be more representative of the early-life buccal microbiota. A metagenomic study would give a larger view of the total microbiota and allow us to assess the impact of the sampling, storage and transport methods on the amount and diversity of the bacterial strains recovered. Secondly, we have used BEAS-2B cells as model of bronchial epithelial cells. While providing several advantages, such as low variability and easy handling, BEAS-2B cells represented a simplification of the bronchial epithelium. Indeed, the monolayered undifferentiated cell culture implies a lack of the different cell types (basal, ciliated, goblet and club cells), which were shown to exert specific roles in the epithelial physiology of the airways. For further analysis, it would be of interest to use primary airway epithelial cells and/or a reconstituted airway epithelia to better understand the effects of these strains on immune homeostasis and especially in a pro-inflammatory context. Finally, it will be important to test these strains in vivo, to investigate their capacity to stimulate the lung immunity and to provide an advantage against the development of chronic or acute respiratory diseases.

Author Contributions: Conceptualization, P.L. and M.T.; data curation, E.M.; formal analysis, E.M., C.W.M. and O.M.; funding acquisition, P.L., T.A.T. and M.T.; investigation, E.M., C.W.M., J.B., O.M. and V.R.; methodology, E.M., C.W.M. and T.A.T.; project administration, E.M. and M.T.; resources, C.W.M., T.A.T. and M.T.; supervision, T.A.T. and M.T.; PhD supervision, T.A.T. and M.T.; validation, T.A.T. and M.T.; visualization, E.M. and V.S.-C.; writing—original draft, E.M.; writing—review and editing, E.M., C.W.M., J.B., O.M., V.S.-C., T.A.T. and M.T. All authors have read and agreed to the published version of the manuscript.

References

1.   Zhang, Y.; Wang, X.; Li, H.; Ni, C.; Du, Z.; Yan, F. Human oral microbiota and its modulation for oral health. *Biomed. Pharmacother.* **2018**, *99*, 883–893. [CrossRef] [PubMed]

2.   Arweiler, N.B.; Netuschil, L. The Oral Microbiota. *Adv. Exp. Med. Biol.* **2016**, *902*, 45–60. [CrossRef] [PubMed]

3.   Rosier, B.T.; Marsh, P.D.; Mira, A. Resilience of the Oral Microbiota in Health: Mechanisms That Prevent Dysbiosis. *Crit. Rev. Oral Biol. Med.* **2018**, *97*, 371–380. [CrossRef]

4.   Escapa, I.F.; Chen, T.; Huang, Y.; Gajare, P.; Dewhirst, F.E.; Lemon, K.P. New insights into human nostril microbiome from the expanded Human Oral Microbiome Database (eHOMD): A resource for species-level identification of microbiome data from the aerodigestive tract. *mSystems* **2018**, *3*. [CrossRef] [PubMed]

5.   The Human Microbiome Project Consortium. Structure, Function and Diversity of the Healthy Human Microbiome. *Nature* **2012**, *486*, 207–214. [CrossRef] [PubMed]

6.   Siqueira, J.F.; Roôças, I.N. The Oral Microbiota in Health and Disease: An Overview of Molecular Findings. *Methods Mol. Biol.* **2017**, *1537*, 127–138. [CrossRef] [PubMed]

7.   Atarashi, K.; Suda, W.; Luo, C.; Kawaguchi, T.; Motoo, I.; Narushima, S.; Kiguchi, Y.; Yasuma, K.; Watanabe, E.; Tanoue, T.; et al. Ectopic colonization of oral bacteria in the intestine drives TH1 cell induction and inflammation. *Science* **2017**, *358*, 359–365. [CrossRef]

8.   Pu, C.Y.; Seshadri, M.; Manuballa, S.; Yendamuri, S. The Oral Microbiome and Lung Diseases. *Current Oral Health Rep.* **2020**, *7*, 79–86. [CrossRef]

9.   Dzidic, M.; Abrahamsson, T.; Artacho, A.; Collado, M.C.; Mira, A.; Jenmalm, M.C. Oral microbiota maturation during the first 7 years of life in relation to allergy development. *Allergy* **2018**, *73*, 2000–2011. [CrossRef]

10.   Heo, S.M.; Haase, E.M.; Lesse, A.J.; Gill, S.R.; Scannapieco, F.A. Genetic Relationships between Respiratory Pathogens Isolated from Dental Plaque and Bronchoalveolar Lavage Fluid from Patients in the Intensive Care Unit Undergoing Mechanical Ventilation. *Clin. Infect. Dis.* **2008**, *47*, 1562–1570. [CrossRef]

11.   Morris, A.; Beck, M.; Schloss, P.D.; Campbell, T.B.; Crothers, K.; Curtis, J.L. Comparison of the respiratory microbiome in healthy nonsmokers and smokers. *Am. J. Respir. Crit. Care Med.* **2013**, *187*, 1067–1075. [CrossRef] [PubMed]

12.   Dickson, R.P.; Huffnagle, G.B. The lung microbiome: New principles for respiratory bacteriology in health and disease. *PLoS Pathog.* **2015**, *11*, e1004923. [CrossRef] [PubMed]

13.   Venkataraman, A.; Bassis, C.M.; Beck, J.M.; Young, V.B.; Curtis, J.L.; Huffnagle, G.B. Application of a neutral community model to assess structuring of the human lung microbiome. *mBio* **2015**, *6*, e02284-14. [CrossRef] [PubMed]

14.   Mathieu, E.; Escribano-Vazquez, U.; Descamps, D.; Cherbuy, C.; Langella, P.; Riffault, S.; Remot, A.; Thomas, M. Paradigms of Lung Microbiota Functions in Health and Disease, Particularly, in Asthma. *Front. Physiol.* **2018** *9*, 1168. [CrossRef] [PubMed]

15. Hilty, M.; Burke, C.; Pedro, H.; Cardenas, P.; Bush, A.; Bossley, C. Disordered microbial communities in asthmatic airways. *PLoS ONE* **2010**, *5*, e8578. [CrossRef] [PubMed]

16. Segal, L.N.; Clemente, J.C.; Tsay, J.C.; Koralov, S.B.; Keller, B.C.; Wu., B.G. Enrichment of the lung microbiome with oral taxa is associated with lung inflammation of a Th17 phenotype. *Nat. Microbiol.* **2016**, *1*, 16031. [CrossRef]

17. Yu, G.; Gail, M.H.; Consonni, D.; Carugno, M.; Humphrys, M.; Pesatori, A.C. Characterizing human lung tissue microbiota and its relationship to epidemiological and clinical features. *Genome Biol.* **2016**, *17*, 163. [CrossRef]

18. Pattaroni, C.; Watzenboeck, M.L.; Schneidegger, S.; Kieser, S.; Wong, N.C.; Bernasconi, E.; Pernot, J.; Mercier, L.; Knapp, S.; Nicod, L.P.; et al. Early-Life Formation of the Microbial and Immunological Environment of the Human Airways. *Cell Host Microb.* **2018**, *24*, 857–865. [CrossRef]

19. Singh, N.; Vats, A.; Sharma, A.; Arora, A.; Kumar, A. The development of lower respiratory tract microbiome in mice. *Microbiome* **2017**, *5*, 61. [CrossRef]

20. Remot, A.; Descamps, D.; Noordine, M.L.; Boukadiri, A.; Mathieu, E.; Robert, V.; Riffault, S.; Lambrecht, B.; Langella, P.; Hammad, H.; et al. Bacteria isolated from lung modulate asthma susceptibility in mice. *ISME J.* **2017**, *11*, 1061–1107. [CrossRef]

21. Gollwitzer, E.S.; Saglani, S.; Trompette, A.; Yadava, K.; Sherburn, R.; McCoy, K.D. Lung microbiota promotes tolerance to allergens in neonates via PD-L1. *Nat. Med.* **2014**, *20*, 642–647. [CrossRef]

22. Segal, L.N.; Rom, W.N.; Weiden, M.D. Lung microbiome for clinicians. New discoveries about bugs in healthy and diseased lungs. *Ann. Am. Thorac. Soc.* **2014**, *11*, 108–116. [CrossRef] [PubMed]

23. Ege, M.J.; Mayer, M.; Normand, A.-C.; Genuneit, J.; Cookson, W.O.C.M.; Phil, D.; Braun-Fahrländer, C.; Heederik, R.; Piarroux, R.; Von Mutius, E.; et al. Exposure to Environmental Microorganisms and Childhood Asthma. *N. Engl. J. Med.* **2011**, *364*, 701–709. [CrossRef] [PubMed]

24. Marsland, B.J. Influences of the microbiome on the early origins of allergic asthma. *Ann. Am. Thorac. Soc.* **2013**, *10*, S165–S169. [CrossRef] [PubMed]

25. Lynch, S.V.; Wood, R.A.; Boushey, H.; Bacharier, L.B.; Bloomberg, G.R.; Kattan, M.; O'Connor, G.T.; Sandel, M.T.; Calatroni, A.; Matsui, E.; et al. Effects of Early Life Exposure to Allergens and Bacteria on Recurrent Wheeze and Atopy in Urban Children. *J. Allergy Clin. Immunol.* **2014**, *134*, 593–601. [CrossRef] [PubMed]

26. Kilpeläinen, M.; Terho, E.O.; Helenius, H.; Koskenvuo, M. Farm environment in childhood prevents the development of allergies. *Clin. Exp. Allergy* **2000**, *30*, 201–208. [CrossRef]

27. Riedler, J.; Eder, W.; Oberfeld, G.; Schreuer, M. Austrian children living on a farm have less hay fever, asthma and allergic sensitization. *Clin. Exp. Allergy* **2000**, *30*, 194–200. [CrossRef]

28. Douwes, J.; Travier, N.; Huang, K.; Cheng, S.; McKenzie, J.; Le Gros, G.; von Mutius, E.; Pearce, N. Lifelong farm exposure may strongly reduce the risk of asthma in adults. *Allergy* **2007**, *62*, 1158–1165. [CrossRef]

29. Zou, J.; Zhou, L.; Hu, C.; Jing, P.; Guo, X.; Liu, S.; Lei, Y.; Yang, S.; Deng, J.; Zhang, H. IL-8 and IP-10 expression from human bronchial epithelial cells BEAS-2B are promoted by Streptococcus pneumoniae endopeptidase O (PepO). *BMC Microbiol.* **2017**, *17*, 187. [CrossRef]

30. Wang, Y.; Bai, C.; Li, K.; Adler, K.B.; Wang, X. Role of airway epithelial cells in development of asthma and allergic rhinitis. *Respir. Med.* **2008**, *102*, 949–955. [CrossRef]

31. Bhowmick, R.; Gappa-Fahlenkamp, H. Cells and Culture Systems Used to Model the Small Airway Epithelium. *Lung* **2016**, *194*, 419–428. [CrossRef] [PubMed]

32. Hammad, H.; Chieppa, M.; Perros, F.; Willart, M.A.; Germain, R.N.; Lambrecht, B.N. House dust mite allergen induces asthma via Toll- like receptor 4 triggering of airway structural cells. *Nat. Med.* **2009**, *15*, 410–416. [CrossRef]

33. Di Stefano, A.; Ricciardolo, F.L.; Caramori, G.; Adcock, I.M.; Chung, K.F.; Barnes, P.J. Bronchial inflammation and bacterial load in stable COPD is associated with TLR4 overexpression. *Eur. Respir. J.* **2017**, *49*, 1602006. [CrossRef]

34. Carlini, F.; Picard, C.; Garulli, C.; Piquemal, D.; Roubertoux, P.; Chiaroni, J.; Chanez, P.; Gras, D.; Di Cristofaro, J. Bronchial Epithelial Cells from Asthmatic Patients Display Less Functional HLA-G Isoform Expression. *Front. Immunol.* **2017**, *8*, 6. [CrossRef] [PubMed]

35. Flynn, J.M.; Niccum, D.; Dunitz, J.M.; Hunter, R.C. Evidence and role for bacterial mucin degradation in cystic fibrosis airway disease. *PLoS Pathog.* **2016**, *12*, e1005846. [CrossRef]

36. Ni, K.; Wang, Y.; Li, D.; Cai, Y.; Pang, H. Characterization, Identification and Application of Lactic Acid Bacteria Isolated from Forage Paddy Rice Silage. *PLoS ONE* **2015**, *10*, e0121967. [CrossRef] [PubMed]

37. Medicine, U.S. National Library of. n.d. National Center for Biotechnology Information. Available online: https://blast.ncbi.nlm.nih.gov/Blast.cgi (accessed on 17 July 2020).

38. MacPherson, C.W.; Shastri, P.; Mathieu, O.; Tompkins, T.A.; Burguieère, P. Genome-Wide Immune Modulation of TLR3- Mediated Inflammation in Intestinal Epithelial Cells Differs between Single and Multi-Strain Probiotic Combination. *PLoS ONE* **2017**, *12*, e0169847. [CrossRef] [PubMed]

39. Dashper, S.G.; Mitchell, H.L.; Leêcao, K.A.; Carpenter, L.; Gussy, M.G.; Calache, H.; Gladman, S.L.; Bulach, D.M.; Hoffmann, B.; Catmull, D.V.; et al. Temporal development of the oral microbiome and prediction of early childhood caries. *Sci. Rep.* **2019**, *9*, 19732. [CrossRef]

40. Komiyama, E.Y.; Lepesqueu, L.S.S.; Yassuda, C.G.; Samaranayake, L.P.; Parahitiyawa, N.B.; Balducci, I.; Koga-Ito, C.Y. Enterococcus Species in the Oral Cavity: Prevalence, Virulence Factors and Antimicrobial Susceptibility. *PLoS ONE* **2016**, *11*, e0163001. [CrossRef]

41. Abranches, J.; Zeng, L.; Kajfasz, J.K.; Palmer, S.R.; Chakraborty, B.; Wen, Z.T.; Richards, V.P.; Brady, L.J.; Lemos, J.A. Biology of Oral Streptococci. *Microbiol. Spectr.* **2018**, *6*, GPP3-0042-201. [CrossRef]

42. Kennedy, B.; Peura, S.; Hammar, U.; Vicenzi, S.; Hedman, A.; Almqvist, C.; Andolf, E.; Pershagen, G.; Dicksved, J.; Bertilsonn, S.; et al. Oral Microbiota Development in early childhood. *Sci. Rep.* **2019**, *9*, 19025. [CrossRef]

43. Dzidic, M.; Collado, M.C.; Abrahamsson, T.; Artacho, A.; Stensson, M.; Jenmalm, M.C.; Mira, A. Oral microbiome development during childhood: An ecological succession influenced by postnatal factors and associated with tooth decay. *ISME J.* **2018**, *12*, 2292–2306. [CrossRef]

44. Kononen, E. Development of oral bacterial flora in young children. *Ann. Med.* **2000**, *32*, 107–112. [CrossRef]

45. Arrieta, M.C.; Stiemsma, L.T.; Dimitriu, P.A.; Thorson, L.; Russell, S.; Yurist-Doutsch, S.; Kuzeljevic, B. Early infancy microbial and metabolic alterations affect risk of childhood asthma. *Sci. Transl. Med.* **2015**, *7*, 307ra152. [CrossRef]

46. Yamaguchi, E.; Nishihira, J.; Shimizu, T.; Takahashi, T.; Kitashiro, N.; Hizawa, N.; Kamishima, K.; Kawakami, Y. Macrophage migration inhibitory factor (MIF) in bronchial asthma. *Clin. Exp. Allergy J. Br. Soc. Allergy Clin. Immunol.* **2000**, *30*, 1244–1249. [CrossRef]

47. Lan, H.; Luo, L.; Chen, Y.; Wang, M.; Yu, Z.; Gong, Y. MIF signaling blocking alleviates airway inflammation and airway epithelial barrier disruption in a HDM-induced asthma model. *Cell. Immunol.* **2020**, *347*. [CrossRef]

48. Jeffrey, M.P.; MacPherson, C.W.; Mathieu, O.; Tompkins, T.A.; Green-Johnson, J.M. Secretome-Mediated Interactions with Intestinal Epithelial Cells: A Role for Secretome Components from Lactobacillus rhamnosus R0011 in the Attenuation of Salmonella enterica Serovar Typhimurium Secretome and TNF- α−Induced Proinflammatory Responses. *J. Immunol. Publ. Online* **2020**, *204*, 2523–2534. [CrossRef]

49. Rossetti, V.; Ammann, T.W.; Thurnheer, T.; Bagheri, H.C.; Belibasakis, G.N. Phenotypic Diversity of Multicellular Filamentation in Oral Streptococci. *PLoS ONE* **2013**, *8*, e76221. [CrossRef]

50. Rawlings, J.S.; Rosler, K.M.; Harrison, D.A. The JAK/STAT signaling pathway. *J. Cell Sci.* **2004**, *117*, 1281–1283. [CrossRef]

51. Kawaguchi, M.; Kokubu, F.; Fujita, J.; Huang, S.K.; Hizawa, N. Role of interleukin-17F in asthma. *Inflamm. Allergy Drug Targets* **2009**, *8*, 383–389. [CrossRef]

52. Dempsey, P.W.; Doyle, S.E.; He, J.Q.; Cheng, G. The signaling adaptors and pathways activated by TNF superfamily. *Cytokine Growth Factor Rev.* **2003**, *14*, 193–209. [CrossRef]

53. Warburton, D.; Bellusci, S.; Del Moral, P.-M.; Kaartinen, V.; Lee, M.; Tefft, D.; Shi, W. Growth factor signaling in lung morphogenetic centers: Automaticity, stereotypy and symmetry. *Respir. Res.* **2003**, *4*, 5. [CrossRef]

54. Been, J.V.; Debeer, A.; Van Iwaarden, J.F.; Kloosterboer, N.; Passos, V.L.; Naulaers, G.; Zimmermann, L.J. Early Alterations of Growth Factor Patterns in Bronchoalveolar Lavage Fluid From Preterm Infants Developing Bronchopulmonary Dysplasia. *Pediatr. Res.* **2010**, *67*, 83–89. [CrossRef]

55. Bird, A.D.; McDougall, A.R.A.; Seow, B.; Hooper, S.B.; Cole, T.J. Glucocorticoid regulation of lung development: Lessons learned from conditional GR knockout mice. *Mol. Endocrinol.* **2014**, *29*, 158–171. [CrossRef]

56. Bolt, R.J.; van Weissenbruch, M.M.; Lafeber, H.N.; Delemarre-van de Waal., H.A. Glucocorticoids and Lung Development in the Fetus and Preterm Infant. *Pediatr. Pulmonol.* **2001**, *32*, 76–91. [CrossRef]

3

The Effect of Selected Dental Materials Used in Conservative Dentistry, Endodontics, Surgery and Orthodontics as Well as during the Periodontal Treatment on the Redox Balance in the Oral Cavity

Izabela Zieniewska [1,*], Mateusz Maciejczyk [2]ⓘ and Anna Zalewska [3,*]ⓘ

[1] Doctoral Studies, Medical University of Bialystok, 24a M. Sklodowskiej-Curie Street, 15-274 Bialystok, Poland
[2] Department of Hygiene, Epidemiology and Ergonomics, Medical University of Bialystok, 15-022 Bialystok, Poland; mat.maciejczyk@gmail.com
[3] Experimental Dentistry Laboratory, Medical University of Bialystok, 24a M. Sklodowskiej-Curie Street, 15-274 Bialystok, Poland
* Correspondence: izazieniewska@gmail.com (I.Z.); azalewska426@gmail.com (A.Z.)

Abstract: Oxidative stress (OS) is a redox homeostasis disorder that results in oxidation of cell components and thus disturbs cell metabolism. OS is induced by numerous internal as well as external factors. According to recent studies, dental treatment may also be one of them. The aim of our work was to assess the effect of dental treatment on the redox balance of the oral cavity. We reviewed literature available in PubMed, Medline, and Scopus databases, including the results from 2010 to 2020. Publications were searched according to the keywords: oxidative stress and dental monomers; oxidative stress and amalgam; oxidative stress and periodontitis, oxidative stress and braces, oxidative stress and titanium; oxidative stress and dental implants, oxidative stress and endodontics treatment, oxidative stress and dental treatment; and oxidative stress and dental composite. It was found that dental treatment with the use of composites, amalgams, glass-ionomers, materials for root canal filling/rinsing, orthodontic braces (made of various metal alloys), titanium implants, or whitening agents can disturb oral redox homeostasis by affecting the antioxidant barrier and increasing oxidative damage to salivary proteins, lipids, and DNA. Abnormal saliva secretion/composition was also observed in dental patients in the course of OS. It is suggested that the addition of antioxidants to dental materials or antioxidant therapy applied during dental treatment could protect the patient against harmful effects of OS in the oral cavity.

Keywords: amalgam; antioxidants; dental resin composites; composites resins; endodontics treatment; glass-ionomer; orthodontics appliances; oxidative stress; periodontal treatment; redox balance; titanium implants; whitening

1. Introduction

Oxidative stress (OS) is defined as an imbalance between the production of oxygen (ROS) and nitrogen (RNS) free radicals and their neutralization by compounds called antioxidants [1]. Interestingly, ROS also act as signaling molecules involved in cell growth, proliferation and survival [2]. ROS/RNS are formed under the influence of external factors, such as ionizing radiation, ultraviolet radiation or ultrasound, as well as produced endogenously [3]. The main non-enzymatic, endogenous source of ROS/RNS in a cell is the mitochondrial respiratory chain. There are also enzymatic sources of ROS/RNS, including: xanthine oxidase (XO), cyclooxygenases (COX), lipoxygenases, myeloperoxidases (MPO), cytochrome P450 monooxygenase, uncoupled nitric oxide synthase (NOS), peroxidases and NADPH oxidase (NOX) [2]. The excess of ROS/RNS leads to the damage of cellular components such as proteins, lipids and nucleic acids as well as to cell death through apoptosis and necrosis [4,5].

Proteins are the main molecules attacked by ROS [6]. Highly reactive radicals cause multi-area damage to the protein side chain and backbone. Less reactive species demonstrate greater selectivity and damage smaller areas. Oxidation of proteins may cause increased hydrophilicity of the protein side chains, fragmentation of the side chains as well as the backbone, aggregation through covalent crosslinking or hydrophobic interactions, and protein conformation [7].

During protein peroxidation, cysteine and—to a lesser extent—methionine residues are oxidized. Usually hydrogen atoms are detached from the C-H or S-H bonds by the radical [7]. The separation of a hydrogen atom from carbon leads to the formation of a stabilized carbon-centered radical, which then reacts with other carbon-centered radicals or with O_2 [8]. These reactions result in protein backbone fragmentation [8].

The side chains of amino acids are also subject to oxidative damage [9]. This mechanism usually leads to the formation of carbon-centered radicals. The amino acid side chains that contain sulfur are the most exposed to the oxidation process. Free amino acids are much less frequently damaged than the side chains, probably due to the fact that there are fewer of them than the side chains [7].

Lipid oxidation occurs in the presence of numerous oxidants, including peroxynitrite, hypochlorite, lipoxygenases, cyclooxygenase, cytochrome P450, and singlet oxygen [10]. Unsaturated lipids are particularly susceptible to oxidation. Under the influence of radical oxidants such as peroxyl radicals, lipid hydroperoxides are produced [11,12].

DNA oxidation usually results in breaks in the DNA thread, modification of bases and rupture of phosphodiester bonds. The consequence of these processes is oxidative damage to DNA. The marker of oxidative damage to nucleic acids is mainly 8-hydroxy-2′-deoxyguanosine (8-OHdG). Increased concentration of 8-OHdG was observed in the course of several systemic diseases caused by oxidative stress, such as cancer or diabetes. The formation of 8-OHdG is triggered by the product in the C8 position of the deoxyguanosine imidazole ring [11].

A special role in maintaining the redox balance is played by enzymatic and non-enzymatic antioxidant systems which protect cells against harmful effects of ROS [13,14]. Antioxidants, when present in low concentrations compared to the content of the oxidized substrate, are intended to inhibit the oxidation of this substrate [15]. The ROS/RNS neutralization process occurs in one or two stages. In the latter case, ROS/RNS are transformed into weak radicals that interact with another weak radical, leading to the formation of an inactive molecule. The most important enzymatic systems include: superoxide dismutase (SOD), catalase (CAT) and glutathione peroxidase (GPx), while the main non-enzymatic antioxidants are, inter alia: the glutathione system, albumins, lactoferrin, ascorbic acid (AS), uric acid and melatonin [16,17].

The oral cavity is the initial part of the digestive tract, a vital place due to the structures it contains, and further sections of the digestive system. It is a place exposed to numerous external factors inducing ROS/RNS production and OS development. Excessive production of ROS/RNS also occurs during the intake of food, drinks, and stimulants or as a result of dental treatment [18]. The cause of redox imbalance in the oral cavity may be pathological changes such as caries, gingivitis, periodontitis, pre-cancerous conditions and cancer, inflammation, and fungal infections [18]. Interestingly, more and more reports show that these diseases and their treatment disturbs the oral redox equilibrium. Evidence showed that the performed dental procedures, such as filling cavities, endodontic, periodontic, orthodontic, and surgical treatment, may increase the production of ROS/RNS, and thus the development of OS. Of course, it should be emphasized that the ROS/RNS generated during dental treatment also positively affects the oral cavity. They promote wound healing, stimulate the immune response, and facilitate the elimination of bacteria [18].

The aim of our study was a literature review of reports on the impact of dental, periodontal, orthodontic, and surgical treatment (in terms of titanium fixation and implants) on redox balance.

2. Materials and Methods

2.1. Search Strategy

A literature review was conducted from 2010 to July 2020. We used the databases of PubMed, Medline and Scopus, and analyzed only international literature in English. Publications were searched according to the entered key words: oxidative stress and dental monomers; oxidative stress and amalgam; oxidative stress and periodontitis, oxidative stress and braces, oxidative stress, and titanium; oxidative stress and dental implants, oxidative stress and endodontics treatment, oxidative stress and dental treatment; oxidative stress and dental composite.

2.2. Inclusion Criteria

Only the works meeting the following criteria were included in this paper:

1. Works on redox disorders related to dental treatment, dental fillings, dental monomers, endodontic treatment, titanium implants, treatment of periodontal diseases, whitening.
2. Results obtained from experiments participated by human subjects, as well as experimental works.
3. Publications in English only.
4. Clinical trials on a group of at least five individuals.

2.3. Exclusion Criteria

1. Works written in languages other than English.
2. Clinical trials on a group of fewer than five individuals.
3. Meta-analyzes.
4. Publications on the redox balance in the treatment of neurocranial diseases and cancer.
5. Publications referring to prosthetic treatment and treatment of functional disorders of the masticatory organ.
6. Case studies.
7. Among the publications based on human material we excluded those that covered subjects with systemic diseases.

3. Data Extraction

The titles and abstracts resulting from this search strategy were evaluated independently by two researchers (I. Z., A. Z). In case of doubt, the given publication was included or excluded after reading its entire text. Cohen's kappa coefficient (κ) was used to measure interexaminer reliability ($\kappa = 0.89$). Each work was initially checked in the scope of its title, then abstract and the full text. When the studies met the inclusion criteria, they were included in this publication.

All works were evaluated in terms of methodology. Every publication had the following variables distinguished: authors, year of publication, study design, size of the study group, inclusion and exclusion criteria, duration of the study and study results.

4. Results

Out of approximately 27,600 publications, 37 were identified as meeting the inclusion and exclusion criteria. The literature review revealed 27,621 works from the MEDLINE (PubMed) library, of which 27,006 were excluded due to their title. A total of 412 summaries were read, 149 of which met the inclusion and exclusion criteria. Of the qualified articles, 112 proved irrelevant to the topic of our review. Therefore, 37 works were eventually included herein (Figure 1).

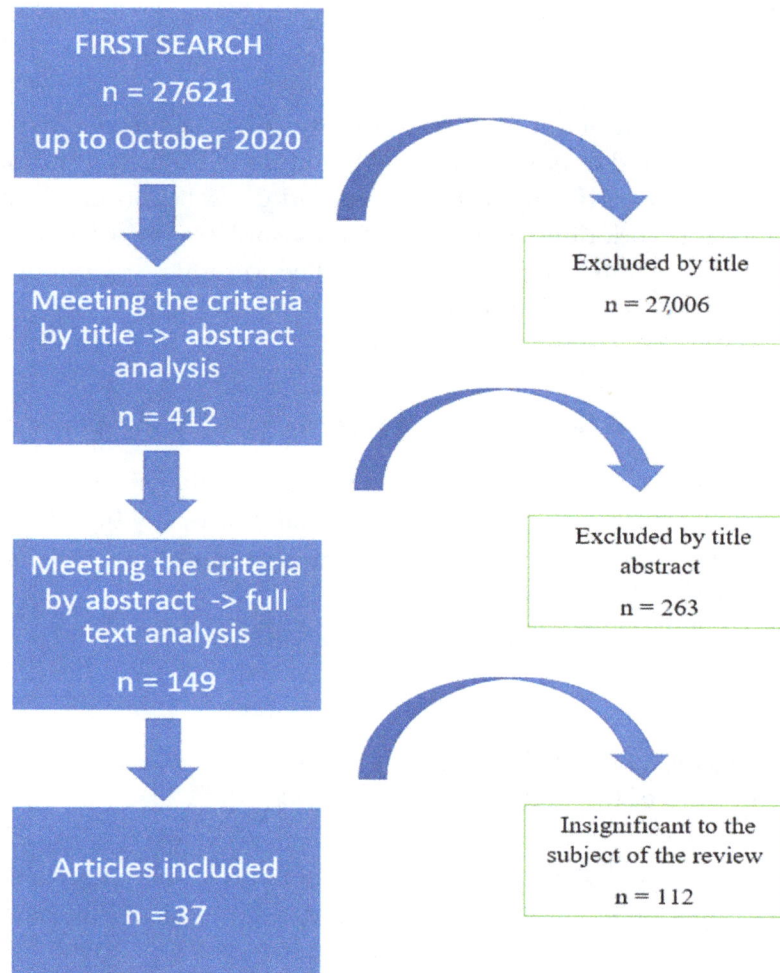

Figure 1. Flow chart of research methodology.

Research included the study are presented in Table 1.

Table 1. Research included in the study.

Experimental Model	Endpoints	References
Amalgam		
Human gingival fibroblast cells (HGFCs) exposed to microhybrid resin-based composite, compomer resin, glass-ionomer cement and amalgam alloy for 7 and 21 days	The levels of total oxidant status (TOS) in the study groups (i.e., samples with the following materials: microhybrid resin-based composite, compomer resin, glass-ionomer cement and amalgam alloy; shaped as a 2-mm-thick disk with a diameter of 10 mm; exposed to light with the wavelength of 430–480 nm and intensity of 1200 mW/cm² were significantly higher in freshly prepared samples compared to the control. After 7 and 21 days, TOS level in the amalgam sample was considerably lower than at the beginning of the study. The highest level of total antioxidant capacity (TAC) was observed after 7 days in the filling with glass-ionomer cement (which prevented TOS increase). In all studied groups, TAC level after 7 days was different than at the initial stage of the study.	[19]
Unstimulated saliva of 48 generally healthy children aged 6–10 (24 males, 24 females) with two class II dental composite or amalgam restorations and the control (caries-free) group	The saliva of patients with composite fillings had significantly higher TAC compared to patients with amalgam fillings as well as caries-free subjects. However, TAC in patients with amalgam restorations was also significantly higher compared to the caries-free control. Patients with composite fillings also demonstrated decreased salivary levels of Ca^{2+} ions.	[20]
Saliva from 60 generally healthy subjects aged 15–40 with class I restorations of: amalgam (20 participants), composite (20 subjects) and glass-ionomer (20 patients), collected before the filling as well as 24 h and 7 and 14 days after the filling	Malondialdehyde (MDA) level in the saliva of patients with an amalgam filling was found to be higher than in patients with a composite or glass-ionomer filling. Significant differences were also observed between MDA concentrations on day 7 and 14, and after 24 h and 7 days in patients with composite fillings. There were no differences in MDA levels before treatment and 7 days after, or before and 14 days after the treatment. In the case of glass-ionomer, a significant difference was found only between 24 h and 7 days after the treatment.	[21]

Table 1. *Cont.*

Experimental Model	Endpoints	References
Urine collected from 106 generally healthy children aged 5–15.5 years with amalgam fillings	It was shown that in children with amalgam filling, there was a reduced excretion of 8-hydroxy-2-deoxyguanosine (8-OHdG) in the urine. It was also shown that the level of NAG in the urine of children with amalgam fillings was significantly higher compared to children without such fillings and was positively correlated with the level of MDA in the urine. There was no correlation between the concentration of 8-OHdG and malondialdehyde (MDA) in the urine of amalgam-filled children. The mercury (Hg) level was also significantly higher in children with amalgam fillings compared to children without amalgam fillings; however, no relationship was found between the Hg level and the number of fillings.	[22]
Hair samples collected from 42 generally healthy women (mean age 44 years) with amalgam fillings applied at least 10 years earlier	An increased activity of SOD-1 and an increase in GSH concentration in the hair of women with amalgam fillings as compared to women without such fillings were observed. A positive correlation was also shown between the concentration of aluminum (Al) and the concentration of GSH, and between the level of mercury (Hg) and the activity of SOD-1.	[23]
Blood collected from 41 generally healthy patients (17–23 years old), which used amalgam (19) and dental resin composite (22) fillings	A significant increase in the level of malondialdehyde (MDA) was observed 24 h after placing amalgam and composite filling. There were no changes in the concentration of 8-OHdG in women 24 h after the placement of the amalgam filling. The 8-OHdG level increased 24 h after placing the dental resin composite filling.	[24]
	Dental Resin Composites—monomers	
Human dental pulp cells (hDPCs) exposed to dental monomers (1 mM HEMA, 5 mM MMA and 1 mM TEGDMA) without and in the presence of 10 mM NAC for 24, 48, 72 and 96 h	In response to 6 h of exposure to dental monomers: 2-hydroxyethyl methacrylate (HEMA), triethylene glycol dimethacrylate (TEGDMA) and methyl methacrylate (MMA), there was a significant increase in ROS production in hDPCs compared to the control group without dental monomers. The addition of N-acetyl cysteine (NAC) decreased ROS production in the monomer-treated group. The presence of monomers also GSH level, which was observed for NAC as well, but to a lesser extent. No significant differences in the content of GSSG (oxidized disulfide) were observed for HEMA and MMA monomers, and a slight GSSG decrease was noted for TEGDMA (triethylene glycol dimethacrylate). In the case of dental monomers, MDA level increased, and after adding NAC—MDA level dropped almost to its level observed in the control group. Moreover, SOD activity decreased in the presence of all dental monomers, which was not observed after the addition of NAC. After 24 h of cell exposure to monomers, CAT activity increased significantly, and decreased after the use of NAC.	[25]
Human dental pulp cells isolated form third molars, exposed to dental monomers (bisphenol-A-glycidyl Methacrylate, Bis-GMA; urethane dimethacrylate, UDMA; and triethylene glycol dimethacrylate, TEGDMA) at concentrations of 10, 30, 100, 300 μm for 48 h	The level of free radicals was measured after 48 h of monomer action by means of 2′,7′-dichlorodihydrofluorescein diacetate (DCF) fluorescent dye, and it was observed that Bis-GMA and UDMA, at high concentrations (30, 100), induced a significant increase in oxidative stress, while the TEGDMA monomer did not trigger OS at any concentration. All monomers reduced the level of GSH.	[26]
Smulow-Glickman (S-G) human gingival epithelial cells and pulp fibroblasts (HPF) exposed to HEMA at the concentrations of 0.01–10 mm for 24 h	Higher HEMA concentrations (1, 2.5, 5, 10) caused a significant increase in the level of intracellular ROS in cells exposed to the monomer.	[27]
Gingival fibroblasts obtained during the extraction of premolars for orthodontic reasons, exposed to TEGDMA at a concentration of 0.6 mM and 1 mM for 15 min to 6 h	15-min exposure to TEGDMA significantly reduced the concentration of intracellular GSH compared to cells not exposed to this monomer. It was also demonstrated that TEGDMA-induced time-dependent increase of thiobarbituric acid reactive substances (TBARS), which indicates increased lipid peroxidation.	[28]
Human dental pulp stem cells (isolated from third molars) exposed to monomer HEMA (at a concentration of 2 mM) and AC (at 50 μg·mL^{-1}) for 24 h	2-hydroxyethyl methacrylate (HEMA) increased the level of reactive oxygen species (ROS), pro-inflammatory mediators such as nuclear factor-κB (NF-kB) and inflammatory cytokines such as interleukin. In the presence of vitamin C, these changes were less noticeable. This indicates a protective effect of vitamin C on the dental pulp cells.	[29]
Human gingival fibroblasts (HGFs) treated with a relatively low level of 2-hydroxyethyl methacrylate (HEMA) for 0, 24 and 96 h	After 24 and 96 h of HGF exposure to the HEMA monomer (3 mmol·L^{-1}), it was observed that ROS levels increased 8 and 11 times compared to the control not exposed to the monomer.	[30]
Primary human gingival fibroblasts (HGFs) and immortalized oral keratinocyte cell line OKF6/TERT2 treated with 2-hydroxyethyl methacrylate (HEMA) at a concentration of 0.5–10 mM	Significantly induced transcription of genes related to defense against oxidative stress was demonstrated for: nuclear factor erythroid 2-related factor 2 (Nrf2), heme oxygenase (HO-1), quinone dehydrogenase 1 (NQO1), superoxide dismutase 1 (SOD1) in both cell types exposed to the HEMA monomer. The transcription of nuclear factor kappa-light-chain-enhancer of activated B cells (NF-κB) and interleukin-6 (IL-6) was repressed in both cell types, while the transcription of tumor necrosis factor α (TNF-α) and interleukin-8 (IL-8) was repressed only in OKF6/TERT-2 cells.	[31]

Table 1. *Cont.*

Experimental Model	Endpoints	References
Primary human dental pulp cells (hDPCs) obtained from healthy patients aged 18–25, during the extraction of healthy third molars, exposed to 1 mM 2-hydroxyethyl methacrylate (HEMA) for 18 and 12 h	It was demonstrated that the expression of NFE2L2 (nuclear factor, erythroid 2 like 2) and HMOX1 (heme oxygenase (decycling) 1) genes encoding the proteins: Nrf2 (nuclear factor erythroid 2-related factor 2) and HO-1 (heme oxygenase 1) in the HEMA-exposed group increased compared to the group not exposed to HEMA.	[32]
Human gingival fibroblasts (HGFs) exposed to 2-hydroxyethyl methacrylate (HEMA) and triethylene glycol dimethacrylate (TEGDMA) at a concentration of 3 mM for 24, 48 and 72 h	It was demonstrated that exposure to HEMA caused autophagy and apoptosis in each of the analyzed periods of time. No signs of autophagia were observed in TEGDMA-exposed cells	[33]
Dental Resin Composites—Cross-linked samples		
Human dental pulp cells exposed to methacrylate-based dental resin composite, including triethylene glycol dimethacrylate and composites free of 2-hydroxyethyl methacrylate and silorane-based composite (5 mm in diameter and 2 mm high) cured with light (780 mW/cm^2) for 40 s in the presence of dental polymers (reduction of free radical polymerization) and absence of polyester film	Flow cytometry showed increased ROS production in cells exposed to dental resin composite materials. A positive correlation was observed between ROS production and cell survival in groups not covered with polyester film. TEGDMA increases ROS production.	[34]
Human dental pulp cells (isolated from third molars) exposed to dental material dental resin composite s for 48 h with IGF-1 i TGF-b	Insulin-like growth factor (IGF-1) and transforming growth factor beta (TGF-β) increased cystine capture, resulting in elevated levels of cellular glutathione in a group of cells exposed to dental resin composite (Flow Line, 9.5 +/− 0.4 mg and Durafill VS, 10.0 +/− 0.4 mg). This provided increased protection against OS effect triggered by dental resin composite.	[35]
Human pulp cells obtained from impacted third molars, exposed to cured bonding agents (Clearfil SE Bond, CB; Prime & Bond 2.1, PB; and Single Bond, SB) at a concentration of 10 µL for 2 days	Dentine bonding agents decrease the level of GSH, which might be the reason for the cytotoxicity of resins. Cytotoxicity decreased when N-acetyl-L-cysteine (NAC) was added to the sample.	[36]
Saliva collected from 52 patients (32 women and 20 men) who had been treated with Filtek Z250 dental resin composite fillings, before the filling and 1 h, 1 day, 7 and 30 days after the filling	Patients with dental resin composite fillings demonstrated a significantly increased MDA level compared to subjects without fillings, but there were no statistical differences between the studied time periods. There was also a significant decrease in SOD activity 7 days after the filling compared to the controls. No significant differences were noted in SOD values between day 7 and 30 in patients with dental resin composite fillings.	[37]
Composite resins		
Human gingival fibroblasts (HGFs) exposed to composite resin (consisting of 45% 2-hydroxyethyl methacrylate—HEMA and 55% bisphenol A-glycidyl dimethacrylate—Bis-GMA) at concentrations of up to 0.25 mM	It was demonstrated that the expression of 8-hydroxyguanine in DNA–hydrolase I, the main enzyme for repairing 8-oxoG damage in composite resin-exposed cells, was elevated compared to cells not exposed to monomers.	[38]
Mouse fibroblast cells (NIH/3T3) exposed to camphorquinone (CQ), CQ and diphenyleneiodonium hexafluorophosphate (DPI), CQ and ethyl 4-dimethylamino benzoate (EDAB), and CQ, EDAB and DPI, with EDAB in high and low concentration, for 10 and 20 s	Increased activity of SOD was observed after 10 s of polymerization vs 20 s in NIH/3T3.	[39]
Orthodontic braces		
L929 mouse fibroblast cell line exposed to six types of orthodontic archiwires (stainless steel, nickel-titanium, copper-nickel-titanium, rhodium-coated nickel-titanium, cobalt-chromium Blue Elgiloy, titanium-molybdenum) in 1-cm-long pieces (1 mL saliva per 0.2 g of the wire)	It was demonstrated that a standard nickel-titanium orthodontic archiwire generates the strongest oxidative stress, while stainless steel and titanium-molybdenum wire triggers the lowest OS in a mouse fibroblast cell culture.	[40]

Table 1. *Cont.*

Experimental Model	Endpoints	References
L929 mouse fibroblast cell line exposed to three conventional (stainless steel, monocrystalline sapphire ceramics, polyurethane) and four self-ligating brackets (stainless steel body with a nickel-titanium clip, aluminum oxide ceramics with a cobalt-chromium clip, aluminum oxide ceramics with a nickel-cobalt clip coated with rhodium, polycarbonate-stainless steel brackets) made of different materials	The assessment of 8-hydroxy-29-deoxyguanosine (8-OHdG) in DNA of L929 murine fibroblast cell line demonstrated that the lowest OS is triggered by a conventional sapphire ceramic bracket. Full metal conventional and self-ligating brackets and conventional polyurethane brackets showed higher OS compared to cells not exposed to these brackets. The highest OS is caused by full metal and polyurethane brackets.	[41]
Saliva of 23 patients aged 12–16 enrolled in the study (12 female, 11 male subjects), treated with multibracket self-ligating vestibular orthodontic appliances	During the first 10 weeks of treatment with multibracket self-ligating vestibular orthodontic appliances, no statistically significant changes in the salivary antioxidant test (SAT) were observed.	[42]
Unstimulated saliva and gingival fluid of 50 generally healthy patients (27 females and 23 males) aged 13–20, treated with permanent brackets, collected before the treatment as well as in the 1st and 6th month of the treatment	There was no increase in oxidative damage (8-OHdG, MDA) in the saliva and gingival fluid of patients treated with permanent brackets compared to pre-treatment results.	[43]
Unstimulated (UWS) and stimulated (SWS) saliva of 37 generally healthy subjects treated with permanent orthodontic brackets, collected immediately after the fitting of the brackets as well as 1 week and 24 weeks after the fitting	There was a significant increase in thiobarbituric acid reactive substance (TBARS) in UWS and SWS one week after braces were fitted. The measured values returned to their initial state 24 weeks after the beginning of the treatment. There were no significant differences between the levels of SOD1, CAT, UA and Px activity in UWS 1 week and 24 weeks after the start of treatment. SOD1 activity was found to be significantly lower in SWS, and Px activity was considerably higher 1 week after the placement of the brackets compared to the values before the treatment and 24 weeks after its commencement. The total antioxidant status (TAS) in UWS and SWS was also found to be considerably lower 24 weeks after the start of the treatment compared to the values before the treatment as well as 1 week after its start. The highest oxidative stress index (OSI) values were observed 1 week after the treatment. 24 weeks after the treatment these values were identical to pre-treatment results.	[44]
	Fixations and dental implants	
Human dental pulp stem cells (DPSC) and murine pre- osteoblast (MC3T3-E1) cells exposed to zirconium and titanium oxide for 24 h	Intracellular oxidation of 5-(and -6)-chloromethyl-2′,7′-dichlorodihydrofluorescein diacetate and acetyl ester (CM-H2DCFDA), a ROS indicator dye, demonstrated relatively higher average ROS levels in both types of cells exposed to zirconium compared to titanium.	[45]
Periosteum of 30 patients (8 women and 22 men) with bilateral fractures of the mandible, treated with Ti6Al4V titanium alloy	The periosteum of patients treated with titanium implants showed significantly higher concentrations of the biomarkers of nitrosative (S-nitrosothiols, peroxynitrite, nitrotyrosine) and oxidative stress (malondialdehyde, protein carbonyls, dityrosine, kynurenine and N-formylkynurenine) compared to the control without titanium fixations. Osteosynthesis patients also demonstrated increased antioxidant protection expressed in elevated levels of reduced glutathione (↑GSH) and glutathione reductase (↑GR). The periosteum of patients with titanium fixations revealed a considerable decrease in the activity of mitochondrial complex I (−77.8%) and CS (citrate synthase) (−166.7%) compared to the control. There were no statistically significant differences in the activity of complex II and cytochrome C oxidase (COX) between patients after osteosynthesis as compared to healthy controls. In the periosteum of osteosynthesis patients, the production of hydrogen peroxide as well as the rate of ROS production were also significantly increased. Titanium implants caused oxidative/nitrosative stress and mitochondrial dysfunction. Moreover, a positive correlation between ROS production rate and GSH concentration was observed, which may suggest increased antioxidant defense in patients after osteosynthesis.	[46]
Whole saliva of patients aged 43–57 with peri-implantitis and five titanium implants (collected from five patients) that were rejected up to 6 months after their implantation (3 from the mandible, 2 from the maxilla); oxidative stress parameters	In the course of peri-implantitis, a significant increase was observed in AGE compared to the control. In the saliva of peri-implantitis patients the level of OS was higher than in healthy individuals.	[47]

Table 1. *Cont.*

Experimental Model	Endpoints	References
Periosteum of 32 patients operated on due to class III dentofacial deformities (21 women and 11 men aged 20–30), who had had titanium implants inserted and then removed 12–30 months after the implantation	Decreased activity of superoxide dismutase-1 (SOD1) ($\downarrow$37%) and tryptophan level ($\downarrow$34%) as well as significantly higher content of advanced oxidation protein products (AOPP) ($\uparrow$25%), total oxidant status (TOS) ($\uparrow$80%) and oxidative stress index (OSI) ($\uparrow$101%) were observed in the maxillary periosteum of osteotomized patients compared to the controls. The mandibular periosteum demonstrated a significant decrease in SOD-1 activity ($\downarrow$55%), total oxidant status (TAC) ($\downarrow$58.6%), advanced glycation end products (AGE) ($\downarrow$60%) and N-formylkynurenine ($\downarrow$34%), and considerably increased content of AOPP ($\uparrow$38%), malondialdehyde (MDA) ($\uparrow$29%), 4-hydroxynonenal (4-HNE) ($\uparrow$114%), TOS ($\uparrow$99%) and OSI ($\uparrow$381%) compared to the controls. Further weakening of the redox economy and increased ROS production were demonstrated in the mandibular periosteum compared to the maxillary periosteum.	[48]
Periosteum of 29 patients (aged 19–29) treated with titanium implants (due to a bilateral mandibular shaft fracture) that were removed 3–5 months after the procedure	The periosteum of patients after osteosynthesis showed significantly higher activity of NADPH and xanthine oxidase, and increased rate of free radical production compared to the control. The periosteum of patients after osteosynthesis also demonstrated a considerable increase in the levels of inflammation markers: interleukin 1 (IL-1), interleukin 6 (IL-6), tumor necrosis factor α (TNF-α), transforming growth factor β (TGF-β) and β-glucuronidase (GLU) as well as markers of apoptosis (Bax, Bax/Bcl-2), caspase-3 (CAS-3) and nitric oxide (NO) compared to the control. Titanium implants increased the production of proinflammatory cytokines and oxygen free radicals. A positive correlation between titanium content and CAS-3 activity was also demonstrated.	[49]
Periosteum, plasma, and erythrocytes collected from 31 generally healthy subjects aged 21–29 (11 women and 20 men) with bilateral mandibular fractures treated with titanium miniplates (Ti4Al4V)	Decreased CAT activity in the mandibular periosteum and its increase in erythrocytes of patients with mandibular fracture treated with titanium miniplates were demonstrated compared to the subjects not exposed to titanium implants. SOD activity and UA concentration were significantly higher in both plasma and periosteum of fracture patients compared to healthy individuals. No differences were found in GPx activity between the studied groups. There was an increase in TAC, FRAP, TOS, AGE, AOPP, 4-HNE and a decrease in OSI level in the maxillary periosteum of patients with fracture compared to healthy subjects. There were no significant differences in plasma TAC, TOS, OSI, FRAP AGE, AOPP, 4-HNE and 8-OHdG levels between patients with a fracture and healthy subjects. A positive correlation was observed between TAC concentration in the mandibular periosteum and plasma UA level in patients with a mandibular fracture. A positive correlation was also found between TOS concentration in the periosteum and CAT activity in erythrocytes, and between 8-OHdG level in the periosteum and GPx activity in erythrocytes.	[50]
Periodontology		
Male adult Wistar rats (2 months of age) with periodontitis, subjected to antimicrobial photodynamic therapy (aPDT)	PDT was shown to increase ROS formation as well as boost the antioxidant response.	[51]
Whole saliva of patients aged 43–57 with peri-implantitis and 5 titanium implants (collected from five patients), which were rejected up to 6 months after their implantation (3 from the mandible, 2 from the maxilla)	In patients with peri-implantitis, the western blot technique revealed a significant increase in AGE compared to healthy controls. By means of TBARS assays, a higher level of OS was also observed in the saliva of peri-implantitis patients compared to healthy subjects.	[47]
Sixteen patients with chronic periodontitis (CP), undergoing non-surgical periodontal therapy alone as well as non-surgical therapy accompanied by antibiotic therapy of Amoxicillin + Metronidazole, 500 mg each, 3 times daily, for 7 days	It was demonstrated that after 3 months OS levels decreased from very high to average during antibiotic therapy, as shown by reduced derivatives of reactive oxygen metabolites (d-ROMs) (from 491.83 ± 134.85 U CARR to 375.58 ± 126.06 U CARR) and reduced glutathione (GSH) (from 48.73 ± 33.89 µmol/L to 46.46 ± 21.59 µmol/L) in plasma.	[52]
Nineteen patients with chronic periodontitis (average age: 46.8 years) examined before the therapy (scaling and root planing) as well as 1 and 2 months after the therapy.	Non-surgical treatment of periodontitis reduced plasma ROM levels compared to pre-treatment levels.	[53]
Tissues and saliva of 10 patients with peri-implantitis and 10 with chronic periodontitis, aged 40–60	In both the saliva and tissues of patients with peri-implantitis and chronic periodontitis, AGE levels more than doubled compared to healthy individuals. A strong positive correlation was also observed between ROS and AGE in the examined patients.	[54]

Table 1. *Cont.*

Experimental Model	Endpoints	References
Peri-implant crevicular fluid (PICF) collected from 31 patients	The concentration of MDA, SOD and TAC in peri-implant crevicular fluid did not differ from that in healthy subjects. However, there was a positive correlation between periodontal pocket depth (PPD) around the implant and MDA and TAC levels.	[55]
	Whitening	
Human primary periodontal ligament fibroblasts (hPDLFs) and Ca9-22 human gingival epithelial cells treated with stable aqueous ozone ultrafine bubble water (OUFBW; ozone concentration: 2.5 ppm) or UV-inactivated OUFBW	OUFBW (30 min of incubation) stimulated ROS production in both cell lines, thus activating the MAPK pathway. OUFBW triggered the activation of c-Fos, a major component of the transcription factor activator protein 1 (AP-1), and also nuclear factor erythroid 2 (NF-E2)-related factor 2 (Nrf2), which demonstrated high sensitivity to oxidative stress.	[56]
One-hundred thirteen patients (60 people using Crest® 3D Whitestrips® premium plus, 10% hydrogen peroxide, 53 subjects in the control group). Oral epithelial cells and saliva samples were collected at the beginning of the study and 30 days later from the control group, and immediately before whitening as well as 15 and 30 days after the completion of the whitening procedure	After the whitening procedure, an elevated level of 8-OHdG in saliva and a positive correlation between oxidative stress produced by hydrogen peroxide and micronuclei were found.	[57]

5. Amalgam

The choice of filling materials is constantly increasing. Despite the dynamic development of cosmetic fillings, amalgam is still commonly used, which is due to its durability as well as low price, immediate availability and ease of use [22].

The influence of amalgam, both on the oral cavity and the entire body, has been discussed for a long time. The harmful effects of amalgam fillings are related to mercury contained in them. Studies demonstrated that mercury interferes with the metabolism of porphyrins which actively participate in numerous metabolic processes, including cellular respiration. The disruption of porphyrin metabolism may result in metabolic diseases, cancer or blood disorders, i.e., anemia or porphyrias [22,23]. Organic mercury, found in the form of methylmercury (MeHg), is considered particularly harmful [23]. Initial oxidative damage caused by MeHg in living organisms occurs as a result of its reaction with thiol (-SH) and/or selenol (-SeH) groups from endogenous molecules, leading to the formation of a very stable complex of type RSHgCH3 or RSeHgCH3 [58]. In proteins and enzymes containing thiol or selenol groups, the formation of S-Hg or Se-Hg bonds leads to the impairment of a given protein function [58–62] or entails the production of protein deposits rich in cysteine residues [63,64]. As mentioned above, due to high reactivity of MeHg to thiols and selenols, mercury occurs in living organisms in a form associated with these groups. In the human body, thiols are more common than selenols [65]; they can be found not only in compounds of low molecular weight (mainly cysteine and reduced glutathione), but also in proteins, whereas selenol groups are present only in a limited group of selenoproteins [66–68]. Considering the fact that both thiol and selenol groups are critical for the catalytic activity of numerous enzymes involved in antioxidant mechanisms and that MeHg reduces the activity of, inter alia, such enzymes (i.e., glucose-6- phosphate dehydrogenase [69], creatine kinase [60], glutathione reductase [70], glutathione peroxidase [59,71], thioredoxin reductase [10,72] there are grounds to postulate that this interaction disturbs the redox balance and results in increased production of ROS and RNS. However, studies by Cabaña-Muñoz et al. [23] revealed a significant boost in the activity of superoxide dismutase 1 (SOD-1) as well as reduced glutathione (GSH) concentration in hair samples collected from women who had amalgam fillings inserted 15 years prior to the study. According to the authors, stimulation of enzymatic antioxidant systems results from MeHg-induced elevated hydrogen peroxide (H_2O_2) concentration. It was shown that MeHg influences the mitochondrial electron transport chain (mainly at the level of complex II–III), which accelerates the formation of H_2O_2 [73]. The observed increased levels of the antioxidant barrier components as well as a positive correlation between mercury concentration and SOD-1 activity may suggest compensatory mechanisms to the chronic presence of mercury in women, aimed at counteracting Hg toxicity in individuals with amalgam fillings [23].

The results of the test for oxidative stress markers in subjects with amalgam fillings are contradictory, which is due to the test methods used, study material and the time that passed between the placement of a filling and the sampling. Al-Saleh et al. [22] observed abnormal concentrations of 8-hydroxy-D-guanosine (8-OHdG) and malondialdehyde (MDA) in the urine of children with amalgam fillings (no time passed from the filling insertion to the sampling was provided), and only 8-OHdG concentration was significantly correlated with the mercury content in the urine of these children. Mercury concentration in urine showed a clear dose-effect relationship with 8-OHdG level, mainly caused by long-term exposure to low Hg concentrations. The authors believe that oxidative damage to DNA of children is a result of exposure to Hg both from amalgam fillings and other sources. What is more, they argue that the presence of amalgam fillings does not exacerbate oxidative damage to DNA, but reduces the body's ability to repair it, leading to a reduction in DNA repair products secreted into the urine compared to children without amalgam fillings. Studies indicated that 8-OHdG concentration in urine is not only a marker of oxidative modifications of the genetic material, but also reflects the efficiency of corrective mechanisms [74–76]. Interestingly, only the MDA concentration in urine was significantly correlated with the activity of urinary N-acetyl-β-D-glucosaminidase (NAG). It is worth mentioning that urinary NAG is used as a marker of renal tubular damage, especially in an environmental exposure to Hg [77]. The multiple regression model also demonstrated a statistically significant interaction between urinary Hg and MDA concentrations. This relationship suggests that exposure to Hg from amalgam fillings may result in renal tubular damage through oxidative stress (OS). In contrast, studies by Yildiz et al. [24] showed increased concentration of lipid peroxidation products (MDA) and no changes in the concentrations of oxidative markers of DNA damage in the plasma of patients 24 h after the placement of amalgam fillings. No correlation with Hg concentration was observed, which was consistent with the results of Daokar et al. [21]. These authors demonstrated a significant increase in MDA concentration in the saliva of patients who had had amalgam fillings inserted 2 weeks earlier.

In the study of Celik et al. [19] amalgam exhibited cytotoxic effect toward the HGF cell line, resulting in higher cell mortality and significantly higher total oxidant status (TOS) in freshly prepared samples compared to samples taken after 7 and 21 days. According to these authors, the decrease in cytotoxicity and TOS over time was caused by a considerable drop in the release of metal ions as the material hardened. Interestingly, amalgam had no significant effect on TOS and total antioxidant capacity (TAC) values compared to the control group. However, samples taken on day 7 and 21 demonstrated a considerably higher TAC compared to fresh samples. However, higher salivary TAC was observed in female and male children with two dental amalgam restorations (the time from the placement of the fillings to the collection of samples was not provided) compared to children who were caries-free and did not have any restorations [20]. Interestingly, females had higher TAC compared to males, which the authors claimed to be caused by hormonal changes typical of early adolescence and indicated more efficient antioxidant systems in girls in response to the increasing level of ROS.

In summary, mercury in amalgams is responsible for the redox imbalance in the system. MeHg modifies the mitochondrial electron transport chain function, which accelerates the formation of H_2O_2 [73]. A strengthening of the antioxidant barrier may suggest compensatory mechanisms to the chronic presence of mercury.

6. Glass-Ionomer Cement

Little is known about glass-ionomer-induced oxidative stress. It was demonstrated that metal ions released from glass-ionomer fillings are not toxic to cells and do not induce ROS formation, whereas polyacrylic acid [19] and fluorine ions released during the first phase of GI filling [19,78] have cytotoxic effects. During the first seven days, ROS production enhances, increasing TAC levels.

The observed increase in TAC is an adaptive reaction of the cells that effectively prevents OS development, shifting the redox balance towards antioxidant reactions [19]. After 21 days, the level of TAC in the cell culture exposed to glass-ionomer filling did not differ from the control culture level, which most likely indicated that glass-ionomer filling was no longer cytotoxic to cells, and it was a sign of achieving redox balance.

7. Dental Resin Composites

In the present paragraph, we want to point out that we do not separate the cytotoxic effect of monomers from the potential toxic effect of dental resin composites once they were properly cross-linked. We take into account such differentiation in Table 1.

Dental resin composite materials are currently the most commonly applied materials for tooth reconstruction in conservative dentistry. In recent years, significant development in the dental materials of this group was observed. They are used especially for esthetic restorations in the front and back sections. It was documented that each resin-based material releases certain amounts of its components into the saliva. The most common of them are bisphenol-A-glycidyl methacrylate (Bis-GMA), urethane dimethacrylate (UDMA), triethylene glycol dimethacrylate (TEGDMA) and 2-hydroxyethyl methacrylate (HEMA). It is believed that HEMA is released in the largest amount from composite materials, and Bis-GMA—in the smallest, which is related to the size of the molecules as well as molecular weight of these monomers [79].

It is known that monomers released from composites contribute to genetic changes at the cellular level, and show cytotoxic effects [80]. It is generally believed that the cytotoxicity of these monomers might be ranked in the decreasing order: Bis-GMA, UDMA, TEGDMA and HEMA [79]. Moreover, studies showed that OS is responsible for monomer cytotoxicity [25,34], whereas silorane-based dental resin composites Hermes III, free of TEGDMA, HEMA and other monomers, does not lead to significant ROS/RNS production, and its cytotoxicity towards pulp cells is low compared to TEGDMA and HEMA-based dental resin composites [34].

A wide range of studies demonstrated that increased ROS/RNS production in resin-exposed cells occurs parallel and simultaneously to the depletion of reduced glutathione resources [27,28,46]. The glutathione system is the most important cellular detoxification mechanism against ROS activity [81]. GSH is a tripeptide (–glutamylcysteinylglycine) with a molecular weight of 307 kDa. GSH enables the removal of free radicals from the body either directly or through the reactions catalyzed by glutathione peroxidase and other peroxidases, thus neutralizing hydrogen peroxide as well as nitrogen peroxides [82]. GSH reacts with electrophiles, creating less reactive conjugates. Interestingly, decreased concentration of GSH in human dental pulp cells (HDPCs) exposed to resin-based composites is not accompanied by increased level of oxidized glutathione (GSSG), which indicates that reduced amount of GSH resources does not result from its oxidation [25]. Studies have shown that carbonyl groups of methacrylates, adjacent to the double carbon-carbon bond, act as electron withdrawing groups. Consequently, carbon in the beta position of the double bond, as a positive charge, can react with nucleophilic centers of amine or thiol groups in small molecules such as GSH in the Michael-type addition reaction [25]. Indeed, Samuelsen et al. [83] observed spontaneous formation of a complex between HEMA and GSH. They concluded that exposure to HEMA leads to a drop in cellular GSH level, probably due to the formation of a complex with HEMA. Nocca et al. [84] found that the kinetics of the formation of GSH-methacrylate adducts depended on the reaction environment. The rate of adduct formation was different when the reaction occurred in human fibroblasts or erythrocytes than when the reaction environment was a mixture of methacrylates and GSH, which suggests that the reaction is strongly correlated with glutathione S-transferase. Studies by Schneider et al. [26] proved that the drop of GSH concentration in pulp cells caused by TEGDMA after 2 h from exposure was comparable to the decrease in GSH concentration caused by Bis-GMA and UDMA after 48 h. Interestingly, the TEGDMA-induced decrease in GSH concentration was a reversible process, and after the exposure to Bis-GMA and UDMA the treatment further decreased. Evidence showed that Bis-GMA and UDMA significantly reduce cystine uptake, while TEGDMA has the opposite effect. The so-called system x_c^- is responsible for the transport of cystine into dental pulp cells in which it is transformed into cysteine that is used for the production of GSH [35]. According to the authors, this explains the observed phenomenon of oxidative stress in the pulp cells exposed to Bis-GMA and UDMA, and its absence in the cells treated with TEGDMA. GSH directs the expression of enzymatic antioxidants that are exposed in cells to monomers, including HEMA. It was demonstrated that HEMA reduces the activity of glutathione peroxidase GPx1/2, but in the presence of L-buthionine sulfoximine (BSO), which inhibits GSH synthesis, this reduction is more intense. Moreover, significantly elevated ROS generation as well as increased catalase (CAT) activity are observed [36,85]. It is noteworthy that the inhibition of GSH synthesis by BSO in cells not treated with monomers boosts GPx1 activity as a result of increased H_2O_2 concentration due to GSH reduction. However, it seems that in cells not treated with monomers the concentration of H_2O_2 is low, because no increase in CAT concentration was observed. It was proven that GPx1/2 regulates lower H_2O_2 level, whereas CAT expression is induced by higher H_2O_2 concentrations observed in HEMA-treated cells [85].

Interestingly, the use of polyester film which reduces the occurrence of oxygen-inhibited free radical polymerization of dental polymers, results in increased monomer conversion and inhibited ROS production in pulp cells exposed to monomers [34].

According to Diomede et al. [29], a significant, spontaneously irreversible increase in ROS concentration in HDPSCs treated with HEMA after 24 h of exposure is not connected with GSH depletion, but results from mitochondrial dysfunction. Confocal microscopy of cells exposed to HEMA indicates 1000 times higher signal from ROS-sensitive indicator in the mitochondrial area compared to control cells. These differences are most likely due to HEMA-induced dysfunction of the respiratory chain dysregulating the oxidative phosphorylation process. The results of Diomede et al. [29] are consistent with the work of Jiao et al. [25,32] who observed morphological disorders of mitochondria, including their elongation and cristae derangements, depolarization of mitochondrial membranes, reduction of oxidative phosphorylation rate in cells exposed to HEMA and decrease of ATP production. Interestingly, mitochondrial dysfunction induced by monomers exacerbates ROS-induced damage to the dental pulp cells through bioenergetic failure and the internal mitochondrial apoptosis pathway [25,86]. The mitochondrial chain, located in the internal mitochondrial membrane, consists of four enzymatic complexes transporting electrons (CI-CIV) and the ATP synthase enzyme. [87]. It is still unknown which of the complexes is damaged in the course of exposure to monomers. A recent study showed CI as the most important toxicity target of TEGDMA [88]. However, in HEMA-exposed cells, the suppression of all four complexes, either by nuclear-encoded mitochondria or mtDNA-encoded transcription, was observed [89]. These discrepancies are certainly due to the method of mitochondrial isolation as well as the type of resin monomer used. It was demonstrated that although both monomers exhibit a similar toxicity mechanism, cells react differently to various resins by differential induction of the cell death (e.g., only HEMA induces autophagy in human gingival fibroblasts) [33]. Jiao et al. [25] demonstrated that NAC reduces monomer-induced oxidative stress in human pulp cells. Styllou et al. [90] found that the addition of NAC to human fibroblasts exposed to TEGDMA and HEMA significantly minimizes double strand breaks and restores cell nucleus integrity. The authors believe that the protective effect of NAC results from the ability of this molecule to neutralize ROS and replenish GSH deficiencies as well as from the direct reaction of NAC with methacrylate groups of monomers in the Michael addition. The presence of ascorbic acid (AS) counteracts the oxidative effects of HEMA, restoring ROS concentration to the level observed in the control group. AS seems to mimic the effect of NAC, because both molecules neutralize HEMA-induced ROS growth in the cytosol, with only AS being able to completely prevent excessive ROS production in mitochondria [29].

Cells have numerous mechanisms to counteract OS. One of them is the activation of the transcription factor: nuclear factor erythroid 2-related factor 2 (Nrf2)-dependent signaling pathway. Under equilibrium conditions, redox Nrf2 is synthesized and quickly degraded. In a situation of increased ROS production, Nrf2 is stabilized and transferred to the cell nucleus in which it activates the transcription of numerous genes by binding the promoter to antioxidant responsive elements (ARE) [91].

The most important genes activated by Nrf2 include heme oxygenase (HO-1), NAD(P)H quinone dehydrogenase 1 (NQO1) and superoxide dismutase 1 (SOD1). These enzymes play an important role in regulating the redox balance and counteracting monomer toxicity. Durante et al. [92] and Gozzelino et al. [93] believe that antioxidant bilirubin, resulting from the catalytic activity of HO-1, is an essential next link in strengthening the antioxidant barrier when exposed to monomers, and directly balance the cellular redox environment. The stimulation of Nrf2 signaling cascade was observed in HEMA-exposed RAW264.7 mouse macrophages [85,94], human fibroblasts [30,31] and the immortalized human oral keratinocyte cell line (OKF6/TERT-2) [31]. Interestingly, in the latter cell line it was noted that Nrf2 has a potential to enhance its own transcription through a positive feedback loop. Perduns et al. [31] observed that even "non-toxic" HEMA concentrations (0.5 mM) induce the expreission of genes of antioxidant enzymes HO-1, NQO1 and SOD1 in human fibroblast and keratinocyte cells. Ramezani et al. [20] showed that dental resin composites significantly enhanced total antioxidant capacity (TAC) in saliva, as TAC level was higher than that of amalgam fillings [31]. Celik et al. [19] obtained increased TAC in gingival fibroblasts (HGFCs) after 7 days of exposure to dental resin composites as well as weakening of the antioxidant barrier on day 21, which was caused by a rapid boost of ROS production from unbound and non-polymerized monomers. The level of HEMA higher than 5 mM enhances ROS production to such an extent that we can observe the occurrence of ROS-induced gene expression disorders associated with inflammation (NF- κB, TNF-α, IL-6, IL-8) and remodeling of the extracellular matrix (COL1A, COL4A, metalloproteinase 9—MMP-9, tissue inhibitor of metalloproteinase 1—TIMP1) [19]. Indeed, studies have revealed that monomer-induced OS acts as a signal for the activation of the pathways controlling cell survival and death, although the exact mechanism of this phenomenon is unknown. It was observed that HEMA significantly increases the number of cells in late phase of apoptosis and necrosis [85]. An additional supply of cysteine, an amino acid essential for the synthesis of GSH by 2-oxothiazolidine-4-carboxylate (OTC), considerably reduces the number of apoptotic and necrotic cells. These observations suggest that HEMA-induced cell death is due to, inter alia, GSH deficiency [85]. These observations are consistent with the study by Lee et al. [95] in which the authors observed increased cell survival after the supplementation of 10 mM NAC. NAC activates GSH reductase, which leads to an increase in GSH concentration.

Yildiz et al. [24] showed that Bis-GMA and TEGDMA, and Jiao et al. [32]—that HEMA and TEGDMA significantly increase MDA concentration in human dental pulp cells. It is noteworthy that the measurement of MDA content at various times after the placement of the dental resin composites revealed its linear increase with the time passed from the material application [37]. Daokar et al. [21] observed that the salivary MDA concentration two weeks after the placement of dental resin composites, the authors did not demonstrate any differences in salivary MDA concentration after the placement of composite and glass-ionomer fillings. In another study, which evaluated TEGDMA and Bis-GMA in dental pulp cells, the increase of 8-OHdG post-application content was noted, and ROS production was correlated with DNA oxidation [24]. Interestingly, the concentration of 8-OHdG was significantly higher in samples after the application of the dental resin composites compared to the amalgam filling group. These observations prove that monomers cause higher oxidation and transformation of the genetic material of dental pulp cells compared to amalgam fillings. It was shown that resin monomers, such as HEMA, lead to the formation of double strand breaks [96–98]. Anteisson et al. [99] demonstrated that HEMA-induced genome damage results in the stimulation of ataxia telangiectasia mutated (ATM) gene and other cell cycle checkpoints, which leads to the activation of kinase signaling networks that impede the progression of the cell cycle and simultaneously activate DNA repair pathways. Similarly, Blasiak et al. [38] found that resin monomers increase the expression of 8-hydroxyguanine in DNA—hydrolase 1, the main enzyme for repairing 8-oxoG damage by trimming alkalis.

The adverse effects of dental resin composites can be attributed to monomers' presence and the influence of the composite once they were properly cross-linked. Glutathione depletion is responsible for GMA, HEMA, TEGDMA-induced OS. Moreover, HEMA and TEGDMA were shown to disrupt the mitochondrial respiratory chain's functioning and disrupt the oxidative phosphorylation process, which contributes to the exacerbation of ROS-induced apoptosis to the dental pulp cells. Interestingly, although dental resin composites increase TAC higher than amalgam fillings, unfortunately, monomers cause higher oxidation and transformation of dental pulp cells' genetic material than amalgam fillings.

8. Composite Resins

Low-viscosity resins are commonly used in restorative dentistry as binding agents connecting dental materials with dental tissue. The inclusion of iodine salts in dental bonding systems was found to be very interesting because they can act as catalysts, reducing activation energy. Due to their ionic nature, they participate in the polymerization of hydrophilic monomers and thus increase the polymerization reaction capacity and percentage of monomer conversion rate. Ferrúa et al. [60] found higher activity of superoxide dismutase (SOD) in 10 s of polymerization vs 20 s, which indicates a slight response of mouse fibroblast cells (NIH/3T3), most probably connected with increased monomer release in the initial phase of polymerization. Significant reduction of lipid peroxidation and oxidation of disulfide groups, after incorporation of iodine salts into bonding systems, was—according to the authors—associated with the inhibition of ROS producing enzymes and proved their protective action towards cell membranes.

Initiators are an essential component of light-hardened composites and dental adhesives. Currently, visible-light photoinitiators, such as phenylbis(2,4,6-trimethylbenzoyl) phosphine oxide (BAPO) and diphenyl(2,4,6-trimethylbenzoyl) phosphine oxide (TPO), are used. Both of these photoinitiators belong to the group of Norrish type I photoinitiators and unlike camphorquinone (CQ) they do not generate ROS. Popal et al. [100] found that both BAPO and TPO used in micromole concentrations do not increase ROS/RNS production in human keratinocytes and V79 fibroblasts during 90 min of exposure. Interestingly, the concentration of ROS/RNS in cells treated with the said photoinitiators was lower compared to the control cells. It is probable that aromatic and phosphine oxide groups serve as electron donors that compete with the fluorescent dye $DCFH_2$ used in the ROS detection method. In the absence of significant changes in ROS/RNS concentration, the alterations in mRNA expression of enzymatic antioxidants in the keratinocyte culture exposed to BAPO and, to a lesser extent, to TPO prove that these cells may be subjected to OS. Within 24 h, BAPO induced a significant increase in HO-1 mRNA and quinone oxidoreductase (NQO1), and TPO only triggered a significant increase in HO-1 mRNA. Yoshino et al. [101] found that long-term irradiation of the human aortic smooth muscle cells (ACBR1716) with blue light (from a quartz-tungsten-halogen lamp) induced the production of H_2O_2 and hydroxy radical (HO·). As a result, increased peroxidation of lipid membrane as well as MDA production were observed. They also proved that treatment with NAC could reduce ROS production and cytotoxicity induced by blue light irradiation. Oktay et al. [102] observed markedly increased TOS in the absence of significant changes in TAS level in rat aorta cells irradiated with blue light (400–520 nm, 1200 mV/cm^2) vs not irradiated cells. Based on the results of these studies, it is difficult to assess whether the rat aorta cells were subjected to OS or whether the antioxidant barrier was efficient enough to balance the emerging ROS/RNS.

Although BAPO and TPO show a dose-dependent cytotoxic effect, unlike CQ, they do not increase the intracellular production of ROS /RNS. Interestingly, dental resin curing blue light alone induces increased peroxidation of membrane lipids.

9. Endodontic Treatment

The complicated morphology of the root canal system of teeth makes instrumentation challenging. One of the most important elements of root canal treatment is the use of irrigating solutions which are designed to neutralize microorganisms as well as dissolve and remove tissue residues, including the smear layer. These solutions come into direct contact with periapical tissues, particularly in teeth with periapical lesions in which the identification of the anatomical apex is difficult, and the physiological opening is virtually non-existent due to periapical microresorption. The most commonly used rinsing solutions include the main ones: sodium hypochlorite (NaOCl) and chlorhexidine (CHX) as well as auxiliary solutions: ethylenediaminetetraacetic acid (EDTA) and citric acid. Botton et al. [103] observed that 2% CHX and 6% citric acid did not cause lipid peroxidation, regardless of the exposure time of human peripheral blood mononuclear cells (PBMCs). The 72-h exposure of PBMCs to both 1% and 2.5% NaOCl resulted in increased lipid peroxidation, which suggests that prolonged contact of the cells with the rinsing solution may result in OS and, consequently, disturbed integrity of cell membranes due to the destruction of the lipid bilayer [104]. The solution of 17% EDTA boosted the process of lipid peroxidation only after 24 h of exposure of the cells, which was not maintained after 72 h (Botton et al. [103]), co Saghiri et al. [104] is the adaptation of cells to environmental conditions. The genetic material appears to be more susceptible to the damaging effects of the rinsing agents, as increased oxidative DNA modifications were observed after both 24 and 72 h of exposure of PBMCs to all the flushing solutions. A similar genotoxic effect was observed by evaluating combinations of major rinsing solutions with auxiliaries after both 24 and 72 h of exposure. Soares et al. [105] observed no DNA damage due to NaOCl (1.25%, 2.5%, 5%), 17% EDTA or citric acid (10.5% and 21%); however, the exposure time in their study was only 3 h.

The effectiveness of the described disinfectants is supported by the so-called photodynamic antibacterial chemotherapy (PACT). PACT uses a light source of the narrow-band wavelength that activates rinsing chemicals [106]. A by-product of this reaction are oxygen free radicals such as ozone and H_2O_2, which on the one hand, help to eliminate infections in the root canal but, on the other, may contribute to cell death.

The final stage of endodontic treatment is filling the canal system. Different materials are chosen depending on whether the roots of primary or permanent teeth are filled. However, the filling materials should not exhibit any cytotoxic effect, but should have antibacterial properties in order to prevent reinfection. In the study by Pires et al. [107] iodoform-based pastes used to fill the root canals of deciduous teeth induced a significant increase in ROS already after 24-h exposure of PBMC cells. Interestingly, after 72 h of exposure to iodoform preparations, further significant increase in ROS concentration in the said cells was not accompanied by intensified lipid peroxidation, which—according to the authors—was due to an efficient antioxidant barrier capable of restoring the redox balance. It should be noted that pastes containing chlorhexidine induced significantly higher ROS production compared to iodoform pastes with neomycin sulfate + bacitracin as well as rifamycin SV sodium + 21 prednisolone acetate. According to Barbin et al. [108], redox imbalance induced by CHX was related to parachloroaniline and ROS-byproducts of the 2% CHX aqueous solution. Parachloroaniline has a high potential to cause oxidative DNA damage [81]. Calcium hydroxide-based pastes triggered the highest ROS increase after 24 h of exposure. After 72 h, only the paste with zinc oxide induced further significant increase in ROS production in the PBMC culture. In the TBARS assay, calcium hydroxide pastes demonstrated a similar increase in lipid peroxidation within 24 h, whereas no calcium hydroxide paste caused oxidative damage to the lipids after 72 h of exposure. All calcium hydroxide pastes and just one of the iodoform pastes (CHX) showed the ability to induce oxidative DNA damage, regardless of the exposure time.

Among the materials applied in endodontics to treat permanent dentition, root canal sealers are sealing materials in most methods based on the use of gutta-percha for canal filling. The most common include AH-Plus pastes (Paste A: bisphenol-A, bisphenol-F, calcium tungstate, zirconium dioxide, silicon monoxide, ferric oxide; Paste B: dibezyl diamine, aminoadamantane, tricyclodecane diamine, calcium tungstate, zirconium dioxide, silicon monoxide, silicone oil), MTA-Fillapex (base paste: salicylate resin, natural resin, calcium tungstate, silica nanoparticles, dyes; catalyst paste: diluted resin, mineral trioxide aggregate, silica nanoparticles, dyes) and materials applied in regenerative endodontics: MTA-Angelus (SiO_2, K_2O, Al_2O_3, Na_2O, Fe_2O_3, SO_3, CaO, Bi_2O_3, MgO and insoluble deposits of CaO, KSO_4, $NaSO_4$ and crystalline silica), Biodentine (tricalcium silicate, zirconium dioxide, calcium carbonate, calcium chloride, polymer) and BioRoot (tricalcium silicate, zirconium dioxide, calcium chloride, polymer). The results of the study by Victoria-Escandell et al. [109] demonstrated that

MTA-Angelus did not induce OS w HDPSCs after 24 h of incubation, while AH-Plus and MTA-Fillapex increased protein carbonyl concentration, which is consistent with the results of Kim et al. [110]. Chang et al. [111] demonstrated that MTA-Angelus is capable of increasing ROS production, but the simultaneously activated antioxidant barrier is strong enough to maintain the redox balance. In HDPSC cells treated with AH-Plus and MTA-Fillapex for 24 h, both CAT and SOD were down-regulated compared to the control and MTA-Angelus-treated cells [109]. Under the conditions of low ROS production, which—according to the authors—occurs during the exposure to MTA-Angelus, cells can respond by activating Nrf2 expression and then the target genes of antioxidant enzymes, e.g., CAT or SOD. In the state of OS that occurs in case of AH-Plus and MTA-Fillapex, the Nrf2 pathway is suppressed and the activity of antioxidant enzymes is decreased. No significant differences were observed in the gene expression of CAT, SOD, glutathione synthase in the human dental pulp cells treated with Biodentine and BioRoot [112]. The authors did not examine oxidative stress markers; therefore, it is difficult to assess the occurrence and possible severity of OS.

Most endodontic materials generate increased amounts of ROS, leading to the development of the OS. However, it should be emphasized that biocompatible materials used in the form of sealers seem to be the most favorable from the point of view of redox balance.

10. Orthodontic Braces

Treatment with braces is becoming more and more popular all over the world. Fixed braces are made of various steel alloys, titanium or Ni-Ti. It was demonstrated that some metals included in the alloys of which braces are made (such as iron, chromium, copper, vanadium) are directly responsible for increased ROS production [60,61], while such metals as cadmium, mercury, nickel or lead generate ROS via the indirect mechanism [60]. Interestingly, nickel increases the activity of intracellular lactate dehydrogenase, which disturbs the redox balance and stimulates apoptosis in human oral epithelium cells [113]. Moreover, it is suspected that titanium elements of dental braces are deprived of their superficial layer of titanium oxide as a result of mechanical friction during treatment, which leads to corrosion and the release of metallic particles into the oral cavity environment. The significance of this phenomenon for the redox balance is explained below. The available research results concerning the influence of orthodontic braces on the oral redox balance are contradictory and, unfortunately, limited to only several scientific studies. Özcan et al. [43] suggest that orthodontic treatment, including the use of braces, does not increase the oxidative damage observed in the saliva and gingival fluid. Kovac et al. [61] observed that both ROS and the ratio of ROS to antioxidants in the blood clearly increased within a short period of time after the fitting of braces (24 h) compared to the control group. These levels normalized 7 days after the beginning of orthodontic treatment. Buczko et al. [44] found significantly elevated levels of TBARS and TOS in the unstimulated and stimulated saliva one week after orthodontic treatment (nickel-chromium archwires) and no OS biomarkers in the saliva of orthodontically treated patients within 24 weeks of wearing dental braces. This initial severity of OS is associated with intensified nickel release, as confirmed by a positive correlation between nickel and TOS concentrations in both unstimulated and stimulated saliva in week 1 of the use of braces. In the 24th week, the salivary nickel concentration was comparable to its content before orthodontic treatment. The authors emphasize that the treated patients maintained perfect oral hygiene and showed no gingivitis. Oral hygiene and periodontal health are crucial for the salivary redox balance. Similar results were obtained by Portelli et al. [42], with measurements taken before as well as 5 and 10 weeks after the start of treatment. The researchers claimed that multi-bracket archwires with vestibular appliances do not induce OS during the first 10 weeks of treatment, which is associated with the fact that this type of braces reduces the forces exerted on the teeth and allows for good oral hygiene. On the other hand, the results of Spalj et al. [40] revealed that nickel-titanium standard braces generated the strongest, while stainless steel and titanium-molybdenum ones the least intensive OS in the L929 mouse fibroblast cell line. The use of copper-nickel-titanium and rhodium-coated nickel-titanium orthodontic appliances resulted in increased production of 8-OHdG, which was lower; however, than in the case of standard nickel-titanium archwires. Cobalt-chromium archwires triggered moderate 8-OHdG production, which was most probably connected with the suppression of mitochondrial activity in the aforementioned cell line. Similar results were obtained by Buljan et al. [41], but the authors observed that the strongest OS expressed in 8-OHdG concentration was induced by polymer brackets, which most likely resulted from the presence of polyether polyol. Moreover, the researchers demonstrated that not only the mentioned polymers, but also zirconium dioxide and synthetic sapphire used in the production of elements of aesthetic braces were not indifferent to salivary redox balance, as expressed by increased 8-OHdG concentration in the L929 murine fibroblast cell line.

All orthodontic appliances induce OS. Its intensity depends on the time and the metal alloys used. Initial severity of OS is believed to be associated with intensified nickel release.

11. Fixations and Dental Implants

Titanium and its alloys are commonly applied for the production of medical implants. They are widely used in maxillofacial surgery and orthopedics as bone fixations, joint prostheses, dental implants, and other devices used in reconstructive surgery. Implants made of titanium and its alloys are very popular due to their good mechanical properties, corrosion resistance and biocompatibility. Their higher biocompatibility in human tissues, compared to other metallic materials, is related to the presence of an inactive layer of titanium dioxide (TiO_2) on the implant surface. However, clinical and experimental studies showed that ions and particles of titanium and its alloys are found in peri-implantation tissues, blood and distant organs after the placement of the implants. Gholinejad et al. [114] observed that titanium dioxide nanoparticles were internalized to HUVECs and induced intracellular ROS production as well as cell membrane oxidative modifications. Borys et al. [48,50] demonstrated that exposure to the titanium alloy Ti-6Al-4V stimulated antioxidative mechanisms in the periosteal cells covering titanium implants in the jaw and mandible. However, this defensive reaction was insufficient as it did not prevent oxidative damage to proteins (↑protein carbonyl) and lipids (↑MDA) in the periosteum-like tissue in the area adjacent to the implants [46]. The results obtained by the authors indicate the persistence of OS phenomena around the fixations of maxillary bones regardless of the time that passed from the surgery of facial bone defects, but these phenomena were not accompanied by any clinical symptoms [48]. Moreover, the authors indicate that the production of ROS results, among others, from mitochondrial dysfunction (decreased activity of complex I and citrate synthase) [46] as well as increased activity of NADPH oxidase and xanthine oxidase [49]. Mitochondrial function disorders in muscle cells and their morphological changes (swelling and vacuolization) were confirmed by the studies of Wang et al. and Pereira et al. [115,116]. Furthermore, Pereira et al. [115] showed that exposure of rat liver mitochondria to TiNPs (titanium nanoparticles) + AgNPs (silver nanoparticles) lowered the respiratory control ratio, which resulted in reduced oxidative phosphorylation efficiency. 21-day exposure of mitochondria to both types of nanoparticles maintained the increased ROS levels and depleted the endogenous antioxidant system. AgNPs and TiNPs acted synergistically: the intensity of the toxic effect on the mitochondrial redox balance was more significant in the presence of both types of nanoparticles. Borys et al. [49] also observed a positive relationship between the production of ROS/RNS and the concentration of titanium, aluminum and vanadium in tissues surrounding the titanium implants, which is explained by the observations of Shanbhag et al. [117] and Mouthuy et al. [118]. These authors demonstrated that the said ions released from the implants stimulate macrophages and osteoclasts to increase ROS and RNS production, and that ROS/RNS boost the release of metal ions from the implant surface through ROS/RNS-induced corrosion. According to these researchers, these observations highlight the need to improve the quality of the applied jawbone fixations by increasing the passive TiO_2 layer thickness in miniplates and screws in the process of hard anodizing, or search for other materials, preferably biodegradable in human tissues, for the production of dental fixations.

In recent years, we witnessed rapid development of implantology as a field of dentistry. Implantation is a more and more common method of filling in missing teeth [63]. The maintenance of an implant in the oral cavity depends on numerous factors. Peri-implantitis has an inflammatory etiology, therefore the effect of OS on the phenomenon of implant rejection is sought. However, the results of these studies are contradictory, depending on the type of the examined material or clinical situation. At the beginning, it is worth mentioning that ROS act as mediators of cytoskeletal remodeling and cell proliferation, while too low intracellular ROS concentration was found to slow down cell adhesion and proliferation. The results of Wei et al. [45] demonstrate that ROS content in DPSC and MC3T3-E1 cells that stuck to the surface of titanium and zirconium after 24 h of incubation is high enough to allow for the correct process of cell adhesion and spreading. These processes are more efficient for the zirconia surface [47]. Pietropaoli et al. [47] believe that both the excessive production of ROS and, consequently, AGEs in the tissues adjacent to the implant are factors that favor the implant rejection process. In the opinion of these authors, ROS-derived AGEs that irreversibly accumulate in the tissues surrounding the implant, disturb the collagen structure and induce inflammation. However, the redox imbalance in the course of peri-implantitis is less severe than in periodontal diseases. Similar results of redox equilibrium changes were obtained by Guo et al. [54]. but it should be emphasized that these observations were found in patients' saliva. Cabaña-Muñoz et al. observed that patients with long-term (10 years) dental titanium and amalgams have systemic oxidative stress expressed as a significant increase in MDA concentration and decrease in Mo/Co and Mo/Fe^{2+} ratios in hair samples than those with amalgam alone [119]. On the other hand, Sánchez-Siles et al. [120] found that salivary concentration of myeloperoxidase and MDA in patients with peri-implantitis and without periodontal diseases did not differ from the healthy control. According to the results of Mousavi et al. [55], there is a positive correlation between periodontal pocket depth (PPD) around the implant and MDA and TAC concentrations. However, the concentration of the tested OS markers (MDA, SOD, TAC) in an osmotically mediated transudate/inflammatory exudate around dental implants (PICF) in diseased implants (PPD $\geq$ 4 mm, gingival index GI $\geq$ 1, bleeding on probing BOP = 1) did not differ from "healthy implants" (PPD < 3 mm, GI = 0, BOP = 0). According to the authors, the study on the aforementioned OS markers does not allow for the differentiation between peri-implant health and disease conditions.

As a result of processes such as friction, titanium implants contribute to the increased production of ROS and increase the carbonyl, MDA, AGE proteins in the tissue around the implant. These observations call into question the safety of leaving titanium implants permanently.

12. Periodontology

Periodontal diseases are a very common problem in dental practice. Interestingly, a key role in periodontitis is played by oxidative stress [121,122]. In response to bacterial microflora and local inflammation, polymorphonuclear leukocytes (but also peripheral blood leukocytes) produce large amounts of ROS, which by oxidizing lipids, proteins, and nucleic acids, lead to the destruction of periodontal connective tissue. Thus, periodontitis may lead to increased tooth mobility and even tooth loss [52].

A question arises: can periodontal treatment influence the intensity of salivary oxidative stress? Tamaki et al. [53] demonstrated that scaling and root planning (SRP) significantly reduced the level of reactive oxygen metabolites (ROMs) in the plasma of patients with chronic periodontitis. Moreover, the rate of ROMs production correlated significantly with the severity of periodontal disease (a positive correlation with bleeding on probing [BOP] and clinical attachment loss [CAL]) both before and after the surgery [53]. SRP also considerably reduced the concentration of salivary malondialdehyde (MDA), which may—to some extent—explain the therapeutic success in patients with non-surgical periodontal treatment [53].

The salivary content of GSH is significantly lower in the saliva of patients with chronic periodontitis [52,123], which is not surprising as this compound is used intensively by periodontal tissues in response to increased ROS production. However, SRP together with 7-day antibiotic therapy (amoxicillin + metronidazole, 500 mg each, 3 times daily) does not change salivary levels of GSH or C-reactive protein (CRP) in patients with periodontitis [52]. Boia et al. [52] demonstrated that non-surgical periodontal therapy lowered ROMs levels in plasma. This parameter correlates positively with CAL, which confirms previous reports on the relationship between ROS production in blood and periodontal inflammation [52,53].

Recently, antimicrobial photodynamic therapy (aPDT) has become a popular method of treatment of periodontitis patients. The term aPDT means a laser therapy in which the photosensitizer produces oxygen free radicals that destroy microorganisms in the gingival pocket biofilm [51]. Indeed, it was demonstrated that laser light in the presence of methylene blue (MB) in 20% ethanol generates significant amounts of ROS, which determines its bactericidal effect. Pillusky et al. [51] also showed that aPDT increases the concentration of erythrocytic GSH, which is the systemic adaptive response to the applied treatment. Photodynamic therapy can be performed as an additional procedure to standard periodontal treatment to enhance the systemic protective response against oxidative stress, boosting and accelerating periodontium healing, particularly when the photosensitizer is dissolved in ethanol (which facilitates its penetration into periodontal tissues) [51].

Ozone (O_3) is also very popular in periodontology. It was demonstrated that O_3 increases ROS production in periodontal tissues, thus leading to the activation of numerous transcription factors such as mitogen-activated protein kinase (MAPK), cellular proto-oncogene encoding the transcription factor FOS (c-Fos), AP-1 (transcription factor activator protein 1) and the nuclear factor erythroid 2 (NF-E2)-related factor 2 (Nrf2). Importantly, Nrf2 is related to the promoter region of metallothionein that participates in the response to OS [56]. Leewananthawet et al. [56] proved that aqueous ozone ultrafine bubble water (OUFBW) increases the antioxidant defense of periodontal ligament fibroblasts, while the stimulation of c-Fos and c-Jun pathways further differentiates osteoblasts involved in periodontal tissue regeneration [56]. A study on an animal model showed that blue light increases the amount of ROS, which results in vasospasm in the aorta. Moreover, researchers suggest that the elevated ROS level under the influence of blue light also occurs in gingival fibroblasts. The alternating vasospasms and vasodilatations due to ROS lead to the subsequent generation of reactive oxygen species, which is called the vicious circle effect [124,125].

The ROS generated in the treatment of periodontal diseases seems to positively affect the healing process: they support the elimination of periopathogenic bacteria and accelerate periodontium healing.

13. Whitening

Tooth whitening is one of the most frequently chosen procedures to restore the esthetics of discolored teeth. Whitening can be performed both in the dental clinic and at home [126,127]. Hydrogen peroxide (H_2O_2) is the most commonly used substance for this purpose due to its low price and high effectiveness [83]. H_2O_2 is characterized by high reactivity, although it is not a free radical. It participates in oxidation reactions, the most biologically significant of which is the oxidation of sulfhydryl groups. [128]. It leads to the formation of disulfide bridges, which changes the conformations as well as biological functions of proteins. H_2O_2 also has the ability to oxidize unsaturated fatty acids during the process of lipid peroxidation. [129]. Moreover, hydrogen peroxide is capable of oxidizing ferrous or copper ions (the proper Fenton reaction: $Fe^{2+} + H_2O_2 \rightarrow Fe^{3+} + \cdot OH + OH^-$, the catalysts for this reaction are also Cu^{2+} ions). During these reactions, hydrogen peroxide is transformed into hydroxyl radical $\cdot OH$. The redox reaction under the influence of H_2O_2 results in the formation of: superoxide anion, hydroxyl radical and singlet oxygen, all of which have an oxidizing effect on the organic components of the enamel, leading to the whitening of tissues [67,72]. It is suggested that low concentrations of hydrogen peroxide do not exhibit a destructive effect on the oral cavity cells [125]. ROS generated during the whitening process induce a sequence of reactions that increase the expression of heme oxygenase 1 (HO-1) in fibroblasts and osteoblasts [83]. Considering the antioxidant and anti-inflammatory properties of this enzyme, it can be concluded that increased expression of HO-1 in cells exposed to H_2O_2 is a defensive mechanism against the adverse effects of whitening.

Del Real Garcia et al. [57] demonstrated that in patients exposed to 10% H_2O_2 contained in whitening strips (Crest® 3D Whitestrips® premium plus), the concentration of salivary 8-OHdG increased compared to non-exposed subjects. Moreover, the positive correlation between the genotoxicity test and 8-OHdG concentration indicates that hydrogen peroxide is the cause of DNA damage in patients using whitening strips. Indeed, in the study group the authors observed chromosome damage, impaired cytokinesis and increased apoptosis of the oral epithelial cells after 15 and 30 days of using whitening strips [57]. Interestingly, no DNA damage was demonstrated after professional whitening treatments with 35% hydrogen peroxide. Whitening procedures are only suggested when performed by qualified dentists [57].

Interestingly, hydrogen peroxide can diffuse through the enamel to a concentration of about 0.01% in the pulp. Recent studies suggested that the higher the content of whitening agents such as hydrogen peroxide, the greater the cytotoxic effect on the pulp [127]. Cytotoxicity increases significantly after using a LED lamp with a wavelength from 400 to 505 nm. In the study group using 0.01% hydrogen peroxide, a considerable increase in ROS production as well as boosted apoptosis on the mitochondrial pathway were demonstrated, which was associated with a decreased number of living cells in this group [127]. However, it was shown that the pulp after whitening undergoes regeneration within 24 to 72 h, which indicated a temporary cytotoxic effect [127]. Lima et al. [130] also demonstrated that the use of antioxidants such as sodium ascorbate (0.25 mM/0.5 mM) reduces ROS production, thus limiting the risk of OS development (85). Vargas et al. observed that the use of alpha-tocopherol (1, 3, 5 and 10 mM) reduced hydrogen peroxide-induced cytotoxicity (0.035%, 0.018%, 0.009% and 0.045%) in odontoblasts and pulp cells [131].

The use of appropriate concentrations of bleaching agents generates ROS while simultaneously induces antioxidant defense systems. Consequently, the whitening process takes place without adverse effects on the redox equilibrium of the oral cavity.

14. Summary

As a result of OS, cell components—mainly proteins, lipids and nucleic acids—are damaged, which leads not only to structural changes of the cell, but also to its death through apoptosis and necrosis. Moreover, oxidative stress is associated with the pathogenesis of numerous systemic diseases, including those related to the oral cavity. Interestingly, not only the diseases of the oral cavity, but also their treatment induce OS. The source of ROS in the oral cavity can be filling materials such as amalgam, composites, glass-ionomer materials, or bonding systems, but also agents used in endodontic treatment, periodontal and surgical procedures, or materials used in orthodontic treatment.

Although some of the listed ROS/RNS sources in the oral cavity are inevitable and, in some situations, beneficial (periodontal treatment), the search for therapeutic solutions to avoid materials and treatment procedures leading to ROS overproduction seems extremely important.

Author Contributions: Conceptualization, A.Z. and M.M.; Data curation, I.Z. and A.Z.; Formal analysis, I.Z. and M.M.; Funding acquisition, A.Z.; Investigation, I.Z., A.Z., and M.M.; Methodology, I.Z., A.Z., and M.M.; Writing—original draft, I.Z. and A.Z.; Writing—review and editing, A.Z. and M.M. All authors have read and agreed to the published version of the manuscript.

References

1. Maciejczyk, M.; Mikoluc, B.; Pietrucha, B.; Heropolitanska—Pliszka, E.; Pac, M.; Motkowski, R.; Car, H. Oxidative stress, mitochondrial abnormalities and antioxidant defense in Ataxia-telangiectasia, Bloom syndrome and Nijmegen breakage syndrome. *Redox Biol.* **2017**. [CrossRef] [PubMed]

2. Chatterjee, S. *Oxidative Stress, Inflammation, and Disease*; Elsevier Inc.: Amsterdam, The Netherlands, 2016; pp. 35–58.

3. Sardaro, N.; della Vella, F.; Incalza, M.A.; Stasio, D.D.I.; Lucchese, A.; Contaldo, M.; Laudadio, C.; Petruzzi, M. Oxidative stress and oral mucosal diseases: An overview. *In Vivo* **2019**, *33*, 289–296. [CrossRef] [PubMed]

4.   Gallorini, M.; Cataldi, A.; di Giacomo, V. HEMA-induced cytotoxicity: Oxidative stress, genotoxicity and apoptosis. *Int. Endod. J.* **2014**, *47*, 813–818. [CrossRef] [PubMed]

5.   Zalewska, A.; Maciejczyk, M.; Szulimowska, J.; Imierska, M.; Błachnio-Zabielska, A. High-fat diet affects ceramide content, disturbs mitochondrial redox balance, and induces apoptosis in the submandibular glands of mice. *Biomolecules* **2019**, *9*, 877. [CrossRef] [PubMed]

6.   Pawlukianiec, C.; Gryciuk, M.E.; Mil, K.M.; Żendzian-Piotrowska, M.; Zalewska, A.; Maciejczyk, M. A New Insight into Meloxicam: Assessment of Antioxidant and Anti-Glycating Activity in In Vitro Studies. *Pharmaceuticals* **2020**, *13*, 240. [CrossRef] [PubMed]

7.   Davies, M.J. Protein oxidation and peroxidation. *Biochem. J.* **2016**, *473*, 805–825. [CrossRef] [PubMed]

8.   Reeg, S.; Grune, T. Protein Oxidation in Aging: Does It Play a Role in Aging Progression? *Antioxid. Redox Signal.* **2015**, *23*, 239–255. [CrossRef] [PubMed]

9.   Maciejczyk, M.; Szulimowska, J.; Taranta-Janusz, K.; Wasilewska, A.; Zalewska, A. Salivary Gland Dysfunction, Protein Glycooxidation and Nitrosative Stress in Children with Chronic Kidney Disease. *J. Clin. Med.* **2020**, 1285. [CrossRef] [PubMed]

10.   Branco, V.; Canário, J.; Holmgren, A.; Carvalho, C. Inhibition of the thioredoxin system in the brain and liver of zebra-seabreams exposed to waterborne methylmercury. *Toxicol. Appl. Pharmacol.* **2011**, *251*, 95–103. [CrossRef] [PubMed]

11.   Morita, M.; Naito, Y.; Yoshikawa, T.; Niki, E. Redox Biology Plasma lipid oxidation induced by peroxynitrite, hypochlorite, lipoxygenase and peroxyl radicals and its inhibition by antioxidants as assessed by diphenyl-1-pyrenylphosphine. *Redox Biol.* **2016**, *8*, 127–135. [CrossRef] [PubMed]

12.   Skutnik-Radziszewska, A.; Maciejczyk, M.; Fejfer, K.; Krahel, J.; Flisiak, I.; Kołodziej, U.; Zalewska, A. Salivary Antioxidants and Oxidative Stress in Psoriatic Patients: Can Salivary Total Oxidant Status and Oxidative Status Index Be a Plaque Psoriasis Biomarker? *Oxid. Med. Cell. Longev.* **2020**. [CrossRef] [PubMed]

13.   Gerreth, P.; Maciejczyk, M.; Zalewska, A.; Gerreth, K.; Hojan, K. Comprehensive Evaluation of the Oral Health Status, Salivary Gland Function, and Oxidative Stress in the Saliva of Patients with Subacute Phase of Stroke: A Case-Control Study. *J. Clin. Med.* **2020**, 2252. [CrossRef] [PubMed]

14.   Sawczuk, B.; Maciejczyk, M.; Sawczuk-Siemieniuk, M.; Posmyk, R.; Zalewska, A.; Car, H. Salivary gland function, antioxidant defence and oxidative damage in the saliva of patients with breast cancer: Does the BRCA1 mutation disturb the salivary redox profile? *Cancers* **2019**, *11*, 1501. [CrossRef] [PubMed]

15.   Waddington, R.J.; Moseley, R.; Embery, G. Reactive oxygen species: A potential role in the pathogenesis of periodontal diseases. *Oral. Dis.* **2000**, *6*, 138–151. [CrossRef] [PubMed]

16.   Zińczuk, J.; Maciejczyk, M.; Zaręba, K.; Romaniuk, W.; Markowski, A.; Kędra, B.; Zalewska, A.; Pryczynicz, A.; Matowicka-Karna, J.; Guzińska-Ustymowicz, K. Antioxidant Barrier, Redox Status, and Oxidative Damage to Biomolecules in Patients with Colorectal Cancer. Can Malondialdehyde and Catalase Be Markers of Colorectal Cancer Advancement? *Biomolecules* **2019**, *9*, 637. [CrossRef] [PubMed]

17.   Maciejczyk, M.; Szulimowska, J.; Skutnik, A.; Taranta-Janusz, K.; Wasilewska, A.; Wiśniewska, N.; Zalewska, A. Salivary Biomarkers of Oxidative Stress in Children with Chronic Kidney Disease. *J. Clin. Med.* **2018**, *7*, 209. [CrossRef]

18.   Żukowski, P.; Maciejczyk, M.; Waszkiel, D. Sources of free radicals and oxidative stress in the oral cavity. *Arch. Oral Biol.* **2018**, *92*, 8–17. [CrossRef]

19.   Celik, N.; Binnetoglu, D.; Ozakar Ilday, N.; Hacimuftuoglu, A.; Seven, N. The cytotoxic and oxidative effects of restorative materials in cultured human gingival fibroblasts. *Drug Chem. Toxicol.* **2019**, *31*, 1–6. [CrossRef]

20.   Ramezani, G.H.; Moghadam, M.M.; Saghiri, M.A.; Garcia-Godoy, F.; Asatourian, A.; Aminsobhani, M.; Scarbecz, M.; Sheibani, N. Effect of dental restorative materials on total antioxidant capacity and calcium concentration of unstimulated saliva. *J. Clin. Exp. Dent.* **2017**, *9*, e71–e77. [CrossRef]

21.   Daokar, S.G.; Shahu, C.; Shikshan, M.; Mustafa, M. Assessment of Oxidative Stress Induced by Various Restorative Materials: An In Vivo Biochemical Study. *J. Int. Oral Health* **2016**, *8*, 1–6.

22.   Al-Saleh, I.; Al-Sedairi, A.; Elkhatib, R. Effect of mercury (Hg) dental amalgam fillings on renal and oxidative stress biomarkers in children. *Sci. Total Environ.* **2012**, *431*, 188–196. [CrossRef] [PubMed]

23.   Cabaña-Muñoz, M.E.; Parmigiani-Izquierdo, J.M.; Bravo-González, L.A.; Kyung, H.M.; Merino, J.J. Increased Zn/glutathione levels and higher superoxide dismutase-1 activity as biomarkers of oxidative stress in women with long-term dental amalgam fillings: Correlation between mercury/aluminium levels (in hair) and antioxidant systems in plasma. *PLoS ONE* **2015**, *10*, 1–11. [CrossRef] [PubMed]

24. Yıldız, M.; Alp, H.H.; Gül, P.; Bakan, N.; Özcan, M. Lipid peroxidation and DNA oxidation caused by dental filling materials. *J. Dent. Sci.* **2017**, *12*, 233–240. [CrossRef] [PubMed]

25. Jiao, Y.; Ma, S.; Wang, Y.; Li, J.; Shan, L.; Liu, Q.; Liu, Y.; Song, Q.; Yu, F.; Yu, H.; et al. N-Acetyl cysteine depletes reactive oxygen species and prevents dental monomer-induced intrinsic mitochondrial apoptosis in vitro in human dental pulp cells. *PLoS ONE* **2016**, *11*, 1–20. [CrossRef] [PubMed]

26. Schneider, T.R.; Hakami-Tafreshi, R.; Tomasino-Perez, A.; Tayebi, L.; Lobner, D. Effects of dental composite resin monomers on dental pulp cells. *Dent. Mater. J.* **2019**, *38*, 579–583. [CrossRef] [PubMed]

27. Chang, H.H.; Guo, M.K.; Kasten, F.H.; Chang, M.C.; Huang, G.F.; Wang, Y.L.; Wang, R.S.; Jeng, J.H. Stimulation of glutathione depletion, ROS production and cell cycle arrest of dental pulp cells and gingival epithelial cells by HEMA. *Biomaterials* **2005**, *26*, 745–753. [CrossRef]

28. Lefeuvre, M.; Amjaad, W.; Goldberg, M.; Stanislawski, L. TEGDMA induces mitochondrial damage and oxidative stress in human gingival fibroblasts. *Biomaterials* **2005**, *26*, 5130–5137. [CrossRef]

29. Diomede, F.; Marconi, G.D.; Guarnieri, S.; D'Attilio, M.; Cavalcanti, M.F.X.B.; Mariggiò, M.A.; Pizzicannella, J.; Trubiami, O. A Novel Role of Ascorbic Acid in Anti-Inflammatory Pathway and ROS Generation in HEMA Treated Dental Pulp Stem Cells. *Materials* **2020**, 130. [CrossRef]

30. Di Nisio, C.; Zara, S.; Cataldi, A.; di Giacomo, V. 2-Hydroxyethyl methacrylate inflammatory effects in human gingival fibroblasts. *Int. Endod. J.* **2013**, *46*, 466–476. [CrossRef]

31. Perduns, R.; Volk, J.; Schertl, P.; Leyhausen, G.; Geurtsen, W. HEMA modulates the transcription of genes relatedto oxidative defense, inflammatory response andorganization of the ECM in human oral cells. *Dent. Mater.* **2019**, *35*, 501–510. [CrossRef]

32. Jiao, Y.; Niu, T.; Liu, H.; Tay, F.R.; Chen, J. Protection against HEMA-Induced Mitochondrial Injury In Vitro by Nrf2 Activation. *Oxid. Med. Cell. Longev.* **2019**, *2019*. [CrossRef] [PubMed]

33. Teti, G.; Orsini, G.; Salvatore, V.; Focaroli, S.; Mazzotti, M.C.; Ruggeri, A.; Mattioli-belmonte, M.; Falconi, M. HEMA but not TEGDMA induces autophagy in human gingival fibroblasts. *Front. Physiol.* **2015**, *6*, 1–8. [CrossRef] [PubMed]

34. Krifka, S.; Seidenader, C.; Hiller, K.A.; Schmalz, G.; Schweikl, H. Oxidative stress and cytotoxicity generated by dental composites in human pulp cells. *Clin. Oral Investig.* **2012**, *16*, 215–224. [CrossRef] [PubMed]

35. Pauly, K.; Fritz, K.; Furey, A.; Lobner, D. Insulin-like Growth Factor 1 and Transforming Growth Factor-β Stimulate Cystine/Glutamate Exchange Activity in Dental Pulp Cells. *J. Endod.* **2011**, *37*, 943–947. [CrossRef]

36. Huang, F.; Li, Y.; Lee, S.; Chang, Y. Cytotoxicity of dentine bonding agents on human pulp cells is related to intracellular glutathione levels. *Int. Endod. J.* **2010**, *43*, 1091–1097. [CrossRef]

37. Gul, P.; Akgul, N.; Hakan, H. Effects of composite restorations on oxidative stress in saliva: An in vivo study. *J. Dent. Sci.* **2015**, *10*, 394–400. [CrossRef]

38. Blasiak, J.; Synowiec, E. Dental methacrylates may exert genotoxic effects via the oxidative induction of DNA double strand breaks and the inhibition of their repair. *Mol. Biol. Rep.* **2012**, *39*, 7487–7496. [CrossRef] [PubMed]

39. Ferrúa, C.P.; Leal, F.B.; de Oliveira Gazal, M.; Ghisleni, G.C.; de Carvalho, R.V.; Demarco, F.F.; Ogliari, F.A.; Nedel, F. Iodonium salt incorporation in dental adhesives and its relation with degree of conversion, ultimate tensile strength, cell viability, and oxidative stress. *Clin. Oral Investig.* **2019**, *23*, 1143–1151. [CrossRef] [PubMed]

40. Spalj, S.; Mlacovic Zrinski, M.; Tudor Spalj, V.; Ivankovic Buljan, Z. In-vitro assessment of oxidative stress generated by orthodontic archwires. *Am. J. Orthod. Dentofac. Orthop.* **2012**, *141*, 583–589. [CrossRef] [PubMed]

41. Buljan, Z.I.; Ribaric, S.P.; Abram, M.; Ivankovic, A.; Spalj, S. In vitro oxidative stress induced by conventional and self-ligating brackets. *Angle Orthod.* **2012**, *82*, 340–345. [CrossRef]

42. Portelli, M.; Militi, A.; Cervino, G.; Lauritano, F.; Sambataro, S.; Mainardi, A.; Nucera, R. Oxidative Stress Evaluation in Patients Treated with Orthodontic Self-ligating Multibracket Appliances: An in Vivo Case-Control Study. *Open Dent. J.* **2017**, *11*, 257–265. [CrossRef] [PubMed]

43. Atuğ Özcan, S.S.; Ceylan, I.; Özcan, E.; Kurt, N.; Dağsuyu, I.M.; Çanakçi, C.F. Evaluation of oxidative stress biomarkers in patients with fixed orthodontic appliances. *Dis. Mark.* **2014**, *2014*. [CrossRef] [PubMed]

44. Buczko, P.; Knaś, M.; Grycz, M.; Szarmach, I.; Zalewska, A. Orthodontic treatment modifies the oxidant–antioxidant balance in saliva of clinically healthy subjects. *Adv. Med. Sci.* **2017**, *62*, 129–135. [CrossRef] [PubMed]

45. Wei, C.; Gong, T.; Pow, E.H.N.; Botelho, M.G. Adhesive and oxidative response of stem cell and pre-osteoblasts on titanium and zirconia surfaces in vitro. *J. Investig. Clin. Dent.* **2019**, *10*, e12407. [CrossRef] [PubMed]

46. Borys, J.; Maciejczyk, M.; Antonowicz, B.; Krętowski, A.; Sidun, J.; Domel, E.; Dąbrowski, J.; Ładny, J.; Morawska, K.; Zalewska, A. Glutathione Metabolism, Mitochondria Activity, and Nitrosative Stress in Patients Treated for Mandible Fractures. *J. Clin. Med.* **2019**, *8*, 127. [CrossRef] [PubMed]

47. Pietropaoli, D.; Ortu, E.; Severino, M.; Ciarrocchi, I.; Gatto, R.; Monaco, A. Glycation and oxidative stress in the failure of dental implants: A case series. *BMC Res. Notes* **2013**, *6*, 1. [CrossRef]

48. Borys, J.; Maciejczyk, M.; Krętowski, A.J.; Antonowicz, B.; Ratajczak-Wrona, W.; Jablonska, E.; Zaleski, P.; Waszkiel, D.; Ladny, J.R.; Zukowski, P.; et al. The redox balance in erythrocytes, plasma, and periosteum of patients with titanium fixation of the jaw. *Front. Physiol.* **2017**, *8*, 386. [CrossRef]

49. Borys, J.; Maciejczyk, M.; Antonowicz, B.; Sidun, J.; Świderska, M.Z.A. Free Radical Production, Inflammation and Apoptosis in Patients Treated With Titanium Mandibular Fixations—An Observational Study. *Front. Immunol.* **2019**, *10*, 1–12. [CrossRef]

50. Borys, J.; Maciejczyk, M.; Antonowicz, B.; Krętowski, A.; Waszkiel, D.; Bortnik, P.; Czarniecka-Bargłowska, K.; Kocisz, M.; Szulimowska, J.; Czajkowski, M.; et al. Exposure to Ti4Al4V titanium alloy leads to redox abnormalities, oxidative stress, and oxidative damage in patients treated for mandible fractures. *Oxid. Med. Cell. Longev.* **2018**, *2018*. [CrossRef]

51. Pillusky, F.M.; Barcelos, R.C.S.; Vey, L.T.; Barin, L.M.; de Mello Palma, V.; Maciel, R.M.; Kantorski, K.Z.; Bürger, M.E.; Danesi, C.C. Antimicrobial photodynamic therapy with photosensitizer in ethanol improves oxidative status and gingival collagen in a short-term in periodontitis. *Photodiagnosis Photodyn. Ther.* **2017**, *19*, 119–127. [CrossRef]

52. Boia, S.; Stratul, Ş.I.; Boariu, M.; Ursoniu, S.; Goţia, S.L.; Boia, E.R.; Borza, C. Evaluation of antioxidant capacity and clinical assessment of patients with chronic periodontitis treated with non-surgical periodontal therapy and adjunctive systemic antibiotherapy. *Rom. J. Morphol. Embryol.* **2018**, *59*, 1107–1113. [PubMed]

53. Tamaki, N.; Tomofuji, T.; Ekuni, D.; Yamanaka, R.; Yamamoto, T. Short—Term Effects of Non-Surgical Periodontal Treatment on Plasma Level of Reactive Oxygen Metabolites in Patients With Chronic Periodontitis. *J. Periodontol.* **2009**, *80*, 901–906. [CrossRef]

54. Guo, M.; Liu, L.; Zhang, J.; Liu, M. Role of Reactive Oxygen Species and Advanced Glycation End Products in the Malfunctioning of Dental Implants. *West. Indian Med. J.* **2015**, *64*, 419–423. [PubMed]

55. Mousavi Jazi, M.; Sadeghi Pour Rodsari, H.R.; Mirmiran, F. Level of Oxidative Stress Markers in Peri-Implant Crevicular Fluid and Their Correlation with Clinical Parameters. *J. Dent.* **2015**, *12*, 340–346.

56. Leewananthawet, A.; Arakawa, S.; Okano, T.; Daitoku Kinoshita, R.; Ashida, H.; Izumi, Y.; Suzuki, T. Ozone ultrafine bubble water induces the cellular signaling involved in oxidative stress responses in human periodontal ligament fibroblasts. *Sci. Technol. Adv. Mater.* **2019**, *20*, 589–598. [CrossRef] [PubMed]

57. Del Real García, J.F.; Saldaña-Velasco, F.R.; Sánchez-de la Rosa, S.V.; Ortiz-García, Y.M.; Morales-Velazquez, G.; Gómez-Meda, B.C.; Zúñiga-González, G.M.; Sánchez-Parada, M.G.; Zamora-Perez, A.L. In vivo evaluation of the genotoxicity and oxidative damage in individuals exposed to 10% hydrogen peroxide whitening strips. *Clin. Oral Investig.* **2019**, *23*, 3033–3046. [CrossRef] [PubMed]

58. Farina, M.; Aschner, M.; Rocha, J.B.T. Oxidative stress in MeHg-induced neurotoxicity. *Toxicol. Appl. Pharmacol.* **2011**, *256*, 405–417. [CrossRef] [PubMed]

59. Franco, J.L.; Posser, T.; Dunkley, P.R.; Dickson, P.W.; Mattos, J.J.; Martins, R.; Bainy, A.C.D.; Marques, M.R.; Dafre, A.L.; Farina, M. Methylmercury neurotoxicity is associated with inhibition of the antioxidant enzyme glutathione peroxidase Jeferson. *Free Radic. Biol. Med.* **2009**, *47*, 449–457. [CrossRef]

60. Glaser, V.; Leipnitz, G.; Raniel, M.; Oliveira, J.; Wannmacher, D.; Fabro, A.; Bem, D.; Valgas, V. Oxidative stress-mediated inhibition of brain creatine kinase activity by methylmercury. *NeuroToxicology* **2010**, *31*, 454–460. [CrossRef]

61. Glaser, V.; Maria, E.; Maria, Y.; Müller, R.; Feksa, L.; Milton, C.; Wannmacher, D.; Batista, J.; Rocha, T.; Fabro, A.; et al. Effects of inorganic selenium administration in methylmercury-induced neurotoxicity in mouse cerebral cortex. *Int. J. Dev. Neurosci.* **2010**, *28*, 631–637. [CrossRef]

62. Rocha, J.B.; Freitas, A.J.; Marques, M.B.; Pereira, M.E.; Emanuelli, T.; Souza, D. Effects of methylmercury exposure during the second stage of rapid postnatal brain growth on negative geotaxis and on delta-aminolevulinate dehydratase of suckling rats. *Braz J. Med. Biol Res.* **1993**, *10*, 1077–1083.

63. Barbosa, A.C.; Jardim, W.; Dórea, J.G.; Fosberg, B.; Souza, J. Hair Mercury Speciation as a Function of Gender, Age, and Body Mass Index in Inhabitants of the Negro River Basin, Amazon, Brazil. *Arch. Environ. Contam. Toxicol.* **2001**, *40*, 439–444. [PubMed]

64. Dorea, J. Environmental contaminants as biomarkers of fish intake: A case for hair mercury concentrations. *Eur. J. Clin. Nutr.* **2011**, *65*, 419–420. [CrossRef] [PubMed]

65. Nogueira, C.W.; Rocha, J.B. Diphenyl Diselenide a Janus-Faced Molecule. *J. Braz. Chem. Soc.* **2010**, *21*, 2055–2071. [CrossRef]

66. Araie, H.; Shiraiwa, Y. Selenium Utilization Strategy by Microalgae. *Molecules* **2009**, *14*, 4880–4891. [CrossRef]

67. Hollenberg, S.M.; Cinel, I. Bench-to-bedside review: Nitric oxide in critical illness—Update 2008. *Crit. Care* **2009**, *9*. [CrossRef]

68. Lobanov, A.V.; Hatfield, D.L.; Gladyshev, V.N. Eukaryotic selenoproteins and selenoproteomes. *Biochim. Biophys. Acta Gen. Subj.* **2012**, *1790*, 1424–1428. [CrossRef]

69. Tsuzuki, Y.Y.T. Inhibitory actions of mercury compounds against glucose-6-phosphate dehydrogenase from yeast. *J. Toxicol. Sci.* **1979**, *4*, 105–113. [CrossRef]

70. Stringari, J.; Nunes, A.K.C.; Franco, J.L.; Bohrer, D.; Solange, C.; Dafre, A.L.; Milatovic, D.; Souza, D.O.; Rocha, J.B.T.; Farina, M. Prenatal methylmercury exposure hampers glutathione antioxidant system ontogenesis and causes long-lasting oxidative stress in the mouse brain. *Toxicol. Appl. Pharmacol.* **2010**, *227*, 147–154. [CrossRef]

71. Farina, M.; Campos, F.; Vendrell, I.; Berenguer, J.; Barzi, M. Probucol Increases Glutathione Peroxidase-1 Activity and Displays Long-Lasting Protection against Methylmercury Toxicity in Cerebellar Granule Cells. *Toxicol. Sci.* **2009**, *112*, 416–426. [CrossRef]

72. Wagner, C.; Sudati, H.; Nogueira, W.; Rocha, J. In vivo and in vitro inhibition of mice thioredoxin reductase by methylmercury. *Biometals* **2010**, *23*, 1171–1177. [CrossRef] [PubMed]

73. Hirayama, N.M.A.Y.K. Comparative study of activities in reactive oxygen species production/defense system in mitochondria of rat brain and liver, and their susceptibility to methylmercury toxicity. *Arch. Toxicol* **2007**, 769–776.

74. Wu, L.L.; Chiou, C.; Chang, P.; Wu, J.T. Urinary 8-OHdG: A marker of oxidative stress to DNA and a risk factor for cancer, atherosclerosis and diabetics. *Clin. Chim. Acta* **2004**, *339*, 1–9. [CrossRef] [PubMed]

75. Kim, J.Y.; Mukherjee, S.; Ngo, L.; Christiani, D.C. Urinary 8-hydroxy-2′-deoxyguanosine as a biomarker of oxidative DNA damage in workers exposed to fine particulates. *Environ. Health Perspect.* **2004**, *112*, 666–671. [CrossRef] [PubMed]

76. Chen, C.; Qu, L.; Li, B.; Xing, L.; Jia, G.; Wang, T.; Gao, Y.; Zhang, P.; Li, M.; Chen, W.; et al. Increased Oxidative DNA Damage, as Assessed by Urinary 8-Hydroxy-2′-Deoxyguanosine Concentrations, and Serum Redox Status in Persons Exposed to Mercury. *Clin. Chem.* **2005**, *767*, 759–767. [CrossRef]

77. Ohno, T.; Sakamoto, M.; Kurosawa, T.; Dakeishi, M. Total mercury levels in hair, toenail, and urine among women free from occupational exposure and their relations to renal tubular function. *Environ. Res.* **2007**, *103*, 191–197. [CrossRef] [PubMed]

78. Selimović-Dragaš, M.; Huseinbegović, A.; Kobašlija, S.; Hatibović-Kofman, Š. A comparison of the in vitro cytotoxicity of conventional and resin modifi ed glass ionomer cements. *Assoc. Basic Med. Sci. FBIH* **2012**, *12*, 273–278. [CrossRef]

79. Van Landuyt, K.L.; Nawrot, T.; Geebelen, B.; De Munck, J.; Snauwaert, J.; Yoshihara, K.; Scheers, H.; Godderis, L.; Hoet, P.; Van Meerbeek, B. How much do resin-based dental materials release? A meta-analytical approach. *Dent. Mater.* **2011**, *27*, 723–747. [CrossRef] [PubMed]

80. Schweikl, H.; Spagnuolo, G.; Schmalz, G. Genetic and cellular toxicology of dental resin monomers. *J. Dent. Res.* **2006**, *85*, 870–877. [CrossRef] [PubMed]

81. Maciejczyk, M.; Heropolitanska-Pliszka, E.; Pietrucha, B.; Sawicka-Powierza, J.; Bernatowska, E.; Wolska-Kusnierz, B.; Pac, M.; Car, H.; Zalewska, A.; Mikoluc, B. Antioxidant defense, redox homeostasis, and oxidative damage in children with ataxia telangiectasia and nijmegen breakage syndrome. *Front. Immunol.* **2019**, *10*, 1–11. [CrossRef]

82. Coelho, A.S.; Laranjo, M.; Gonçalves, A.C.; Paula, A.; Paulo, S.; Abrantes, A.M.; Caramelo, F.; Ferreira, M.M.; Silva, M.J.; Carrilho, E.; et al. Cytotoxic effects of a chlorhexidine mouthwash and of an enzymatic mouthwash on human gingival fibroblasts. *Odontology* **2020**, *108*, 260–270. [CrossRef] [PubMed]

83. Samuelsen, J.T.; Kopperud, H.M.; Holme, J.A.; Dragland, I.S.; Christensen, T.; Dahl, J.E. Role of thiol-complex formation in 2-hydroxyethyl- methacrylate-induced toxicity in vitro. *J. Biomed. Mater. Res.* **2010**, *96*, 395–401. [CrossRef] [PubMed]

84. Nocca, G.; De Palma, F.; Minucci, A.; De Sole, P.; Martorana, G.E.; Callà, C.; Morlacchi, C.; Gozzo, M.L.; Gambarini, G.; Chimenti, C.; et al. Alterations of energy metabolism and glutathione levels of HL-60 cells induced by methacrylates present in composite resins. *J. Dent.* **2007**, *35*, 187–194. [CrossRef] [PubMed]

85. Krifka, S.; Hiller, K.; Spagnuolo, G.; Jewett, A.; Schmalz, G.; Schweikl, H. The influence of glutathione on redox regulation by antioxidant proteins and apoptosis in macrophages exposed to 2-hydroxyethyl methacrylate (HEMA). *Biomaterials* **2012**, *33*, 5177–5186. [CrossRef] [PubMed]

86. Schweikl, H.; Petzel, C.; Bolay, C.; Hiller, K.; Buchalla, W.; Krifka, S. 2-Hydroxyethyl methacrylate-induced apoptosis through the ATM- and p53-dependent intrinsic mitochondrial pathway. *Biomaterials* **2014**, *35*, 2890–2904. [CrossRef] [PubMed]

87. Zalewska, A.; Szarmach, I.; Żendzian-Piotrowska, M.; Maciejczyk, M. The effect of N-acetylcysteine on respiratory enzymes, ADP/ATP ratio, glutathione metabolism, and nitrosative stress in the salivary gland mitochondria of insulin resistant rats. *Nutrients* **2020**, 458. [CrossRef]

88. Mikulás, K.; Hermann, P.; Gera, I.; Komlódi, T. Triethylene glycol dimethacrylate impairs bioenergetic functions and induces oxidative stress in mitochondria via inhibiting respiratory Complex. *Dent. Mater.* **2018**, 1–16. [CrossRef]

89. Gomes, A.P.; Price, N.L.; Ling, A.J.Y.; Moslehi, J.J.; Montgomery, M.K.; Rajman, L.; Teodoro, S.; Wrann, C.D.; Hubbard, B.P.; Mercken, E.M.; et al. Declining NAD+ Induces a Pseudohypoxic State Disrupting Nuclear-Mitochondrial Communication during Aging. *Cell* **2013**, *155*. [CrossRef]

90. Styllou, P.; Styllou, M.; Hickel, R.; Högg, C.; Reichl, F.X.; Scherthan, H. NAC ameliorates dental composite-induced DNA double-strand breaks and chromatin condensation. *Dent. Mater. J.* **2017**, *36*, 638–646. [CrossRef]

91. Ma, Q. Role of Nrf2 in Oxidative Stress and Toxicity. *Annu. Rev. Pharmacol. Toxicol.* **2013**, *53*, 401–426. [CrossRef]

92. Durante, W. Protective Role of Heme Oxygenase-1 against Inflammation in Atherosclerosis. *Front. Biosci* **2018**, *16*, 2372–2388. [CrossRef] [PubMed]

93. Gozzelino, R.; Jeney, V.; Soares, M.P. Mechanisms of Cell Protection by Heme Oxygenase-1. *Annu. Rev. Pharmacol. Toxicol.* **2010**, *50*, 323–354. [CrossRef] [PubMed]

94. Gallorini, M.; Petzel, C.; Bolay, C.; Hiller, K.; Cataldi, A.; Buchalla, W.; Krifka, S.; Schweikl, H. Biomaterials Activation of the Nrf2-regulated antioxidant cell response inhibits HEMA-induced oxidative stress and supports cell viability. *Biomaterials* **2015**, *56*, 114–128. [CrossRef] [PubMed]

95. Lee, D.H.; Lim, B.S.; Lee, Y.K.; Ahn, S.J.; Yang, H.C. Involvement of oxidative stress in mutagenicity and apoptosis caused by dental resin monomers in cell cultures. *Dent. Mater.* **2006**, *22*, 1086–1092. [CrossRef] [PubMed]

96. Krifka, S.; Spagnuolo, G.; Schmalz, G.; Schweikl, H. A review of adaptive mechanisms in cell responses towards oxidative stress caused by dental resin monomers. *Biomaterials* **2013**, *34*, 4555–4563. [CrossRef] [PubMed]

97. Jones, R.M.; Petermann, E. Replication fork dynamics and the DNA damage response. *Biochem. J.* **2012**, *26*, 13–26. [CrossRef]

98. Ansteinsson, V.; Solhaug, A.; Samuelsen, J.T.; Holme, J.A.; Dahl, J.E. DNA-damage, cell-cycle arrest and apoptosis induced in BEAS-2B cells by 2-hydroxyethyl methacrylate (HEMA). *Mutat. Res. Genet. Toxicol. Environ. Mutagen.* **2011**, *723*, 158–164. [CrossRef] [PubMed]

99. Ansteinsson, V. In Vitro Toxicity of Filler Particles and Methacrylates Used in Dental Composite Materials Cytokine Release and Cell Death. Ph.D. Thesis, The University of Bergen, Bergen, Norway, 2013.

100. Popal, M.; Volk, J.; Leyhausen, G.; Geurtsen, W. Cytotoxic and genotoxic potential of the type I photoinitiators BAPO and TPO on human oral keratinocytes and V79 fibroblasts. *Dent. Mater.* **2018**, *34*, 1783–1796. [CrossRef] [PubMed]

101. Yoshino, F.; Yoshida, A.; Okada, E.; Okada, Y.; Maehata, Y.; Miyamoto, C.; Kishimoto, S.; Otsuka, T.; Nishimura, T.; Lee, M.C. Il Dental resin curing blue light induced oxidative stress with reactive oxygen species production. *J. Photochem. Photobiol. B Biol.* **2012**, *114*, 73–78. [CrossRef] [PubMed]

102. Oktay, E.A.; Tort, H.; Yıldız, O.; Ulusoy, K.G.; Topcu, F.T.; Ozer, C. Dental resin curing blue light induces vasoconstriction through release of hydrogen peroxide. *J. Photochem. Photobiol. B Biol.* **2018**, *185*, 41–45. [CrossRef]

103. Botton, G.; Pires, C.W.; Cadoná, F.C.; Machado, A.K.; Azzolin, V.F.; Cruz, I.B.M.; Sagrillo, M.R.; Praetzel, J.R. Toxicity of irrigating solutions and pharmacological associations used in pulpectomy of primary teeth. *Int. Endod. J.* **2016**, *49*, 746–754. [CrossRef] [PubMed]

104. Saghiri, M.A.; Delvarani, A.; Mehrvarzfar, P.; Nikoo, M.; Lotfi, M.; Karamifar, K.; Asgar, K.; Dadvand, S. The impact of pH on cytotoxic effects of three root canal irrigants. *Saudi Dent. J.* **2011**, *23*, 149–152. [CrossRef] [PubMed]

105. Soares, J.; Marins, R.; Sassone, L.M.; Fidel, S.R.; Ribeiro, D.A. In Vitro Genotoxicity and Cytotoxicity in Murine Fibroblasts Exposed to EDTA, NaOCl, MTAD and Citric Acid. *Braz. Dent. J.* **2012**, *23*, 527–533.

106. Singh, H.; Khurana, H.; Singh, H.; Singh, M. Photodynamic therapy: Truly a marriage between a drug and a light. *Muller J. Med. Sci. Res.* **2014**, *5*, 48–55. [CrossRef]

107. Pires, C.W.; Botton, G.; Cadoná, F.C.; Machado, A.K.; Azzolin, V.F.; da Cruz, I.B.M.; Sagrillo, M.R.; Praetzel, J.R. Induction of cytotoxicity, oxidative stress and genotoxicity by root filling pastes used in primary teeth. *Int. Endod. J.* **2016**, *49*, 737–745. [CrossRef] [PubMed]

108. Barbin, L.E.; Estrela, C.; Guedes, D.F.C.; Spanó, J.C.E.; Sousa-Neto, M.D.; Pécora, J.D. Detection of para-chloroaniline, reactive oxygen species, and 1-chloro-4-nitrobenzene in high concentrations of chlorhexidine and in a mixture of chlorhexidine and calcium hydroxide. *J. Endod.* **2013**, *5*, 664–668. [CrossRef]

109. Victoria-Escandell, A.; Ibañez-Cabellos, J.S.; De Cutanda, S.B.; Berenguer-Pascual, E.; Beltrán-García, J.; García-López, E.; Pallardó, F.V.; García-Giménez, J.L.; Pallarés-Sabater, A.; Zarzosa-López, I.; et al. Cellular Responses in Human Dental Pulp Stem Cells Treated with Three Endodontic Materials. *Stem. Cells Int.* **2017**, *2017*. [CrossRef] [PubMed]

110. Kim, T.G.; Lee, Y.H.; Lee, N.H.; Bhattarai, G.; Lee, I.K.; Yun, B.S.; Yi, H.K. The Antioxidant Property of Pachymic Acid Improves Bone Disturbance against AH Plus–induced Inflammation in MC-3T3 E1 Cells. *J. Endod.* **2013**, *39*, 461–466. [CrossRef]

111. Chang, S.-W.; Lee, S.-Y.; Ann, H.-J.; Kum, K.-Y.; Kim, E.-C. Effects of Calcium Silicate Endodontic Cements on Biocompatibility and Mineralization-inducing Potentials in Human Dental Pulp Cells. *J. Endod.* **2014**, *40*, 1194–1200. [CrossRef]

112. Loison-robert, L.S.; Tassin, M.; Bonte, E. In vitro effects of two silicate-based materials, Biodentine and BioRoot RCS, on dental pulp stem cells in models of reactionary and reparative dentinogenesis. *PLoS ONE* **2018**, *13*, 1–19. [CrossRef]

113. Trombetta, D.; Mondello, M.R.; Cimino, F.; Cristani, M.; Pergolizzi, S.; Saija, A. Toxic effect of nickel in an in vitro model of human oral epithelium. *Toxicol. Lett.* **2005**, *159*, 219–225. [CrossRef] [PubMed]

114. Gholinejad, Z.; Ansari, M.H.K.; Rasmi, Y. Titanium dioxide nanoparticles induce endothelial cell apoptosis via cell membrane oxidative damage and p38, PI3K/Akt, NF-κB signaling pathways modulation. *J. Trace Elem. Med. Biol.* **2019**, *54*, 27–35. [CrossRef] [PubMed]

115. Pereira, L.C.; Pazin, M.; Franco-Bernardes, M.F.; Martins, C.; Barcelos, R.M.; Pereira, C.M.; Rodrigues, J.L.; Barbosa, F., Jr.; Dorta, D.J. A Perspective of Mitochondrial Dysfunction in Rats Treated with Silver and Titanium Nanoparticles (AgNPs and TiNPs). *J. Trace Elem. Med. Biol.* **2018**. [CrossRef] [PubMed]

116. Wang, G.; Xu, Y.; Zhang, L.; Ye, D.; Feng, X.; Fu, T. Enhancement of Apoptosis by Titanium Alloy Internal Fixations during Microwave Treatments for Fractures: An Animal Study. *PLoS ONE* **2015**. [CrossRef] [PubMed]

117. Shanbhag, A.S.; Macaulay, W.; Stefanovic-racic, M.; Rubash, H.E. Nitric oxide release by macrophages in response to particulate wear debris. *J. Biomed. Maters Res.* **1998**, *3*, 497–503. [CrossRef]

118. Mouthuy, P.; Snelling, S.J.B.; Dakin, S.G.; Milković, L.; Gašparović, Č.; Carr, A.J.; Žarković, N. Biocompatibility of implantable materials: An oxidative stress viewpoint. *Biomaterials* **2016**. [CrossRef]

119. Cabaña-Muñoz, M.E.; Parmigiani-Izquierdo, J.M.; Alonso, F.C.; Merino, J. Increased Systemic Malondialdehyde Levels and Decreased Mo/Co, Mo/Hg^{2+}, Co/Fe^{2+} Ratios in Patients with Long-Term Dental Titanium Implants and Amalgams. *J. Clin. Med.* **2019**, *8*, 86. [CrossRef]

120. Sánchez-Siles, M.; Lucas-Azorin, J.; Salazar-Sánchez, N.; Carbonell-Meseguer, L.; Camacho-Alonso, F. Salivary Concentration of Oxidative Stress Biomarkers in a Group of Patients with Peri-Implantitis: A Transversal Study. *Clin. Implant. Dent.* **2015**, *18*, 1015–1022. [CrossRef] [PubMed]

121. Toczewska, J.; Maciejczyk, M.; Konopka, T.; Zalewska, A. Total Oxidant and Antioxidant Capacity of Gingival Crevicular Fluid and Saliva in Patients with Periodontitis: Review and Clinical Study. *Antioxidants* **2020**, *9*, 450. [CrossRef] [PubMed]

122. Toczewska, J.; Konopka, T.; Zalewska, A. Nitrosative Stress Biomarkers in the Non-Stimulated and Stimulated Saliva, as well as Gingival Crevicular Fluid of Patients with Periodontitis: Review and Clinical Study. *Antioxidants* **2020**, *9*, 259. [CrossRef]

123. Yeung, S.Y.; Huang, C.S.; Chan, C.P.; Lin, C.P.; Lin, H.N.; Lee, P.H.; Jia, H.W.; Huang, S.K.; Jeng, J.H.; Chang, M.C. Antioxidant and pro-oxidant properties of chlorhexidine and its interaction with calcium hydroxide solutions. *Int. Endod. J.* **2007**, *40*, 837–844. [CrossRef] [PubMed]

124. Yoshida, A.; Iwata, S.; Iizuka, J.; Takahashi, S.; Wada-takahashi, S.; Miyamoto, C.; Maehata, Y.; Ogura, Y.; Lee, M.; Yo, F. Blue Light from Dental Resin Curing Unit Causes Light-Induced Vasocon- striction in Isolated Rat Aorta. *OHDM* **2014**, *13*, 1147–1151.

125. Jha, N.; Ryu, J.J.; Choi, E.H.; Kaushik, N.K. Generation and Role of Reactive Oxygen and Nitrogen Species Induced by Plasma, Lasers, Chemical Agents, and Other Systems in Dentistry. *Oxid. Med. Cell. Longev.* **2017**, *2017*. [CrossRef] [PubMed]

126. Wu, T.T.; Li, L.F.; Du, R.; Jiang, L.; Zhu, Y.Q. Hydrogen peroxide induces apoptosis in human dental pulp cells via caspase-9 dependent pathway. *J. Endod.* **2013**, *39*, 1151–1155. [CrossRef]

127. Marto, C.M.; Laranjo, M.; Paula, A.; Coelho, A.S.; Abrantes, A.M.; Casalta-Lopes, J.; Gonçalves, A.C.; Sarmento-Ribeiro, A.B.; Ferreira, M.M.; Cabrita, A.; et al. Cytotoxic effects of zoom® whitening product in human fibroblasts. *Materials* **2020**, *13*, 1491. [CrossRef]

128. Zalewska, A.; Ziembicka, D.; Zendzian-Piotrowska, M.; MacIejczyk, M. The impact of high-fat diet on mitochondrial function, free radical production, and nitrosative stress in the salivary glands of wistar rats. *Oxid. Med. Cell. Longev.* **2019**. [CrossRef]

129. Matczuk, J.; Zendzian-Piotrowska, M.; Maciejczyk, M.; Kurek, K. Salivary lipids: A review. *Adv. Clin. Exp. Med.* **2017**. [CrossRef]

130. Lima, A.F.; Lessa, F.C.; Hebling, J.; de Souza Costa, C.A.; Marchie, G.M. Protective Effect of Sodium Ascorbate on MDPC-23 Odontoblast-Like Cells Exposed to a Bleaching Agent. *Eur. J. Dent.* **2010**, *4*, 238–244.

131. Vargas, S.; Soares, D.G.; Paula, A.; Ribeiro, D.; Hebling, J.; Alberto, C.; Costa, D.S. Protective Effect of Alpha-Tocopherol Isomer from Vitamin E against the H_2O_2 Induced Toxicity on Dental Pulp Cells. *Biomed. Res. Int.* **2014**, *2014*, 1–5. [CrossRef]

4

IL-1β Damages Fibrocartilage and Upregulates MMP-13 Expression in Fibrochondrocytes in the Condyle of the Temporomandibular Joint

Hessam Tabeian [1,†], Beatriz F. Betti [1,2,3,†], Cinthya dos Santos Cirqueira [4], Teun J. de Vries [5], Frank Lobbezoo [2], Anouk V. ter Linde [1], Behrouz Zandieh-Doulabi [1], Marije I. Koenders [6], Vincent Everts [1] and Astrid D. Bakker [1,*]

[1] Oral Cell Biology, Academic Centre for Dentistry Amsterdam, University of Amsterdam and Vrije Universiteit Amsterdam, 1081 LA Amsterdam, The Netherlands; h.tabeian@acta.nl (H.T.); b.f.betti@acta.nl (B.F.B.); anouk.terlinde@student.auc.nl (A.V.t.L.); b.zandiehdoulabi@acta.nl (B.Z.-D.); v.everts@acta.nl (V.E.)

[2] Oral Kinesiology, Academic Centre for Dentistry Amsterdam, University of Amsterdam and Vrije Universiteit Amsterdam, 1081 LA Amsterdam, The Netherlands; f.lobbezoo@acta.nl

[3] Orthodontics, Academic Centre for Dentistry Amsterdam, University of Amsterdam and Vrije Universiteit Amsterdam, 1081 LA Amsterdam, The Netherlands

[4] Núcleo de Anatomia Patológica, Instituto Adolfo Lutz, São Paulo 01246-000, Brazil; cinthyaquiron@gmail.com

[5] Periodontology, Academic Centre for Dentistry Amsterdam, University of Amsterdam and Vrije Universiteit Amsterdam, 1081 LA Amsterdam, The Netherlands; teun.devries@acta.nl

[6] Rheumatology, Radboud University Medical Center, 6525 GA Nijmegen, The Netherlands; marije.koenders@radboudumc.nl

* Correspondence: a.bakker@acta.nl

† These authors contributed equally to this work.

Abstract: The temporomandibular joint (TMJ), which differs anatomically and biochemically from hyaline cartilage-covered joints, is an under-recognized joint in arthritic disease, even though TMJ damage can have deleterious effects on physical appearance, pain and function. Here, we analyzed the effect of IL-1β, a cytokine highly expressed in arthritic joints, on TMJ fibrocartilage-derived cells, and we investigated the modulatory effect of mechanical loading on IL-1β-induced expression of catabolic enzymes. TMJ cartilage degradation was analyzed in 8–11-week-old mice deficient for IL-1 receptor antagonist (IL-1RA$^{-/-}$) and wild-type controls. Cells were isolated from the juvenile porcine condyle, fossa, and disc, grown in agarose gels, and subjected to IL-1β (0.1–10 ng/mL) for 6 or 24 h. Expression of catabolic enzymes (ADAMTS and MMPs) was quantified by RT-qPCR and immunohistochemistry. Porcine condylar cells were stimulated with IL-1β for 12 h with IL-1β, followed by 8 h of 6% dynamic mechanical (tensile) strain, and gene expression of MMPs was quantified. Early signs of condylar cartilage damage were apparent in IL-1RA$^{-/-}$ mice. In porcine cells, IL-1β strongly increased expression of the aggrecanases ADAMTS4 and ADAMTS5 by fibrochondrocytes from the fossa (13-fold and 7-fold) and enhanced the number of MMP-13 protein-expressing condylar cells (8-fold). Mechanical loading significantly lowered (3-fold) IL-1β-induced MMP-13 gene expression by condylar fibrochondrocytes. IL-1β induces TMJ condylar cartilage damage, possibly by enhancing MMP-13 production. Mechanical loading reduces IL-1β-induced MMP-13 gene expression, suggesting that mechanical stimuli may prevent cartilage damage of the TMJ in arthritic patients.

Keywords: ADAMTS4; ADAMTS5; fossa; cartilage degradation; arthritis; mechanical loading; MMP-13; IL1β; temporomandibular joint; juvenile idiopathic arthritis

1. Introduction

The temporomandibular joint (TMJ) is a unique joint, consisting of a fossa, disc, and condyle that is essential for mastication, speech, and deglutition [1]. The major difference between the TMJ and other synovial joints is that the TMJ contains fibrocartilage rather than hyaline cartilage, i.e., it contains collagen type I in addition to collagen type II and proteoglycans [2]. More precisely, the matrix of all three anatomical structures of the TMJ contained collagen type I. The condyle and the fossa stained positive for collagen type II and proteoglycans, but the condyle contained considerably more collagen type II and proteoglycans than the fossa. The disc did not contain collagen type II, and the disc did not stain positive for proteoglycans [2]. The TMJ is an under-recognized joint in arthritic disease, while it is one of the most commonly affected joints in patients with juvenile idiopathic arthritis (JIA) [3]. It has been suggested that at the time of diagnosis, approximately 75% of JIA patients have problems with the TMJ [3]. JIA, the most prevalent type of arthritis of unknown cause in young children, is initiated before the age of 16 years old and is characterized by chronic inflammation of the joints, which can result in joint degradation. Affected children suffer from jaw pain but also jaw dysfunction, which can manifest in malocclusion [4] and a reduced maximum mouth opening [5]. How the cartilage of the TMJ is affected by inflammation in JIA and in other arthritic diseases with involvement of the TMJ remains elusive.

One of the most potent inflammatory factors involved in hyaline cartilage degradation in many forms of arthritis is interleukin (IL)-1β [6]. This cytokine is responsible for hyaline cartilage matrix degradation by inducing expression of matrix metalloproteinases (MMPs) and disintegrin and metalloproteinase with thrombospondin motifs (ADAMTS) by chondrocytes [7,8]. The importance of IL-1β in the pathogenesis of systemic arthritic diseases is demonstrated by the success of treatment with IL-1 receptor antagonist (IL-1RA) [9]. However, it is unknown whether IL-1β also affects the integrity of the cartilaginous structures of the TMJ.

Since the TMJ is a secondary growth center, damage induced by catabolic factors during JIA can introduce growth abnormalities, resulting in asymmetric growth of the mandible [10] undersized jaw, and abnormal positioning of the maxilla [11]. Therefore, strategies to prevent TMJ joint damage, particularly in JIA patients, are highly desirable. Preferably, a non-invasive treatment should be deployed that inhibits the catabolic effect of inflammatory factors on TMJ cartilage. Mechanical loading of inflamed joints can be a promising approach towards achieving this. Moderate exercise has been shown to have a systematic anti-inflammatory effect by reducing the disease activity in rheumatoid arthritis (RA) patients [12]. Furthermore, mechanical loading reduced the expression of MMP-13 in synovial cells from RA patients [13]. However, it is not known whether mechanical loading will also reduce IL-1β-induced expression of catabolic factors in cells derived from the TMJ condyle, which is especially susceptible to damage in JIA [14].

We hypothesize that IL-1β plays an important role in inducing degradation of the TMJ cartilage, that it enhances expression of catabolic factors such as MMPs and ADAMTSs, and that mechanical stimuli can revert IL-1β-induced expression of catabolic factors. We have used different model systems to investigate this hypothesis. First of all, an IL1RA knock-out mouse model was used to investigate whether overactive IL-1β signaling induces histological signs of damage in the fibrocartilage tissue of the temporomandibular joint. The second and third part of the hypothesis was challenged using pig TMJ-derived cells. Pigs were chosen to isolate cells because they will yield more cells than mice and because the TMJ of this species is comparable with that of humans in cellular composition [15–19].

2. Results

2.1. IL-1βRA$^{-/-}$ Mice Showed Early Signs of Condylar Cartilage Damage

To investigate the role of IL-1β in TMJ damage, we assessed whether young mice that lack IL1-RA develop arthritis in the TMJ. Discs were barely visible in sections of mouse TMJ. Because of the similar histological appearance of fossa and disc tissue in both wild-type (WT) and IL-1RA$^{-/-}$ mice, only the condyles were quantified. Safranin O staining was more intense in IL-1RA$^{-/-}$ condyles compared to WT condyles (Figure 1A,B). In addition, the most superficial layer of the cartilage in IL-1RA$^{-/-}$ condyles was positive for Safranin O staining (Figure 1B), which was not the case in WT mice (Figure 1A). The IL-1RA$^{-/-}$ TMJ samples had a significantly higher Mankin score compared to the joints of the WT mice ($p < 0.01$) (Figure 1C). The IL-1RA$^{-/-}$ condyles contained 11-fold more empty lacunae than the WT mice ($p < 0.001$) (Figure 1D).

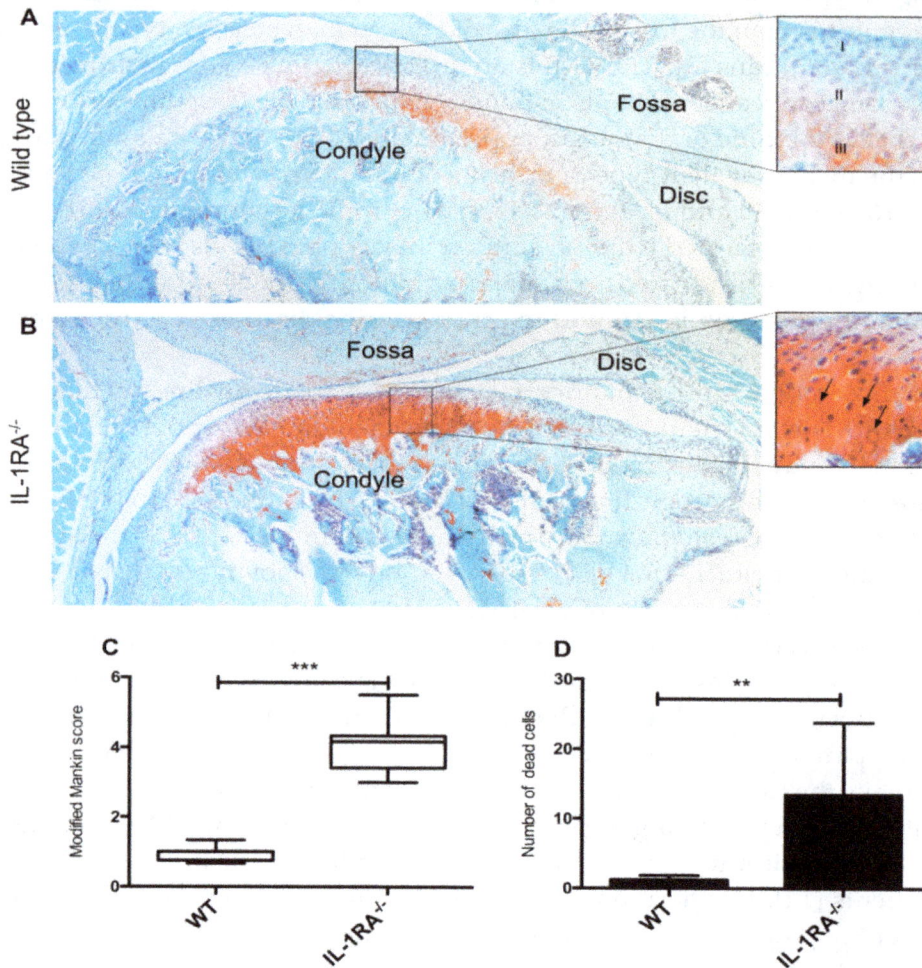

Figure 1. Histologic assessment of the temporomandibular joint (TMJ) of IL-1 receptor antagonist (IL-1RA$^{-/-}$) and wild-type (WT) mice. Sagittal section of the condyles of IL-1RA$^{-/-}$ and WT mice stained with Safranin O. (**A**) WT TMJ, original magnification 10×. The condyle cartilage can be divided into the fibrous, proliferative, and hypertrophic zones, indicated in the figure as I, II, III, respectively. In the WT sample the modest red staining is limited to zone III. (**B**) The IL-1R$^{-/-}$ mice condyle showed a higher level of Safranin O staining in comparison to WT. In the IL-1R$^{-/-}$ mice, Safranin O staining was not limited to the hypertrophic and the proliferative zone of the condyle but extended to the fibrous layer. Empty lacunae were frequently seen (arrows). (**C**) The Mankin score of the IL-1RA$^{-/-}$ mice was higher than the WT. (**D**) The number of empty lacunae in the condyles of the IL-1RA$^{-/-}$ mice was higher than in the WT. ** Significant difference between IL-1RA$^{-/-}$ and WT mice, $p < 0.01$; *** significant difference between IL-1R$^{-/-}$ and WT mice, $p < 0.001$, a t-test is used.

2.2. Cells from the Fossa, Disc, and Condyle Expressed IL-1 Receptors

The ability of the cells isolated from porcine fossa, disc, and condyle cartilaginous structures to react to IL-1β was assessed by measuring gene expression of receptors for IL-1β. All cells from the three types of TMJ cartilage displayed similar gene expression levels for IL-1RI as well as of the mock receptor of IL-1β, IL-1RII (Figure 2A,B). The ratio of IL-1RI to IL-1RII gives a rough indication of the effectiveness of IL-1β to elicit downstream signaling. The three cartilaginous structures displayed similar IL-1RI/IL-1RII ratios (Figure 2C). Expression of IL-1RA and IL-1β was in most cases undetectable, and therefore no statistical analysis could be performed.

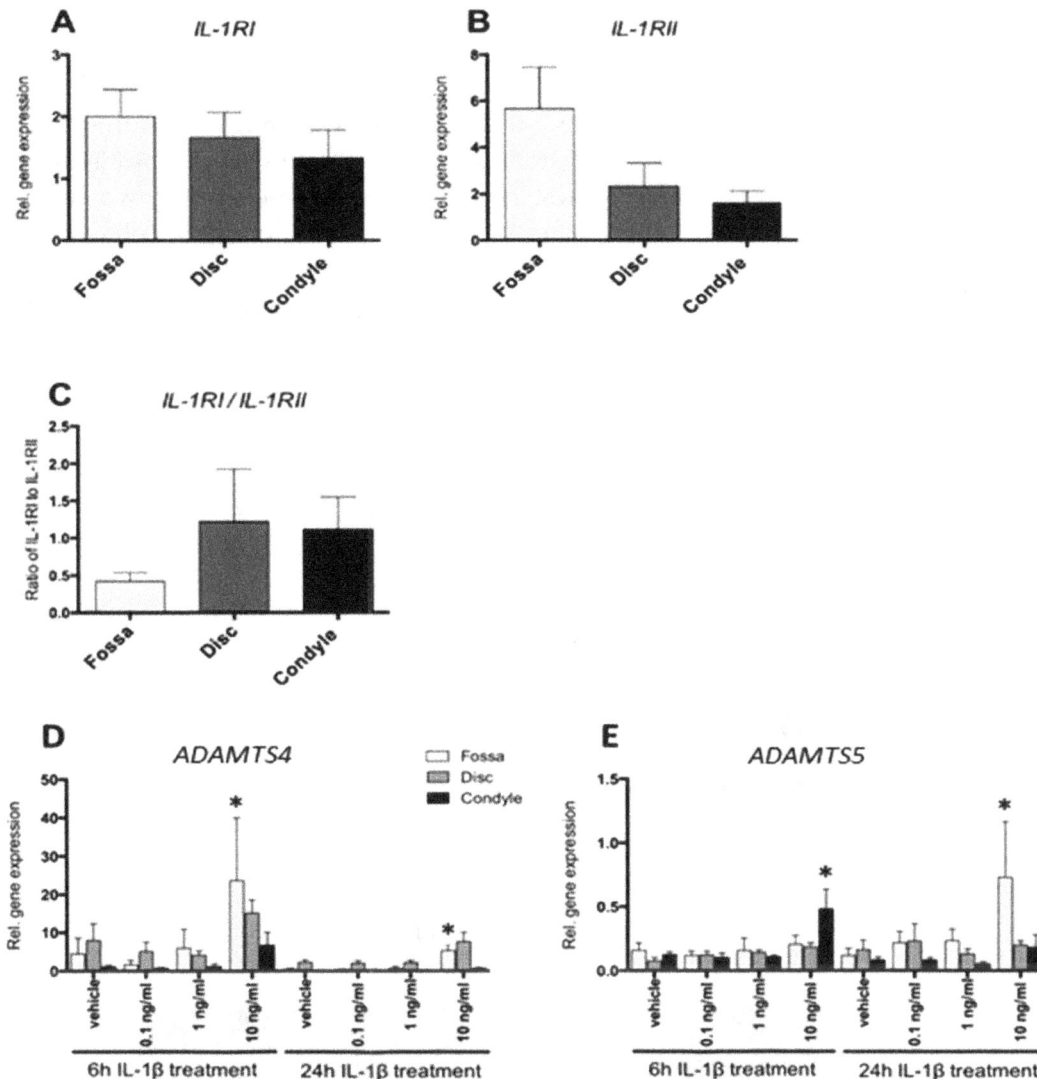

Figure 2. Relative gene expression of IL-1 receptor (IL-1R)I, IL-1RII, disintegrin and metalloproteinase with thrombospondin motifs (ADAMTS)4 and ADAMTS5 by porcine fossa, condyle and disc cells. (**A**) IL-1RI and (**B**) IL-1RII expression of the cells from fossa, disc, and condyle. All cells expressed IL-1RI and RII gene at similar levels. (**C**) The ratio between *IL-1RI* and *IL-1RII*. The ratio IL-1RI/IL-1RII was comparable for all cells. (**D**) *ADAMTS4* expression in the cells from the fossa, disc, and condyle. IL-1β incubation for 6 h enhanced ADAMTS4 expression in condyle cells. After 24 h of incubation with 10 ng/mL IL-1β, both fossa and discs showed an increase in ADAMTS4 expression in comparison to the vehicle-treated cells. (**E**) *ADAMTS5* expression in the cells from the fossa, disc, and condyle. Six hours of 10 ng/ml IL-1β treatment enhanced ADAMTS5 gene expression in condyle cells. After 24 h of 10 ng/mL IL-1β, the fossa cells showed an increased *ADAMTS5* expression. * Significant effect of treatment with IL-1β relative to vehicle, $p < 0.05$.

2.3. IL-1β Increased ADAMTS4 and ADAMTS5 Gene Expression

IL-1β at 10 ng/mL enhanced ADAMTS4 gene expression by 5-fold after 6 h in cells from the fossa ($p < 0.01$) (Figure 2D). After 24 h incubation, fossa cells showed a 13-fold increased expression of ADAMTS4 in response to 10 ng/mL IL1β ($p < 0.01$) (Figure 2D).

Six hours of IL-1β stimulation (10 ng/mL) also enhanced ADAMTS5 by 4-fold, but only in condylar cells ($p < 0.01$) (Figure 2E). After 24 h incubation with 10 ng/mL IL-1β, only fossa cells demonstrated enhanced ADAMTS5 gene expression (7-fold) in comparison to vehicle-treated cells ($p < 0.017$) (Figure 2E).

2.4. MMP-2 Activity Was Higher in Condyle Than Disc and Fossa Cells; MMP9 mRNA Upregulated in Condyle by IL-1β

Six hours of IL-1β treatment did not affect MMP-9 gene expression in any of the TMJ-derived cell types (Figure 3B). After 24 h of stimulation with 10 ng/mL IL-1β, there was a 3-fold increase of MMP-9 gene expression by condyle cells ($p < 0.01$, Figure 3B). MMP-9 enzyme activity was undetectable by zymographic analysis of the conditioned medium of fossa, disc, and condyle cells, regardless of the IL-1β treatment (Figure 3C), suggesting that the mRNA for MMP-9 was not sufficiently converted into active protein. Though not statistically significant at the mRNA level (Figure 3A), MMP-2 enzyme activity appeared higher in condyle cells than in the disc and fossa (Figure 3C). IL-1β did not visibly affect the level of MMP-2 activity in any of the cells (Figure 3C).

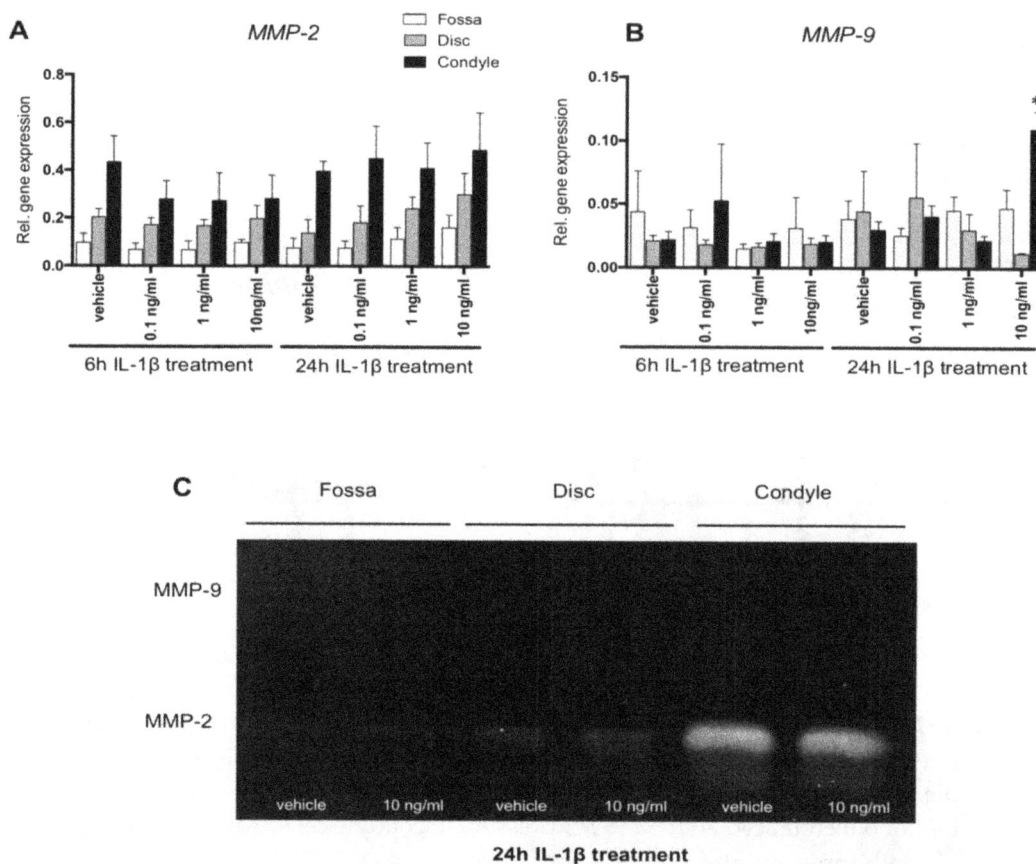

Figure 3. Matrix metalloproteinase (MMP)-2 and MMP-9 gene expression and activity. (**A**) IL-1β did not affect *MMP-2* expression by the cells from the fossa, disc, and condyle at any time point tested. (**B**) After 24 h of 10 ng/mL IL-1β incubation, the *MMP-9* gene expression of the disc and condyle cells were higher than that of the vehicle-treated samples. (**C**) Zymogram of the conditioned medium from fossa, disc, and condyle cells after 24 h of incubation with IL-1β. There was no MMP-9 activity detected. The condyle showed strong MMP-2 activity, but no effect of IL-1β was apparent. * Significant effect of treatment with IL-1β, relative to vehicle, $p < 0.05$. Results are shown from one out of three identical experimental replicates.

2.5. IL-1β Induced MMP-13 Expression by Condylar Cells Only

After 6 and 24 h of 10 ng/mL IL-1β stimulation, MMP-13 gene expression by cells of the condyle was up-regulated by 3.4- and 9-fold, respectively ($p < 0.001$ and $p < 0.0001$, respectively) (Figure 4A). MMP-13 gene expression was almost undetectable in the cells from the disc and fossa and remained low after IL-1β incubation (Figure 4A).

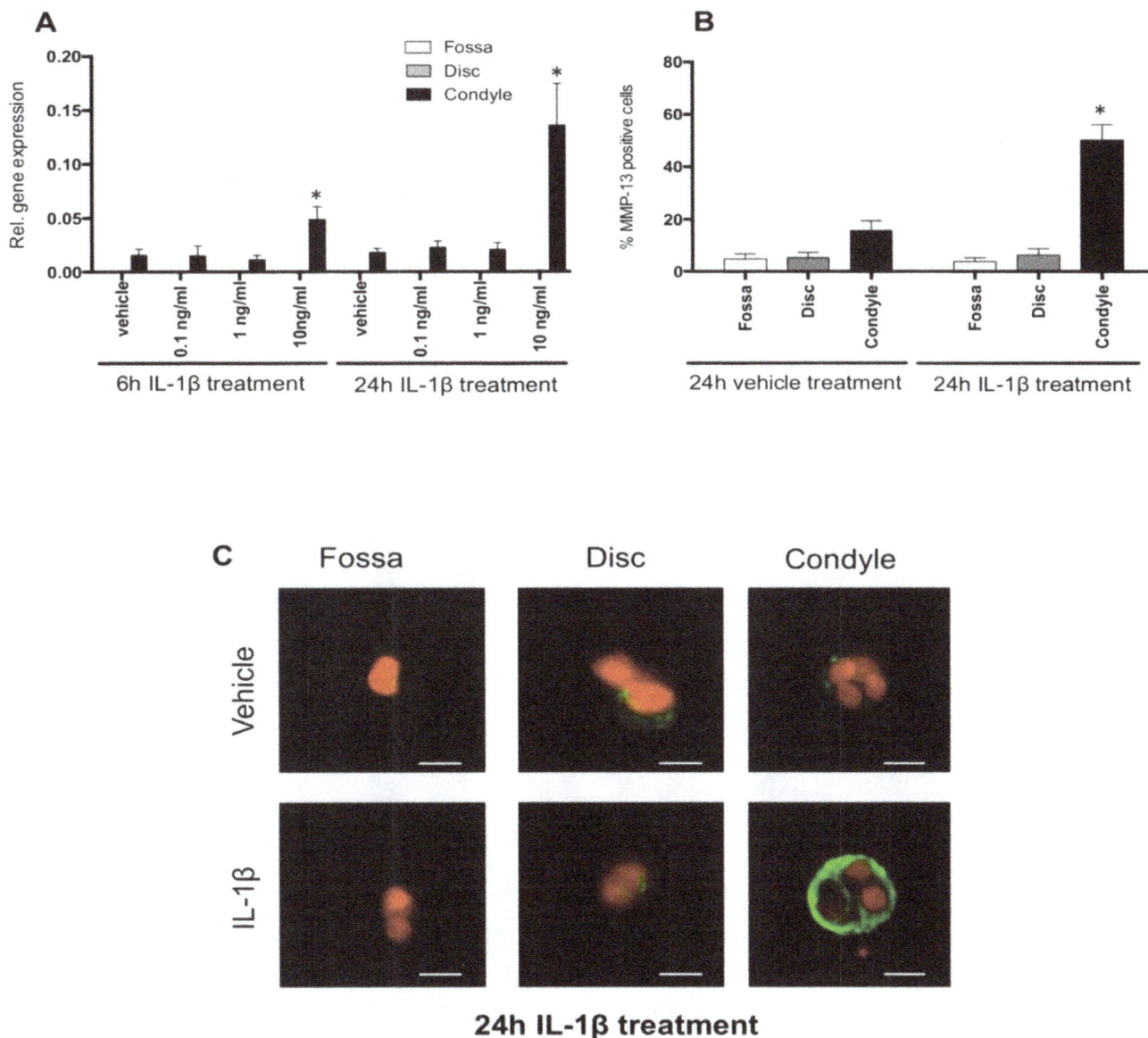

Figure 4. MMP-13 gene and protein expression. (**A**) MMP-13 gene expression by the cells from the fossa, disc, and condyle. IL-1β for 6 h and 24 h at 10 ng/mL increased MMP-13 expression in condyle cells in comparison to vehicle. (**B**) Number of MMP-13-positive cells. Condylar cells incubated with 10 ng/mL IL-1β for 24 h showed the highest number of MMP-13-positive cells. (**C**) Image of MMP-13-positive cells after 24 h of 10 ng/mL IL-1β treatment. The green label indicates the presence of MMP-13, and the nuclei are red. * Significant effect of treatment with IL-1β relative to vehicle treatment, $p < 0.05$. Scale bar represents 5 μm.

Next, we analyzed the number of cells expressing MMP-13 by immunostaining. Twenty-four hours of 10 ng/mL IL-1β incubation increased the percentage of MMP-13-positive condylar cells (3.5-fold increase, $p < 0.001$) (Figure 4B). The number of MMP-13-positive cells derived from the condyle compared to the fossa and disc was remarkably higher (Figure 4C).

2.6. Cyclic Tensile Strain Reduced IL-1β-Induced MMP-13 Expression

Six percent cyclic tensile strain (CTS) reduced IL-1β-induced MMP-13 gene expression by 3-fold ($p < 0.05$) (Figure 5B). CTS neither affected expression of MMP-2, IL-12RI, IL-1RII nor the ratio of IL-1RI and IL-1RII in control condylar cells or in those incubated with IL-1β (Figure 5A,C,D).

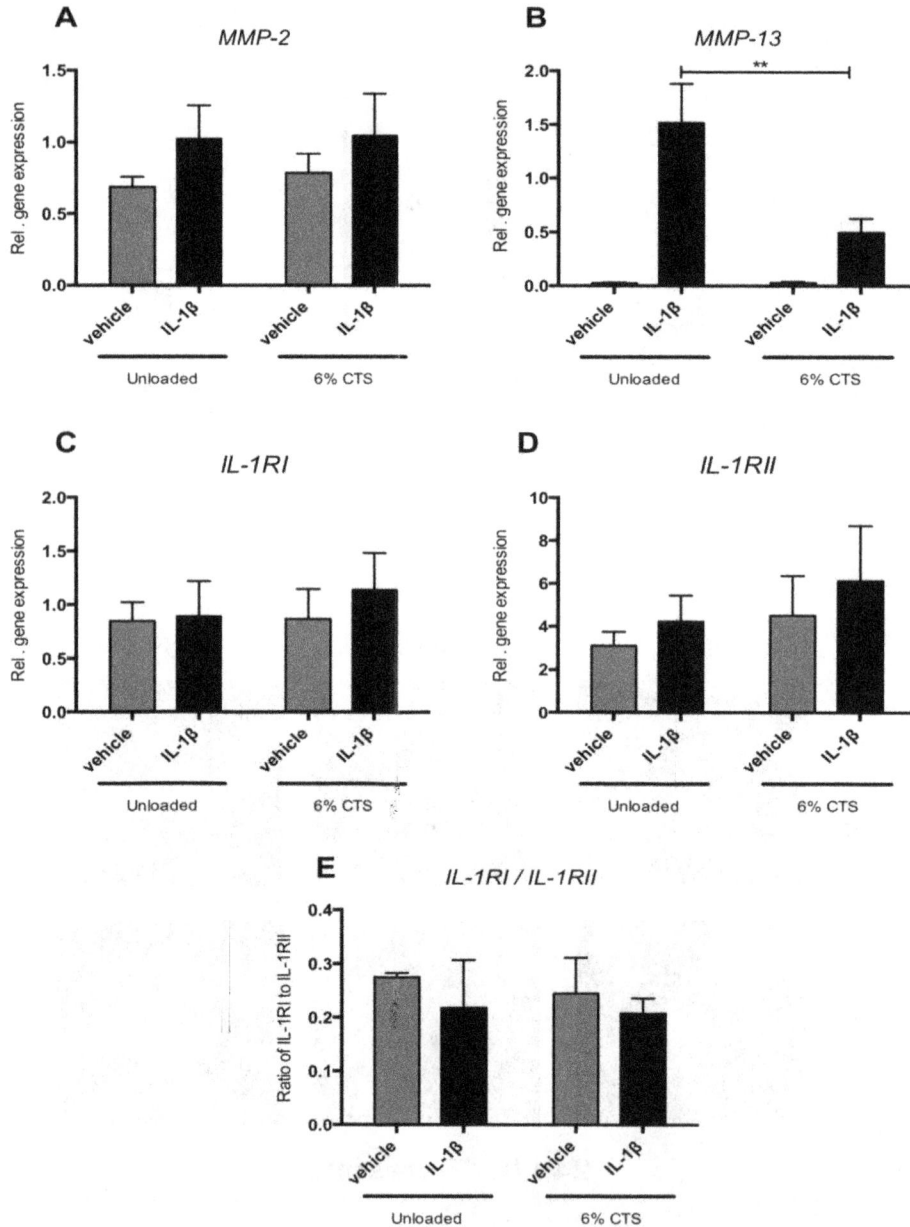

Figure 5. Mechanical strain reduces MMP-13 expression of condylar cells incubated with IL1-β. Gene expression of (**A**) MMP-13, (**B**) MMP-2, (**C**) IL1-RI, and (**D**) IL1-RII. (**E**) Ratio between IL-1RI and IL-1RII by condylar cells. Mechanical loading reduced IL-1β-induced gene expression of MMP-13. ** Significant effect of mechanical loading, $p < 0.01$.

3. Discussion

The TMJ is frequently affected in patients with chronic inflammation, which can result in permanent damage to the joint, especially in young patients. Since biological sampling of the TMJ of children for research purposes is unethical, the role of specific inflammatory factors in the degradation of the TMJ of young individuals remains elusive. In the present study, we made use of relatively young mice and juvenile porcine TMJs to investigate the effect of the inflammatory cytokine IL-1β on its three cartilaginous structures. Our findings strongly suggest that excess IL-1β induces degradation of TMJ cartilage. Young mice deficient for IL-1RA showed early histological signs of TMJ degradation, an effect preferentially found in the condyle. In culture, porcine cells isolated from the three cartilaginous structures expressed different catabolic enzymes in response to IL-1β, e.g., IL-1β at 10 ng/mL induced the expression of ADAMTS4 and ADAMTS5 by cells from the fossa, while cells isolated from the condyle responded to IL-1β with an increased expression of MMP-9, and MMP-13. Mechanical loading reduced MMP-13 expression in IL-1β-treated condylar fibrochondrocytes.

Horai et al. previously demonstrated that IL-RA$^{-/-}$ mice developed spontaneous arthritis due to unopposed excess of IL-1 signaling. In this systemic arthritis model, between 5–20% of the front paws developed arthritis, which depended on, for instance, the microbiological status of the animal facility [20]. We used these mice to investigate whether an excess of IL-1 signaling could result in TMJ damage. We did indeed find some remarkable changes in the condyle. A high level of staining for proteoglycans was seen around the condyles and also in the fibrous areas of the condyle. This area normally does not contain proteoglycans. Condyles of the IL-RA$^{-/-}$ mice showed, overall, more clustering of cells, more intense proteoglycan staining, and higher Mankin score in comparison to WT mice. Over-production of proteoglycans and cluster formation of chondrocytes may represent signs of local repair of articular cartilage, an indication of the onset of the cartilage degradation process. Proteoglycans are unlike collagen in a continuous turnover [20], therefore overshoot in matrix synthesis might occur more easily with proteoglycans. Other studies have also found an increased level of proteoglycans in the early phases of condyle cartilage degradation [21–23]. In these studies, at later stages, a gradual loss of proteoglycans occurred together with cleaving of collagen fibrils. This pattern of degeneration implies that there may be a common chain of molecular events underlying degeneration [21]. Further studies in older IL-1RA$^{-/-}$ mice should indicate whether these mice will undergo loss of proteoglycans together with cleaving of the collagen fibrils in their TMJ by, for instance, MMP-13, which was upregulated in the porcine model. Taken together, our results with IL-1RA$^{-/-}$ mice suggest that overactive IL-1β signaling induces damage in the fibrocartilage tissue of the condyle of the TMJ.

We assumed initially that the fossa and disc cells would not express the genes of the receptors related to IL-1β signaling, since these cartilage parts seemed to be unaffected in the inflamed joint of JIA patients [14]. However, we found that the cells from the fossa and disc expressed mRNA for these receptors, and cells from the fossa responded to IL-1β with an enhanced expression of ADAMTS4 and ADAMTS5. This shows that the receptors are present and functional in the fossa and disc, even though these structures are damaged to a lesser extent than the condyle in JIA patients. Increased ADAMTS5 expression in response to IL-1β in combination with lack of tissue damage was also observed in articular cartilage from knees of Sox9 knockout animals [24]. In addition, very limited numbers of proteoglycans are present in the fossa and disc. Therefore, with ADAMTS4 and ADAMTS5 being the catalytic enzymes that degrade proteoglycans, damage by these aggrecanases would be limited in comparison to the condyle.

Condylar cells responded to IL-1β by increasing the expression of the catabolic enzymes ADAMTS5, MMP-9 and MMP-13. These cells also expressed constitutively active MMP-2. These enzymes are able to cleave the matrix proteins of the condylar cartilage. The aggrecanases ADSMTS5, MMP-13 and MMP-2 are capable of cleaving proteoglycans [25,26], and both MMP-13 and MMP-2 are able to unwind and cleave collagen fibrils [27]. The resulting fragments will form an excellent substrate for the gelatinase MMP-2. This enzyme is also able to cleave the pro-MMP-13, thereby activating this collagenase [28]. We found that IL-1β enhanced MMP-13 expression in cells isolated from the porcine condyle. The isolated cells constitute a mix of more fibroblast-like cells from the upper layer of the condyle and chondrocyte-like cells from the deeper layers. It is possible that only one of these subtypes of cells responds to IL-1β with increased MMP-13 expression. We found in a limited set of histological slides that MMP-13 protein was mostly expressed by chondrocyte-like cells of the deeper layers of mouse condyles (data not shown). It is thus possible that the response to IL-1β was most pronounced in the chondrocyte-like cells within our mix of isolated condyle cells. The importance of MMP-13 in cartilage degradation in arthritis was demonstrated in transgenic mice overexpressing MMP-13 [29] and elevated levels of MMP-13 were found in synovial fluid of arthritic patients [30]. Therefore, MMP-13 can be considered as one of the prime suspects in the degradation of condylar cartilage in JIA. Taken together, we found that IL-1β enhances the expression of catabolic enzymes by TMJ-derived cells, thereby possibly explaining cartilage damage as observed after overactive IL-1 signaling.

One limitation of this study is that we cannot be certain that histological changes indicative of degeneration in the condylar fibrocartilage of the TMJ of IL-1R$^{-/-}$ mice can be attributed to MMP-13 over-expression. Studies using IL-1R$^{-/-}$ mice treated with MMP-13 inhibitors could provide clarity, but such experiments were beyond the scope of the current study. In addition, our in vitro studies showing the effect of IL-1β on MMP-13 expression in condyle-derived fibrochondrocytes were performed with cells from pig TMJs but not mice, and species differences can occur. We have performed immunohistochemistry for MMP-13 on sections of mouse TMJs, but the resulting quality prevented accurate quantitative assessment, though roughly 60% of the condylar cells seemed positive in wildtype animals and nearly 100% in IL-RA knock-out mice (data not shown), which indicates that the effects of overactive IL-1β with regards to MMP-13 expression is similar between pig and mouse. Another limitation is the selection of only one mechanical loading regime of tensile forces, whereas compressive forces are also occurring in the moving jaw.

Since MMP-13 plays an important role in many biological processes, including growth and development [31], inhibition of activity of this enzyme could have severe, undesirable side-effects in the children with JIA that are still growing. This important role of MMP-13 in many biological processes [31] requires a *direct* inhibition. Pharmaceutical intervention should therefore be based on tempering IL-1β's destructive effects [32,33]. A potential non-invasive, non-pharmaceutical approach to inhibit inflammation-induced MMP-13 expression is exercise or physical therapy of inflamed joints. We found that 6% cyclic tensile strain exerted on the condylar cells significantly reduced the IL-1β-induced MMP-13 gene expression, similar to our previous finding that tensile strain exerted on condylar cells significantly reduced TNFα-induced MMP-13 gene expression [34]. These findings are in line with several other studies, in which the anti-catabolic capacity of cyclic strain was analyzed [34–36]. In our study, the cells maintained their pericellular matrix when they were embedded in an agarose gel, thereby allowing proper transmission of mechanical forces to the cells. The condylar cartilage undergoes considerable tensile forces due to compression and shear [37]. For this reason, we used 6% cyclic tensile strain. This percentage was calculated by using the following literature data. Deschner et al. used 20% of strain to stimulate rat disc cells [35], but Chain et al. calculated that the maximal tensile strain that the condyle cartilage would experience would be 3.7-fold lower than the disc [38]. Further in vivo studies are needed to assess whether 6% tensile strain is effective in downregulating catabolic enzymes induced by inflammation.

In conclusion, overactive IL-1 signaling can induce changes in condyle cartilage metabolism indicative of degeneration, and cells from the three cartilaginous structures of the TMJ react to exposure to the inflammatory cytokine IL-1β, whereby the condyle seems particularly sensitive in terms of catabolic enzyme expression. This might explain why only the condyle is disproportionately degraded in children with JIA. MMP-13 induced by IL-1β might be a prime suspect in causing degradation of the condyle in JIA patients, and mechanical loading could inhibit expression. Future studies should confirm whether a direct link exists between JIA, IL-1β and MMP-13 over-expression, and whether controlled exercise can reduce MMP-13 expression in the condyle of the TMJ in vivo. These are important future steps with high clinical relevance because controlled physical exercise could provide a therapeutic intervention in children with JIA, potentially preventing serious effects of TMJ inflammation such as pain, dysfunction, and even malformations. Non-invasive studies, for instance using MRI, could be useful to monitor the effect of motion on the progression of JIA.

4. Materials and Methods

4.1. Mice

IL-1RA-deficient (IL-1RA$^{-/-}$) mice on a BALB/c background were kindly supplied by Martin Nicklin (Sheffield, UK). Wild-type control mice were 8–10 weeks old and were purchased from Charles River (Sulzfeld, Germany). Before the age of 12 weeks, mice were sacrificed, heads were dissected and fixed in 4% formaldehyde for 6–12 weeks. Ethical permission was obtained in July 2013 at the Radboud University Nijmegen, RU-DEC 2013-096.

4.2. Histological Analysis of Murine TMJ

Mouse heads (four mice per strain) were decalcified for 6 days in 10% formic acid and 10% sodium citrate solution. The heads were then dehydrated, embedded in paraffin, and 5 μm-thick sagittal sections were cut. Safranin O-fast green and hematoxylin and eosin staining were performed. Mouse TMJ cartilage was evaluated by a blinded observer based on pericellular staining, chondrocyte arrangement, and structural appearance of the articular cartilage, using a modified Mankin score [21] (Table 1).

Table 1. Modified Mankin score.

1) Pericellular Safranin O staining	
a. Normal	0
b. Slightly enhanced	1
c. Intensely enhanced	2
2) Background Safranin O staining	
a. Normal	0
b. Slight decrease/increase	1
c. Severe decrease/increase	2
d. No staining	3
3) Arrangement of Chondrocytes	
a. Normal	0
b. Appearance of clustering	1
b. Hypocellularity	2
4) Cartilage Structure	
a. Normal	0
b. Fibrillation in superficial layer	1
c. Fibrillation beyond superficial layer	2
d. Missing articular cartilages	3

4.3. Cell Isolation and Culture

Because mouse TMJs only contain few cells, all in vitro studies were performed with cells isolated from pig TMJs. Heads of Dutch Landrace pigs (*Sus scrofa*), with a body weight in the range of 70–80 kg and aged 6–8 months old, were obtained from a local abattoir (Westford, Gorinchem, The Netherlands). Approval by the Animal Ethics Committee of the VU University was not required as the animals were not sacrificed for the purpose of the experiment. Within 4 h after sacrifice, the entire articular cartilage of the fossa and condyle and the whole disc were dissected. The cells were isolated as previously described [39,40]. The medium containing the cells was mixed 1:1 with 6% ultrapure low melting point agarose (Invitrogen, Carlsbad, CA, USA) to a final concentration of 1×10^6 cells/mL, 3% agarose, 1× DMEM supplemented with 50 μg/mL ascorbic acid (Merck, Darmstadt, Germany), 10% fetal bovine serum (FBS) (Thermo Fisher Scientific, Waltham, MA, USA), and 1% penicillin/streptomycin/fungizone (Invitrogen). The non-solidified gel was poured in a 2 mL syringe with a diameter of 8 mm of which the needle end was cut off, leaving a cylinder with an open needle-end. After gelation, the cell-gel construct was gently pressed out using the plunger and was cut into slices with a 2 mm thickness and transferred into a 24-wells plate. The 3D constructs were cultured for 6 days (Table 2) using a previously described protocol that is suitable for culturing chondrocytes [41]. On day 6, the cells were incubated with vehicle (PBS) or with 0.1, 1, or 10 ng/mL (7) recombinant porcine IL-1β (R&D Systems, Minneapolis, MN, USA) for 6 or 24 h.

Table 2. Timetable of progressive substitution of serum for ITS in the cell-agarose construct.

	Fetal Bovine Serum (%)	ITS (%)	Ascorbic Acid ($\mu g\ mL^{-1}$)	PSF (%)
Day 0	10	-	50	2
Day 1	5	-	50	2
Day 2	1	1	50	1
Day 4	-	1	50	1
Day 6	-	1	50	1

For mechanical loading experiments, the cell-gel solution was poured on the silicone membrane of a Flexcell tissue train plate (Dunn Labortechnik, Asbach, Germany) on which two Velcro strips were glued. The Velcro strips ensured that the agarose cell-gel constructs would stick to the membrane of the tissue train plate. The rectangular shape of the cell-gel construct was confined by a 3D-printed mold to match the standard dimensions of gels on a tissue train plate. The cell-gel constructs were cultured as described in Table 2 for 6 days before performing tensile strain experiments. In the cyclic tensile strain experiments, the cells were incubated first for 12 h with IL-1β (10 ng/mL, R&D Systems), followed by 6% of sinusoidal mechanical strain at 0.5 Hz for 8 h, which was applied using the Flexcell system. Cells were post-incubated without strain for 24 h with IL-1β.

4.4. RNA Extraction and Real-Time Quantitative PCR

After 6 and 24 h of incubation with IL-1β, the cell-gel constructs were snap-frozen, and the RNA was extracted according to the protocol developed by Bougault and co-workers [41], cDNA was made using SuperScript® VILO™ cDNA Synthesis Kit according to the manufacturer's instructions (Life Technologies, Carlsbad, CA, USA). Real-time PCR reactions were performed according to the manufacturer's instructions in a LightCycler480® (Roche Diagnostics, Switzerland). The sequences of the primer pairs are presented in Table 3.

Table 3. Primers used for real-time PCR.

Genes	Primers	Primer Sequences [a]
YWHAZ (reference gene)	Forward: Reverse:	GATGAAGCCATTGCTGAAACTTG CTATTTGTGGGACAGCATGGA
HPRT (reference gene)	Forward: Reverse:	GCTGACCTGCTGGATTACAT CTTGCGACCTTGACCATCT
IL-1RI	Forward: Reverse:	CATGACTGCCCATTGTTGAG AGGGCAGAAGCCTAGGAAG
IL-1RII	Forward: Reverse:	GTGCCTGTTGAGCCTCATT GGCCTTCATGGGCAAATGTCA
ADAMTS4	Forward: Reverse:	CATCCTACGCCGGAAGAGTC GGATCACTAGCCGAGTCACCA
ADAMTS5	Forward: Reverse:	GTGGAGGAGGAGTCAGTTTG TTCAGTGCCATCGGTCACCTT
MMP-2	Forward: Reverse:	CCGTGGTGAGATCTTCTTCTTC GCGGTCAGTGGCTGGGGTA

Table 3. *Cont.*

Genes	Primers	Primer Sequences [a]
MMP-9	Forward: Reverse:	ACAGGCAGCTGGCAGAGGA GCCGGCAAGTCTTCCGAGTA
MMP-13	Forward: Reverse:	GGAGCATGGCGACTTCTAC GAGTGCTCCAGGGTCCTT

[a] Only primers with equal efficacy were used.

4.5. Zymography

MMP-2 and MMP-9 activities in the conditioned medium of IL-1β-treaded cells (10 ng/mL for 24 h) were analyzed by zymography. The medium was lyophilized and concentrated three times. Novex® 10% Zymogram (Gelatin) Protein Gels, 1.0 mm, 15-wells (Life Technologies) were used for electrophoresis. After 1.5 h of electrophoresis, the gel was incubated for 30 min at room temperature in renaturing buffer (Life Technologies) with gentle agitation. The buffer was replaced with developing buffer (Life Technologies) for 30 min at room temperature and subsequently replaced for fresh buffer. After overnight incubation, the gels were washed with demi water and stained for 1 h with SimplyBlue SafeStain (Life Technologies). MMP-2 and MMP-9 activity was displayed as unstained bands.

4.6. Immunohistochemistry

Cell-gel constructs were fixed with formaldehyde and incubated for 2 h at room temperature with blocking buffer. Immunolocalization of MMP-13 was performed by using rabbit polyclonal anti-human MMP-13 (1:1000) (ab84594; Abcam, Cambridge, MA, USA) overnight at 4 °C. The secondary antibody alexa-555 goat anti-rabbit (1:2000 dilution) (A31630; Invitrogen) was incubated for 2 h at room temperature. Negative control staining was performed with Dako rabbit negative control (Dako, Glostrup, Denmark). Nuclei were stained with 4′,6-diamidino-2-phenylindole (DAPI).

Six μm optical sections were made of the gels with an Axio ZoomV16 microscope (Zeiss, Munich, Germany). The micrographs were then superimposed, and the number of positive cells was counted. With this technique, we were able to scan through 200 μm gel and count the MMP-13-positive cells in these areas.

4.7. Statistical Analysis

Prism (GraphPad Software Inc., San Diego, CA, USA) was used for statistical analyses. Mean values and standard errors of the mean (SEM) were calculated and depicted in the figures throughout the manuscript. Differences in pericellular staining of extracellular matrix (proteoglycans), chondrocyte arrangement, and structural appearance of the articular cartilage between four wild-type and four IL-1RA$^{-/-}$ mice were tested using the Mann–Whitney U test ($n = 4$). For each parameter measured, the null hypothesis was that cartilage damage-related changes scored equally in TMJs from WT and IL-1RA$^{-/-}$ mice. Experiments with pig cells were performed at three separate occasions. Data obtained at one separate occasion were considered $n = 1$ (thus, total $n = 3$). At each separate occasion, a *new* cell pool (derived from three pig heads) per anatomical region was created. Cell pools derived from the condyle, fossa, and disc were kept separate, and all were treated with or without IL-1β. To determine whether IL-1β (0.1, 1, or 10 ng/mL) significantly affected gene expression of ADAMTS4, ADAMTS5, MMP-2, MMP-9 and MMP-13, as well as protein expression for MMP-13, and activity of MMP-2 and MMP-9, compared to vehicle, in TMJ-derived cell populations, Dunnett's multiple comparison test was performed. Bonferoni correction was applied, as three tests were performed per parameter (one for fossa, one for disc and one for condyle) at the 6 h and at the 24 h time point, separately. At a $p < 0.017$, the null hypothesis, i.e., IL-1β (at either 0.1, 1, or 10 ng/mL) did not affect gene or protein expression of the catabolic factor of interest in pig TMJ cells, was rejected. To test the effect of mechanical strain on IL-1β-induced gene expression by pig condylar fibrochondrocytes, one-way ANOVA was performed. Differences were regarded significant at values of $p < 0.05$.

Author Contributions: H.T. performed most of the practical work, and supervised A.V.t.L. B.F.B. was involved in experiments concerning mechanical loading, B.Z.-D. was involved in the protein analysis and zymography, C.d.S.C. performed immunohistochemistry. M.I.K. contributed on the IL1-RA$^{-/-}$ part, T.J.d.V. and A.D.B. were the daily PhD supervisors of H.T., F.L. and V.E. the formal PhD supervisors. All work was discussed on a weekly basis between H.T., T.J.d.V., A.D.B., F.L. and V.E. H.T. initiated writing, all authors have contributed to the writing of the submitted version.

Acknowledgments: We thank Jolanda Hogervorst for her assistance with the qPCR; Rebecca Rogier and Debbie Roeleveld for collecting the mouse heads; Regina Maria Catarino for help with MMP-13 immunostaining; and Ben Nelemans and Manual Schmitz for their assistance with the Axio-zoom.

References

1. Mercuri, L.G. Temporomandibular joint reconstruction. *Alpha Omegan* **2009**, *102*, 51–54. [CrossRef] [PubMed]
2. Tabeian, H.; Bakker, A.D.; De Vries, T.J.; Zandieh-Doulabi, B.; Lobbezoo, F.; Everts, V. Juvenile porcine temporomandibular joint: Three different cartilaginous structures? *Arch. Oral Boil.* **2016**, *72*, 211–218. [CrossRef]
3. Weiss, P.F.; Arabshahi, B.; Johnson, A.; Bilaniuk, L.T.; Zarnow, D.; Cahill, A.M.; Feudtner, C.; Cron, R.Q. High prevalence of temporomandibular joint arthritis at disease onset in children with juvenile idiopathic arthritis, as detected by magnetic resonance imaging but not by ultrasound. *Arthritis Rheum.* **2008**, *58*, 1189–1196.
4. Hu, Y.; Billiau, A.D.; Verdonck, A.; Wouters, C.; Carels, C. Variation in dentofacial morphology and occlusion in juvenile idiopathic arthritis subjects: A case-control study. *Eur. J. Orthod.* **2009**, *31*, 51–58. [CrossRef] [PubMed]
5. Ringold, S.; Torgerson, T.R.; Egbert, M.A.; Wallace, C.A. Intraarticular corticosteroid injections of the temporomandibular joint in juvenile idiopathic arthritis. *J. Rheumatol.* **2008**, *35*, 1157–1164.
6. McInnes, I.B.; Schett, G. Cytokines in the pathogenesis of rheumatoid arthritis. *Nat. Rev. Immunol.* **2007**, *7*, 429–442. [CrossRef]
7. Ge, X.; Ma, X.; Meng, J.; Zhang, C.; Ma, K.; Zhou, C. Role of Wnt-5A in interleukin-1β-induced matrix metalloproteinase expression in rabbit temporomandibular joint condylar chondrocytes. *Arthritis Rheum.* **2009**, *60*, 2714–2722.
8. Su, S.-C.; Tanimoto, K.; Tanne, Y.; Kunimatsu, R.; Hirose, N.; Mitsuyoshi, T.; Okamoto, Y.; Tanne, K. Celecoxib exerts protective effects on extracellular matrix metabolism of mandibular condylar chondrocytes under excessive mechanical stress. *Osteoarthr. Cartil.* **2014**, *22*, 845–851. [CrossRef]
9. Pascual, V.; Allantaz, F.; Arce, E.; Punaro, M.; Banchereau, J. Role of interleukin-1 (IL-1) in the pathogenesis of systemic onset juvenile idiopathic arthritis and clinical response to IL-1 blockade. *J. Exp. Med.* **2005**, *201*, 1479–1486. [CrossRef] [PubMed]
10. Kjellberg, H. Craniofacial growth in juvenile chronic arthritis. *Acta Odontol. Scand.* **1998**, *56*, 360–365. [CrossRef] [PubMed]
11. Twilt, M.; Schulten, A.J.; Nicolaas, P.; Dulger, A.; van Suijlekom-Smit, L.W. Facioskeletal changes in children with juvenile idiopathic arthritis. *Ann. Rheum. Dis.* **2006**, *65*, 823–825. [CrossRef] [PubMed]
12. Sun, H.B. Mechanical loading, cartilage degradation, and arthritis. *Ann. N. Y. Acad. Sci.* **2010**, *1211*, 37–50. [CrossRef]
13. Tani-Ishii, N.; Tsunoda, A.; Teranaka, T.; Umemoto, T. Autocrine regulation of osteoclast formation and bone resorption by IL-1 alpha and TNF alpha. *J. Dent.* **1999**, *78*, 1617–1623.
14. Svensson, B.; Larsson, A.; Adell, R. The mandibular condyle in juvenile chronic arthritis patients with mandibular hypoplasia: A clinical and histological study. *Int. J. Oral Surg.* **2001**, *30*, 300–305. [CrossRef]
15. Herring, S.W. The dynamics of mastication in pigs. *Arch. Oral Boil.* **1976**, *21*, 473–480. [CrossRef]

16. Bermejo, A.; González, O.; Gonzalez, J. The pig as an animal model for experimentation on the temporomandibular articular complex. *Oral Surg. Oral Med. Oral Pathol.* **1993**, *75*, 18–23. [CrossRef]

17. Wang, L.; Detamore, M.S. Effects of growth factors and glucosamine on porcine mandibular condylar cartilage cells and hyaline cartilage cells for tissue engineering applications. *Arch. Oral Biol.* **2009**, *54*, 1–5. [CrossRef] [PubMed]

18. Springer, I.N.; Fleiner, B.; Jepsen, S.; Acil, Y. Culture of cells gained from temporomandibular joint cartilage on non-absorbable scaffolds. *Biomaterials* **2001**, *22*, 2569–2577. [CrossRef]

19. Vapniarsky, N.; Aryaei, A.; Arzi, B.; Hatcher, D.C.; Hu, J.C.; Athanasiou, K.A. The Yucatan Minipig Temporomandibular Joint Disc Structure–Function Relationships Support Its Suitability for Human Comparative Studies. *Tissue Eng. Part. C Methods* **2017**, *23*, 700–709. [CrossRef] [PubMed]

20. Horai, R.; Tanioka, H.; Nakae, S.; Okahara, A.; Ikuse, T.; Iwakura, Y.; Saijo, S.; Sudo, K.; Asano, M. Development of Chronic Inflammatory Arthropathy Resembling Rheumatoid Arthritis in Interleukin 1 Receptor Antagonist-Deficient Mice. *J. Exp. Med.* **2000**, *191*, 313–320. [CrossRef]

21. Xu, L.; Polur, I.; Lim, C.; Servais, J.M.; Dobeck, J.; Li, Y.; Olsen, B.R. Early-onset osteoarthritis of mouse temporomandibular joint induced by partial discectomy. *Osteoarthr. Cartil.* **2009**, *17*, 917–922. [CrossRef]

22. Hu, K.; Xu, L.; Cao, L.; Flahiff, C.M.; Brussiau, J.; Ho, K.; Setton, L.A.; Youn, I.; Guilak, F.; Olsen, B.R.; et al. Pathogenesis of osteoarthritis-like changes in the joints of mice deficient in type IX collagen. *Arthritis Rheum.* **2006**, *54*, 2891–2900.

23. Lam, N.P.; Li, Y.; Waldman, A.B.; Brussiau, J.; Lee, P.L.; Olsen, B.R.; Xu, L. Age-dependent increase of discoidin domain receptor 2 and matrix metalloproteinase 13 expression in temporomandibular joint cartilage of type IX and type XI collagen-deficient mice. *Arch. Oral Biol.* **2007**, *52*, 579–584. [CrossRef] [PubMed]

24. Henry, S.P.; Liang, S.; Akdemir, K.C.; De Crombrugghe, B. The Postnatal Role of Sox9 in Cartilage. *J. Bone* **2012**, *27*, 2511–2525. [CrossRef]

25. Fosang, A.J.; Last, K.; Neame, P.J.; Murphy, G.; Knäuper, V.; Tschesche, H.; Hughes, C.E.; Caterson, B.; Hardingham, T.E. Neutrophil collagenase (MMP-8) cleaves at the aggrecanase site E373–A374 in the interglobular domain of cartilage aggrecan. *Biochem. J.* **1994**, *304*, 347–351. [CrossRef] [PubMed]

26. Takaishi, H.; Kimura, T.; Dalal, S.; Okada, Y.; D'Armiento, J. Joint Diseases and Matrix Metalloproteinases: A Role for MMP-13. *Pharm. Biotechnol.* **2008**, *9*, 47–54. [CrossRef]

27. Aimes, R.T.; Quigley, J.P. Matrix metalloproteinase-2 is an interstitial collagenase. Inhibitor-free enzyme catalyzes the cleavage of collagen fibrils and soluble native type I collagen generating the specific 3/4- and 1/4-length fragments. *J. Biol. Chem.* **1995**, *270*, 5872–5876. [CrossRef]

28. Mort, J.S.; Billington, C. Articular cartilage and changes in arthritis: Matrix degradation. *Arthritis Res.* **2001**, *3*, 337–341. [CrossRef]

29. Neuhold, L.A.; Killar, L.; Zhao, W.; Sung, M.-L.A.; Warner, L.; Kulik, J.; Turner, J.; Wu, W.; Billinghurst, C.; Meijers, T.; et al. Postnatal expression in hyaline cartilage of constitutively active human collagenase-3 (MMP-13) induces osteoarthritis in mice. *J. Clin. Investig.* **2001**, *107*, 35–44. [CrossRef]

30. Yoshihara, Y.; Nakamura, H.; Obata, K.; Yamada, H.; Hayakawa, T.; Fujikawa, K.; Okada, Y. Matrix metalloproteinases and tissue inhibitors of metalloproteinases in synovial fluids from patients with rheumatoid arthritis or osteoarthritis. *Ann. Rheum. Dis.* **2000**, *59*, 455–461. [CrossRef]

31. Inada, M.; Wang, Y.; Byrne, M.H.; Rahman, M.U.; Miyaura, C.; López-Otín, C.; Krane, S.M. Critical roles for collagenase-3 (Mmp13) in development of growth plate cartilage and in endochondral ossification. *Proc. Natl. Acad. Sci. USA* **2004**, *101*, 17192–17197. [CrossRef]

32. Cheleschi, S.; Pascarelli, N.A.; Valacchi, G.; Di Capua, A.; Biava, M.; Belmonte, G.; Giordani, A.; Sticozzi, C.; Anzini, M.; Fioravanti, A. Chondroprotective effect of three different classes of anti-inflammatory agents on human osteoarthritic chondrocytes exposed to IL-1β. *Int. Immunopharmacol.* **2015**, *28*, 794–801. [CrossRef]

33. Bai, X.; Guo, A.; Li, Y. Protective effects of calcitonin on IL-1 stimulated chondrocytes by regulating MMPs/TIMP-1 ratio via suppression of p50-NF-κB pathway. *Biosci. Biotechnol. Biochem.* **2019**, *83*, 598–604. [CrossRef]

34. Tabeian, H.; Bakker, A.D.; Betti, B.F.; Lobbezoo, F.; Everts, V.; de Vries, T.J. Cyclic Tensile Strain Reduces TNF-alpha Induced Expression of MMP-13 by Condylar Temporomandibular Joint Cells. *J. Cell. Physiol.* **2017**, *232*, 1287–1294. [CrossRef]

35. Deschner, J.; Rath-Deschner, B.; Agarwal, S. Regulation of matrix metalloproteinase expression by dynamic tensile strain in rat fibrochondrocytes. *Osteoarthr. Cartil.* **2006**, *14*, 264–272. [CrossRef]

36. Agarwal, S.; Long, P.; Gassner, R.; Piesco, N.P.; Buckley, M.J. Cyclic tensile strain suppresses catabolic effects of interleukin-1β in fibrochondrocytes from the temporomandibular joint. *Arthritis. Rheum.* **2001**, *44*, 608–617. [CrossRef]

37. Singh, M.; Detamore, M.S. Tensile properties of the mandibular condylar cartilage. *J. Biomech. Eng.* **2008**, *130*, 011009. [CrossRef] [PubMed]

38. Chen, J.; Akyuz, U.; Xu, L.; Pidaparti, R. Stress analysis of the human temporomandibular joint. *Med. Eng. Phys.* **1998**, *20*, 565–572. [CrossRef]

39. Lee, G.M.; Poole, C.A.; Kelley, S.S.; Chang, J.; Caterson, B. Isolated chondrons: A viable alternative for studies of chondrocyte metabolism in vitro. *Osteoarthr. Cartil.* **1997**, *5*, 261–274. [CrossRef]

40. Vonk, L.A.; Doulabi, B.Z.; Huang, C.; Helder, M.N.; Everts, V.; Bank, R.A. Preservation of the chondrocyte's pericellular matrix improves cell-induced cartilage formation. *J. Cell. Biochem.* **2010**, *110*, 260–271. [CrossRef]

41. Bougault, C.; Paumier, A.; Aubert-Foucher, E.; Mallein-Gerin, F. Investigating conversion of mechanical force into biochemical signaling in three-dimensional chondrocyte cultures. *Nat. Protoc.* **2009**, *4*, 928–938. [CrossRef] [PubMed]

5

Quercetin Enhances the Thioredoxin Production of Nasal Epithelial Cells In Vitro and In Vivo

Yukako Edo [1], Amane Otaki [2] and Kazuhito Asano [3,*]

[1]   Graduate School of Health Sciences, Showa University Graduate School, Yokohama 226-8555, Japan; yukakoeddy18@gmail.com

[2]   Division of Nursing, Showa University School of Nursing and Rehabilitation Sciences, Yokohama 226-8555, Japan; aotaki@nr.showa-u.ac.jp

[3]   Division of Physiology, Showa University School of Nursing and Rehabilitation Sciences, Yokohama 226-8555, Japan

*   Correspondence: asanok@med.showa-u.ac.jp

Abstract: Background: Thioredoxin (TRX) acts as both a scavenger of reactive oxygen species (ROS) and an immuno-modulator. Although quercetin has been shown to favorably modify allergic rhinitis (AR) symptoms, its influence on TRX production is not well defined. The present study was designed to examine whether quercetin could favorably modify AR symptoms via the TRX production of nasal epithelial cells in vitro and in vivo. **Methods**: Human nasal epithelial cells (HNEpCs) were stimulated with H_2O_2 in the presence of quercetin. TRX levels in 24-h culture supernatants were examined with ELISA. BALB/c male mice were intraperitoneally sensitized to ovalbumin (OVA) and intranasally challenged with OVA every other day, beginning seven days after the final sensitization. The mice were orally administered quercetin once a day for five consecutive days, beginning seven days after the final sensitization. Nasal symptoms were assessed by counting the number of sneezes and nasal rubbing behaviors during a 10-min period immediately after the challenge. TRX levels in nasal lavage fluids obtained 6 h after the challenge were examined by ELISA. **Results**: Treatment with 1.0 nM quercetin increased H_2O_2-induced TRX levels. The oral administration of 20.0 mg/kg of quercetin significantly inhibited nasal symptoms after the challenge. The same dose of quercetin significantly increased TRX levels in nasal lavage fluids. **Conclusions**: Quercetin's ability to increase TRX production may account, at least in part, for its clinical efficacy toward AR.

Keywords: allergic rhinitis; mice; quercetin; thioredoxin; nasal epithelial cell; production; increase; in vitro; in vivo

1. Introduction

Allergic rhinitis (AR) is a well-known type of chronic allergic inflammation that occurs in the nasal mucosa and is characterized by multiple symptoms such as sneezing, itching, and watery rhinorrhea [1,2]. Although AR is not life-threatening, it places a significant burden on patients and society because its symptoms lead to inconveniences in daily life. These clinical symptoms also exert adverse effects on industrial work productivity and school learning performance, resulting in increased medical costs and lower quality of life [1,2].

AR treatment can be divided into three main categories: allergen avoidance, drug therapy, and immunomodulating therapy [3]. Allergen avoidance is the safest mode of treatment, but it is often insufficient to obtain satisfactory results [3]. Although histamine H1 receptor antagonists and topical steroids can significantly ease the associated symptoms, they require repeated treatment sessions over the patient's lifetime [3,4]. Moreover, the currently available therapeutic agents cause adverse effects, including dizziness, dry mouth, and constipation [3,4]. Although immunotherapy induces immunological tolerance through the subcutaneous injection of or sublingual application of allergens, it has several disadvantages: it requires several years of therapy, is expensive, and contains a risk of anaphylaxis [5]. Furthermore, many patients dislike taking daily medication merely for prevention [3]. Therefore, the development of new medications for the treatment of allergic diseases, including AR, is desired.

Quercetin is a dietary flavonoid found in red wine, tea, many fruits, and onions [6]. For many years, the possible healthy biological activities of quercetin have been studied, with anti-pollinosis, anti-diabetic, and anti-viral activity reported [7]. Moreover, quercetin acts as a scavenger of free radicals, which damage cell membranes, tamper with DNA, and even cause cell death [8–10]. Quercetin also plays a role in allergic inflammatory responses by inhibiting mast cells and eosinophils from producing chemical mediators (e.g., histamine and leukotriene) and inflammatory cytokines, which are responsible for the induction and persistence of allergic reactions [11,12]. Furthermore, the oral administration of quercetin can alleviate ocular and nasal symptoms observed in patients with pollinosis [13]. Quercetin's attenuating effect on the clinical symptoms of allergic reactions has also been observed in experimental animal models of allergic asthma and AR [14–16]. Although these reports strongly suggest that quercetin is a good dietary supplement candidate for preventing the development of allergic diseases such as AR, the precise mechanisms by which quercetin modulates the clinical symptoms of allergic diseases remain unknown.

It is currently accepted that inflammatory cells including eosinophils, which are the most important effector cells in the development of inflammatory diseases, produce several types of toxic granule proteins and reactive oxygen species (ROS), such as O_2 and H_2O_2 [17,18]. Although the physiological production of ROS is generally considered essential in host defense and to maintain homeostasis, the overproduction of ROS and their metabolites are harmful and cause oxidative stress responses, which are implicated in the pathogenesis of allergic inflammatory airway diseases, including AR [17,19]. Conversely, under normal physiological conditions, several types of endogenous antioxidants, such as glutathione and superoxide dismutase, prevent the development of oxidative stress responses [19]. Among these, thioredoxin (TRX) has attracted attention as an endogenous antioxidant protein. TRX is a 12-kDa protein with two redox (reduction/oxidation) active half-cysteine residues [20,21]. In addition to its anti-oxidative activity, TRX is reported to exert immunomodulatory effects. The administration of exogenous TRX suppresses airway hyperresponsiveness induced by specific allergens by inhibiting eosinophil accumulation in the airways of asthmatic mouse models [22,23]. TRX has also been reported to augment the production of Th1-type cytokines, such as IL-12 and IFN-γ, which prevent allergic responses. These reports suggest that manipulating TRX production may be a good target for the treatment of chronic airway allergic diseases, including AR [22,23]. However, the influence of quercetin on the production of TRX is currently unclear. Therefore, the present study investigated the influence of quercetin on the TRX system by examining the ability of agents from human nasal epithelial cells (HNEpCs) to affect TRX production in vitro and in vivo.

2. Materials and Methods

2.1. Mice

Specific 5-week-old pathogen-free BALB/c male mice were purchased from CLEA Japan Co., Ltd. (Tokyo, Japan). The mice were maintained in our animal facility at 25 °C $\pm$ 2 °C with 55% $\pm$ 10% humidity under a 12-h dark/light cycle and were allowed free access to tap water and standard laboratory rodent chow (Oriental Yeast Co., Ltd., Tokyo, Japan) throughout the experiments. Each control and experimental group consisted of five mice. All animal experiments were approved by the Ethics Committee for Animal Experiments of Showa University (Approved No. 54011). Date of approval: 1 April 2018.

2.2. Reagents

Quercetin was purchased from Sigma-Aldrich Co., Ltd. (St. Louis, MO, USA) as a preservative-free pure powder. Quercetin was first dissolved in dimethyl sulfoxide (DMSO) at a concentration of 10.0 mM. This solution was then diluted with Airway Epithelial Cell Growth Media (AECG medium; PromoCell GmbH, Heidelberg, Germany) at appropriate concentrations for the experiments; then, the solution was sterilized by passing through 0.2-μm filters and was stored at 4 °C until use. To assess in vivo use, quercetin was mixed with 5% tragacanth gum solution at a concentration of 7.5 mg/mL [13]. Chicken ovalbumin (OVA; grade V) and $Al(OH)_3$ (alum) were obtained from Sigma-Aldrich Co. Ltd. as preservative-free pure powders.

2.3. Cell Culture

HNEpCs, purchased from PromoCell GmbH, were suspended in AECG medium (PromoCell GmbH) at a concentration of 5×10^5 cells/mL and used as target cells. The HNEpCs (5×10^5 cells/mL) were stimulated with 12.5–100.0 μM H_2O_2 for 24 h in a final volume of 2.0 mL. To examine the influence of quercetin on TRX production, the HNEpCs (5×10^5 cells/mL) were stimulated with 50.0 μM H_2O_2 in the presence of 0.1–10.0 nM quercetin for 24 h in a final volume of 2.0 mL. To examine TRX mRNA expression, the cells were stimulated with 50.0 μM H_2O_2 in the presence of 0.1–10.0 nM quercetin for 12 h. Quercetin was added to the cell cultures 2 h before H_2O_2 stimulation.

2.4. Assay to Assess Cytotoxicity of H_2O_2 and Quercetin

HNEpCs (5×10^5 cells/mL) were cultured with either 12.5–100.0 μM H_2O_2 or 0.1–10.0 nM quercetin for 24 h. The cells were then collected, and cell viability was assessed by the trypan blue dye exclusion test. The dead cells were stained with trypan blue, and the proportion of dead cells was determined by counting 300 total cells.

2.5. Assay to Assess TRX mRNA Expression

TRX mRNA expression was examined by the methods described previously (24). Briefly, Poly A^+ mRNA was extracted from cultured cells with oligo(dT)-coated magnetic micro beads (Milteny Biotec, Bergisch Gladbach, Germany). The first-strand cDNA was synthesized from 1.0 μg of Poly A^+ mRNA using a Superscript cDNA synthesis kit (Invitrogen Corp., Carlsbad, CA, USA) according to the manufacturer's recommendations. Polymerase chain reaction (PCR) was then performed using a GeneAmp 5700 Sequence Detection System (Applied Biosystems, Forster City, CA, USA). The PCR mixture consisted of 2.0 μL of sample cDNA solution (100 ng/μL), 25.0 μL of SYBR-Green Mastermix (Applied Biosystems), 0.3 μL of both sense and antisense primers, and distilled water for a final volume of 50.0 μL. The conditions used for the reaction was as follows: 4 min at 94 °C, followed by 40 cycles of 15 s at 95 °C and 60 s at 60 °C. GAPDH was used as an internal control. TRX mRNA levels were calculated using the comparative parameter threshold cycle and normalized to GAPDH. The primers used for real-time RT-PCR were as follows: 5'-GCCTTGCAAAATGATTCAAGC-3' (Sense) and 5'-TTGGCTCCAGAAAATTCACC-3' (Antisense) for TRX [24], and 5'-TGTTGCCATCAATGACCCCTT-3' (Sense) and 5'-CTCCACGACGTACTCAGCG-3' (Antisense) for GAPDH [24].

2.6. Sensitization and Treatment of Mice

BALB/c mice were sensitized with an intraperitoneal injection of 20.0 μg/mL OVA in phosphate-buffered saline (PBS) combined with 1.0 mg of alum in a total volume of 200.0 μL on days 0, 7, and 14 [3,4]. On days 21, 23, and 25, the mice were intranasally instilled with 100 μg of OVA (5.0 μL in PBS) [3,4]. The mice were orally administered 10, 15, 20, or 25 mg/kg of quercetin using a stomach tube in a volume not exceeding 0.5 mL once a day for five consecutive days, beginning on day 21 relative to the sensitization.

2.7. Collection of Nasal Lavage Fluids

The mice were anesthetized by intraperitoneal injection with 50.0 mg/kg sodium pentobarbital (Kyoritsu Seiyaku Co., Ltd., Tokyo, Japan) 6 h after the OVA nasal challenge. The trachea was exposed and cannulated to introduce 1.0 mL of PBS [16]. The lavage fluid from the nares was collected and centrifuged at 3000 rpm for 15 min at 4 °C. After measuring IgA levels with ELISA (Bethyl Lab., Inc., Montgomery, TX, USA), the fluids were stored at −40 °C until use [16].

2.8. Assessment of Nasal Symptoms

Nasal allergy symptoms were assessed by counting the number of sneezes and nasal rubbing movements for 10 min immediately after the OVA nasal instillation. The experimental mice were placed into plastic animal cages (35 × 20 × 30 cm) for approximately 10 min to acclimate. After the nasal instillation of 0.1% OVA solution in PBS in a volume of 5.0 μL, the mice were placed into plastic cages (two animals/cage), and the number of sneezes and nasal rubbing movements were counted for 10 min [16].

2.9. TRX Assay

The TRX levels in the culture supernatants and nasal lavage fluids were examined using human and mouse TRX ELISA test kits (CUSABIO TECHNOLOGY LLC., Huston, TX, USA) according to the manufacturer's recommendations. The minimum detectable levels of the ELISA test kits were 1.172 ng/mL and 0.078 ng/mL for humans and mice, respectively.

2.10. Oxidative Stress Assay

The oxidative stress responses in the nasal mucosa were evaluated by measuring lipid peroxide levels in nasal lavage fluids using d-ROM tests (DIACRON, Via Zircone, Italy) according to the manufacturer's recommendations. The results were expressed as mean Carratelli Units (CARR U) ± SE.

2.11. Statistical Analysis

The statistical significance between the control and experimental groups was assessed with an ANOVA followed by Dunette's multiple comparison test. A P value of less than 0.05 was considered significant.

3. Results

3.1. Influence of H_2O_2 Stimulation on TRX Production from HNEpCs in Vitro

The first experiments were performed to examine whether H_2O_2 stimulation could increase TRX production from HNEpCs and to determine the optimal concentration of H_2O_2 for stimulation. Thus, the cells were stimulated with various concentrations of H_2O_2 for 24 h, and the TRX levels in the culture supernatants were determined via ELISA. As shown in Figure 1, the stimulation of cells with H_2O_2 caused a significant increase in the ability of cells to produce TRX. As little as 2.5 μM H_2O_2 caused a strong stimulation in TRX production. Maximum production was observed with 25.0–75.0 μM H_2O_2 whereas 100.0 μM H_2O_2 was inhibitory (Figure 1).

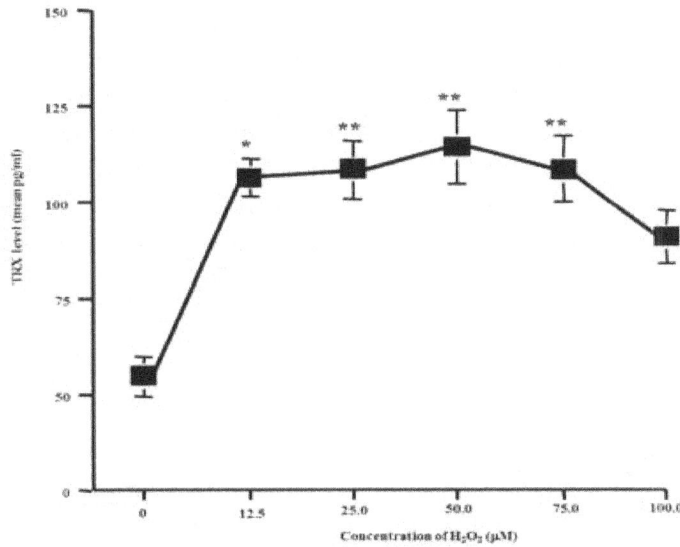

Figure 1. Influence of H_2O_2 on thioredoxin (TRX) production from HNEpCs in vitro. Nasal epithelial cells (5×10^5 cells) were stimulated with various concentrations of H_2O_2. After 24 h, TRX levels in culture supernatants were examined with ELISA. The data are expressed as the mean pg/mL $\pm$ SE of triplicate cultures. One representative experiment of two is shown in this figure. *: $P < 0.05$ versus control (0); ** $P > 0.05$ versus 12.5 μM H_2O_2.

3.2. In Vitro Influence of Quercetin on H_2O_2-Induced TRX Production from HNEpCs

The second set of experiments was designed to examine the influence of quercetin on the TRX production of HNEpCs after H_2O_2 stimulation. The cells were stimulated with 50.0 μM H_2O_2 in the presence or absence of quercetin for 24 h. TRX levels in the culture supernatants were examined by ELISA. As shown in Figure 2, the treatment of cells with quercetin at concentrations of both 0.1 nM and 0.5 nM barely affected the ability of the cells to produce TRX: the TRX levels in the culture supernatants were nearly identical (not significant) to those detected in the controls. At concentrations greater than 1.0 nM, however, quercetin induced significantly increased TRX levels in culture supernatants compared to those levels in the controls.

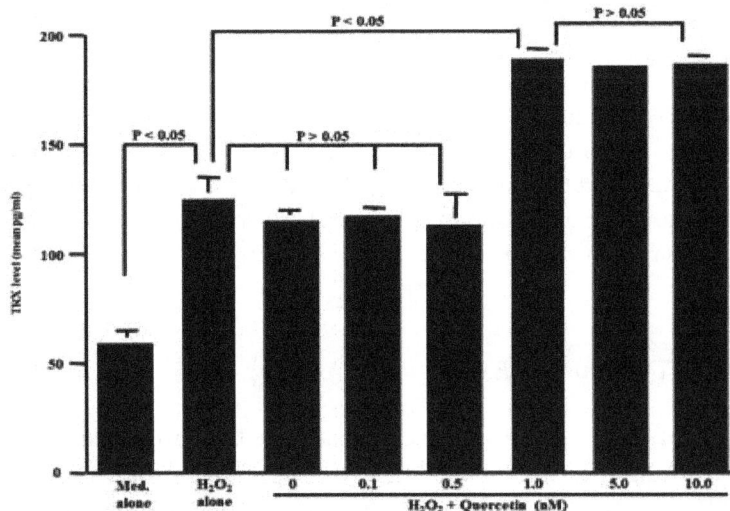

Figure 2. Influence of quercetin on thioredoxin (TRX) production from HNEpCs induced by H_2O_2 stimulation in vitro. Nasal epithelial cells (5×10^5 cells) were stimulated with 50 μM H_2O_2 in the presence of various concentrations of quercetin for 24 h. TRX levels in culture supernatants were examined with ELISA. The data are expressed as the mean pg/mL $\pm$ SE of triplicate cultures. One representative experiment of two is shown in this figure. Med. alone: Medium alone.

3.3. Influence of H_2O_2 and Quercetin on Cell Viability

The third set of experiments was performed to examine the influence of H_2O_2 and quercetin on cell viability. HNEpCs were cultured with either H_2O_2 or quercetin for 24 h, and cell viability was examined via the trypan blue dye exclusion test. Although the cells cultured with H_2O_2 concentrations less than 50.0 µM did not display reduced cell viability, 100.0 nM H_2O_2 caused significant cell death (Figure 3A). We then examined the influence of quercetin on cell viability. Quercetin did not exert cytotoxic effects on HNEpCs; the number of dead cells observed in cells cultured with 100.0 nM quercetin was nearly identical to that observed in controls (Figure 3B).

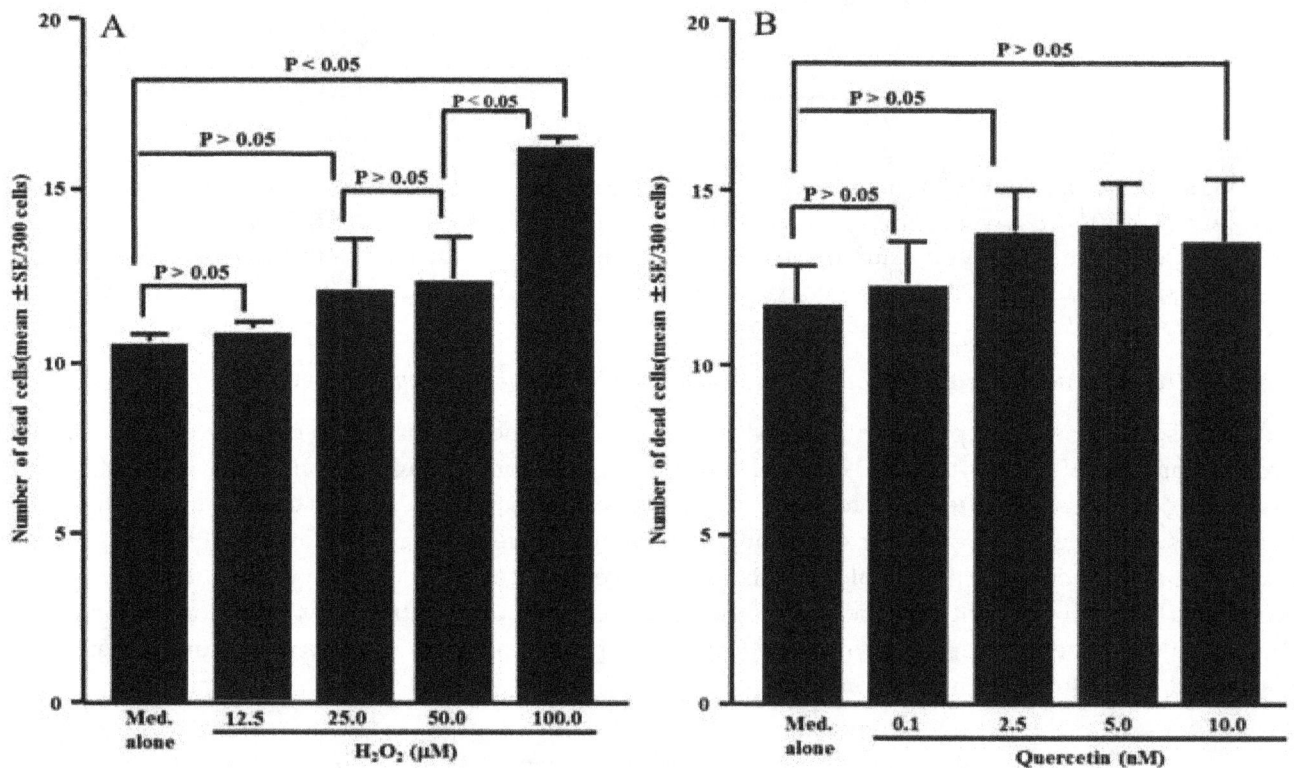

Figure 3. Influence of H_2O_2 (**A**) and quercetin (**B**) on cell viability. Nasal epithelial cells (5×10^5 cells) were stimulated with various concentrations of either H_2O_2 or quercetin for 24 h. The trypan blue exclusion test was performed, and the number of dead cells was counted out of 300 total cells. The data are expressed as the mean number of dead cells $\pm$ SE of triplicate cultures. One representative experiment of two is shown in this figure. Med. alone: Medium alone.

3.4. Influence of Quercetin on TRX mRNA Expression

The fourth set of experiments was performed to examine the influence of quercetin on TRX mRNA expression in HNEpCs stimulated with 50.0 µM H_2O_2. The stimulation of HNEpCs with H_2O_2 caused significant increases in TRX mRNA expression compared to the non-stimulated (Med. alone) controls (Figure 4). However, TRX mRNA expression was significantly suppressed in HNEpCs treated with more than 1.0 nM quercetin but not in HNEpCs treated with less than 0.5 nM, whereas TRX mRNA expression was increased by stimulation with H_2O_2 (Figure 4).

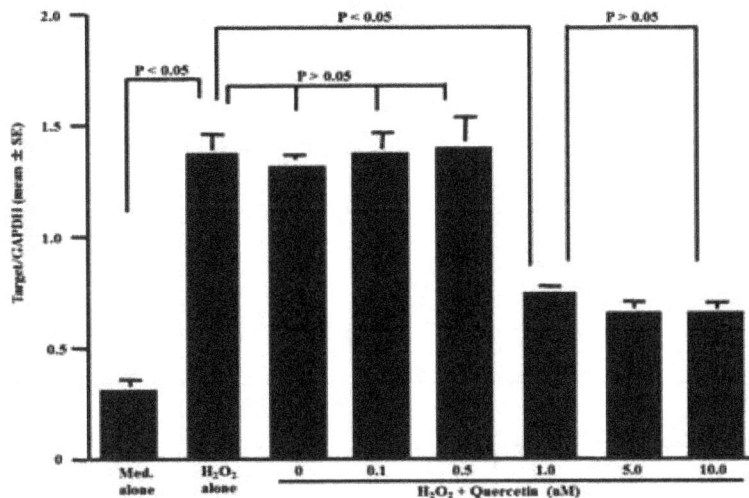

Figure 4. Influence of quercetin on TRX mRNA expression in HNEpCs. Nasal epithelial cells (5×10^5 cells) were stimulated with 50 μM H_2O_2 in the presence or absence of quercetin for 12 h. TRX mRNA levels in the cultured cells were examined by RT-PCR. The data are expressed as the mean Target/GAPD ± SE of triplicate cultures. One representative experiment of two is shown in this figure. Med. alone: Medium alone.

3.5. Influence of Quercetin on Oxidative Stress Responses in Nasal Mucosa

The fifth set of experiments was performed to examine whether oxidative stress responses were occurred in OVA-sensitized mice and whether quercetin administration into OVA-sensitized mice could modulate oxidative stress responses. Therefore, OVA-sensitized mice were orally administered 10.0–25.0 mg/kg of quercetin at days 21–25 after sensitization. Nasal lavage fluids were obtained 6 h after the final nasal OVA challenge, and lipid peroxide levels in nasal secretions were examined by the d-ROM test. Quercetin treatment significantly decreased lipid peroxide levels in the nasal lavage fluids of the mice, whereas the OVA nasal challenge increased lipid peroxide levels (Figure 5).

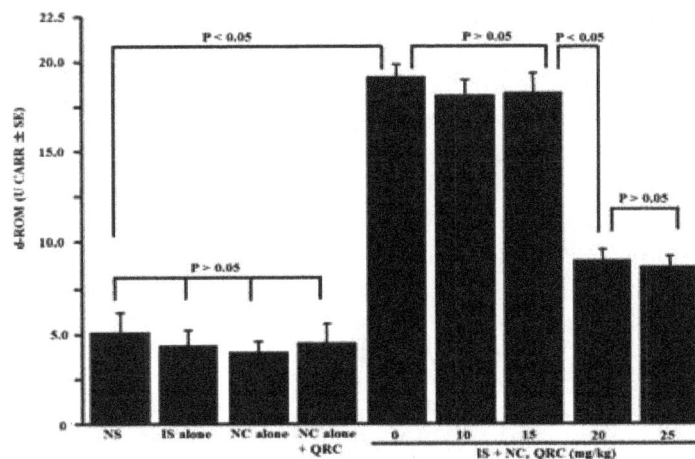

Figure 5. Influence of quercetin on the appearance of lipid peroxide in nasal lavage fluids after ovalbumin (OVA) sensitization in mice. BALB/c mice were sensitized by an intraperitoneal injection of OVA on days 0, 7, and 14. Seven days after the final sensitization, the OVA-sensitized mice were intranasally challenged with OVA on days 21, 23, and 25, and various concentrations of quercetin were administered orally once a day for five consecutive days. Nasal lavage fluids were obtained from mice 6 h after the OVA nasal challenge. Lipid peroxide levels were measured using the d-ROM test. The data are expressed as the mean CARR U ± SE of five mice. NS: non-sensitized; IS: intraperitoneal sensitization; NC: nasal challenge alone; QRC: quercetin.

3.6. Influence of Quercetin on the Appearance of TRX in Nasal Lavage Fluids

The sixth set of experiments was designed to examine the influence of quercetin on the appearance of TRX in nasal lavage fluids obtained from sensitized mice after the OVA nasal challenge. The OVA-sensitized mice were orally administered 10.0–25.0 mg/kg of quercetin at days 21–25 after sensitization. Nasal lavage fluids were obtained 6 h after the final nasal OVA challenge. As shown in Figure 6, the oral administration of 20.0 and 25.0 mg/kg of quercetin, but not 10.0 and 15.0 mg/kg, could increase TRX levels in nasal lavage fluids.

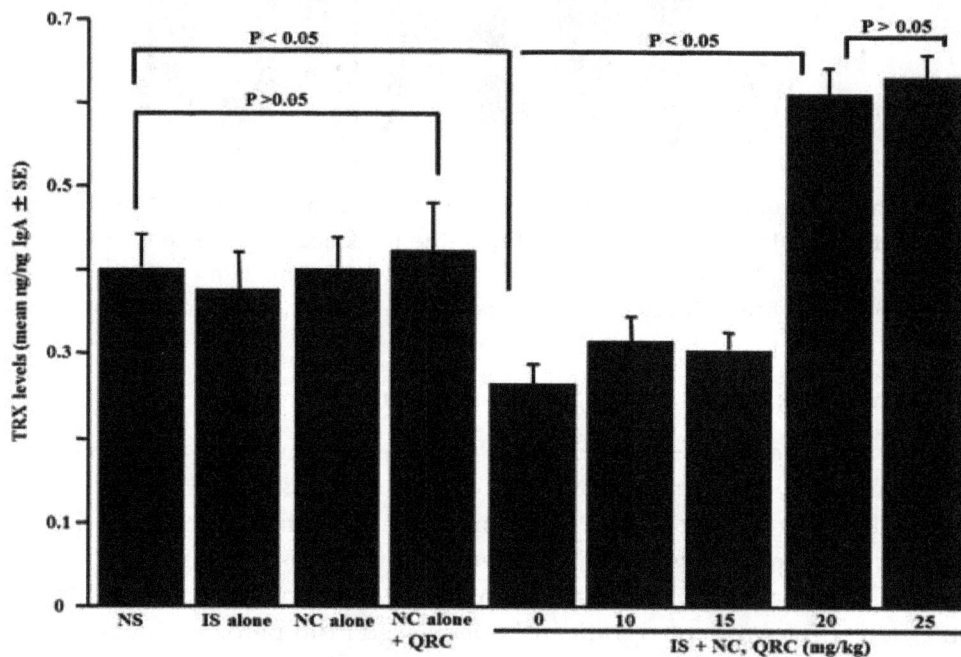

Figure 6. Influence of quercetin on the appearance of thioredoxin (TRX) in nasal lavage fluids obtained from OVA-sensitized mice after the OVA nasal challenge. BALB/c mice were sensitized by an intraperitoneal injection of OVA on days 0, 7, and 14. Seven days after the final sensitization, the OVA-sensitized mice were intranasally challenged with OVA on days 21, 23, and 25, and various concentrations of quercetin were administered orally once a day for five consecutive days. Nasal lavage fluids were obtained from the mice 6 h after the nasal antigenic challenge. TRX levels were examined by an ELISA. The data are expressed as the mean ng/ng IgA ± SE of five mice. NS: non-sensitized; IS: intraperitoneal sensitization; NC: nasal challenge alone; QRC: quercetin.

3.7. Influence of Quercetin on the Development of OVA-Induced Nasal Allergy-Like Symptoms

The final set of experiments was performed to examine whether the oral administration of quercetin in OVA-sensitized mice could inhibit the development of nasal allergy-like symptoms, which were induced by the nasal antigenic challenge. Nasal symptoms were assessed by counting the number of sneezes and nasal rubbing movements for 10 min immediately after the OVA nasal challenge. As shown in Figure 7, treating the OVA-sensitized mice with less than 15.0 mg/kg of quercetin could not inhibit the development of nasal allergy-like symptoms: the number of sneezes and nasal rubbing movements were nearly identical (not significant) to those observed in the non-treated controls. Conversely, the oral administration of more than 20.0 mg/kg of quercetin attenuated the development of nasal allergy-like symptoms, and the number of sneezes and nasal rubbing movements was significantly lower than those observed in the non-treated controls (Figure 7).

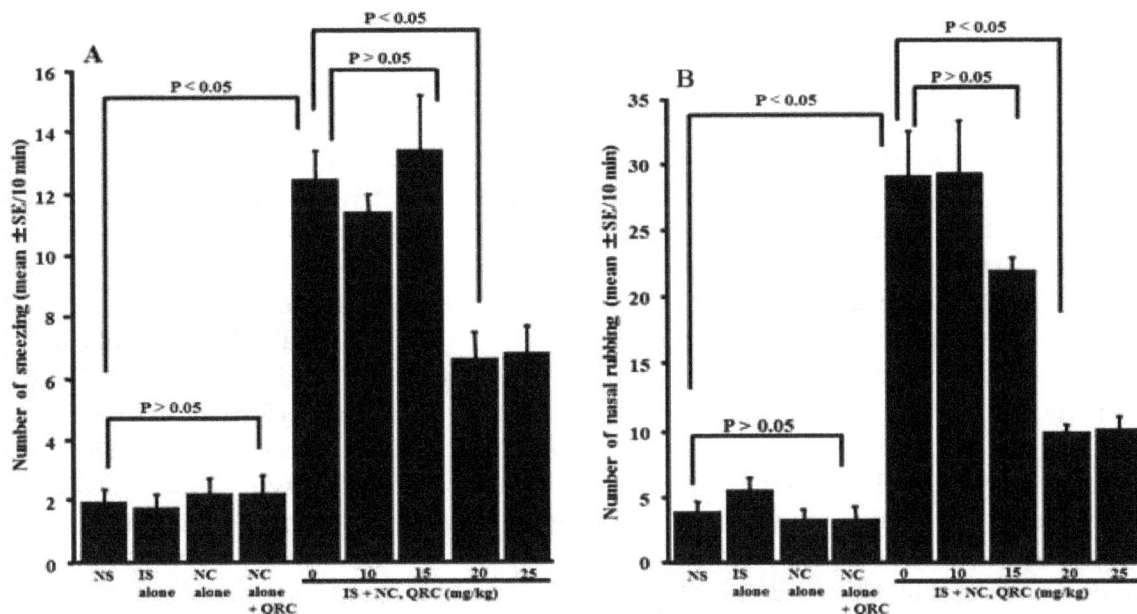

Figure 7. Influence of quercetin on the development of nasal allergy-like symptoms in OVA-sensitized mice after the OVA nasal challenge. BALB/c mice were sensitized by an intraperitoneal injection of OVA on days 0, 7, and 14. Seven days after the final sensitization, the OVA-sensitized mice were intranasally challenged with OVA on days 21, 23, and 25, and various concentrations of quercetin were administered orally once a day for five consecutive days. Nasal allergy-like symptoms, the number of sneezes (**A**), and nasal rubbing behaviors (**B**) were counted for 10 min immediately after the final nasal antigenic challenge. The data are expressed as the mean $\pm$ SE of five mice. NS: non-sensitized; IS: intraperitoneal sensitization; NC: nasal challenge alone; QRC: quercetin.

4. Discussion

The results obtained from the in vitro experiments clearly show that quercetin can increase the ability of HNEpCs to produce TRX in response to H_2O_2 stimulation. The minimum concentration that caused a significant increase in TRX production was 1.0 nM.

After the oral administration of 64 mg of quercetin to humans, quercetin plasma levels gradually increased and attained peak at 650 nM, with a half-life elimination of 17–24 h [25]. Although there is no standard recommended dosage of quercetin, a dose of 1200 to 1500 mg per day is commonly used [26] as a supplement. It is also observed that a 1200 mg dose could lead to a plasma concentration of up to 12 μM [25], which is higher than the concentration necessary to induce the increase in the ability of HNEpCs to produce TRX in vitro. Based on these reports, the findings of the present in vitro study may reflect the biological function of quercetin in vivo. At present, we cannot exclude the possibility that the stimulation of thioredoxin production at higher concentrations of hydrogen peroxide and quercetin may be cellular protective mechanism against the cytotoxicity induced by these agents. Further experiments are needed to test this possibility.

AR is defined as an allergic inflammation of the nasal mucosa and is characterized by a symptom complex that consists of any combination of sneezing, nasal congestion, and nasal itching, among others [1,2]. These symptoms are primarily induced by chemical mediators from mast cells, such as histamine, tryptase, and kinin [1,2]. These mediators also recruit other inflammatory cells, including neutrophils and eosinophils, to the mucosa [1]. These polymorphonuclear leukocytes secrete harmful granular proteins and ROS, which cause tissue remodeling and persistent AR [18,27]. Because ROS are necessary for life, the body initiates several mechanisms to decrease ROS-induced tissue damage and to repair damage that occurs, including several enzymes and proteins [19]. Among these mechanisms, TRX attracts attention as not only an important anti-oxidative factor but also as a protective factor in the development of various inflammatory diseases, including AR [22,23]. TRX is reported to suppress eosinophil chemotaxis induced by CC chemokine stimulation through the suppression of both the activation of extracellular signal-regulated kinase 1/2 and p38 mitogen-activated protein kinase pathways [28]. Treating mice with TRX inhibits the development of airway inflammation and the overproduction of macrophage inflammatory protein (MIP)-1, RANTES, IL-4, and IL-5, which are responsible for the development of allergic inflammatory responses [22,23]. Furthermore, airway remodeling and eosinophilic inflammation induced by chronic antigen exposure were prevented in TRX transgenic mice that displayed overproduction of TRX [23]. Together with these reports, the present results obtained in in vivo experiments suggest that quercetin increases TRX production in the nasal mucosa and results in a favorable modification of the clinical conditions of AR. However, before concluding that the oral administration of quercetin in AR patients increases the ability of nasal cells, particularly epithelial cells, to produce TRX and attenuate the development of AR, we must examine the influence of quercetin on TRX production in vivo. Therefore, the second half of the study was performed to examine whether quercetin could also increase the ability of nasal cells to produce TRX after specific allergen inhalation and whether this activity was related to the development of nasal allergy-like symptoms in OVA-sensitized mice. The present in vivo data showed that nasal lavage fluids obtained from sensitized-non-treated mice contained higher levels of lipid peroxide compared to those from non-sensitized mice. Moreover, the oral administration of quercetin decreased lipid peroxide levels and increased TRX levels in nasal lavage fluids. Furthermore, the oral administration of quercetin to OVA-sensitized mice inhibited the development of nasal allergy-like symptoms after the OVA nasal challenge. The minimum concentration that caused significant changes in these parameters was 20 mg/kg. From these results, it can be reasonably interpreted that the actions of quercetin on TRX production may represent a possible mechanism that can explain the favorable effects of quercetin on AR.

The present data clearly show that quercetin enhances the ability of nasal cells to produce TRX in response to stimulation with either H_2O_2 or specific allergens in vitro and in vivo, despite the suppression of TRX mRNA expression. Furthermore, our previous report clearly showed that quercetin inhibited the production of chemokines, such as eotaxin and macrophage inflammatory protein-1beta (MIP-1β), by suppressing the mRNA expression of chemokines in eosinophils after stem cell factor simulation [29]. Furthermore, quercetin exerts suppressive effects on the activation of transcription factors, which are essential for several types of endogenous immune-modulatory proteins [30]. Synthesis of proteins in cells requires two quite different steps: in transcription, the first step, specific mRNA is synthetized from DNA in the nucleus. The newly synthetized mRNA travels through the nuclear membrane into the cytoplasm where it binds to mRNA-binding sites on ribosomes and initiates protein synthesis, which is called translation. From these established concepts, there is a possibility that quercetin increases the translatable activity of TRX mRNA and results in the production and secretion of large amounts of TRX from nasal epithelial cells after stimulation. Although glucocorticoids, which are considered first-line therapeutic agents in the treatment of AR [2], are accepted to exert their immune-modulatory effects by suppressing inflammatory mediator mRNA expression, they can increase the ability of cells to produce an immune-modulatory peptide, uteroglobin, after inflammatory stimulations by enhancing the translation of uteroglobin mRNA [31,32]. These reports support the speculation that the translation of TRX mRNA is enhanced by quercetin and results in the appearance of a large amount of TRX in both culture supernatants and nasal secretions.

Oral allergy syndrome (OAS), also recognized as pollen-food syndrome, is an allergic response in the oral cavity following the ingestion of fruits, vegetables, or nuts. OAS reportedly occurs in approximately 20–70% of patients with AR and atopy [33]. Pollen-specific IgE antibodies in AR patients recognize homologous dietary allergens that share the same epitopes of pollen and trigger the cross-reaction between allergens in pollens and those in foods, resulting in the development of OAS [33]. OAS includes several allergic reactions that occur very rapidly, within minutes of eating a trigger food. The most common symptoms are itchy mouth, scratchy throat, or swelling of the lips, tongue, and throat [33,34]. Although no standard treatment for OAS exists, antihistamines and oral steroids can help relieve symptoms [33], which suggests that quercetin will be a good candidate to supplement the treatment of OAS.

5. Conclusions

The results obtained from the present experiments strongly suggest that quercetin increases the ability of nasal epithelial cells, to produce TRX after stimulation with oxidants or allergens. Moreover, quercetin results in the attenuation of development of the clinical symptoms of AR by suppressing oxidative stress responses in nasal mucosa.

Author Contributions: Cell culture and assay for thioredoxin and lipid peroxide, Y.E.; animal experiments, statistical analysis of the data, and drawing figures, A.O.; conceptualization, study design, and manuscript writing, K.A.

References

1. Pawankar, R.; Mori, S.; Ozu, C.; Kimura, S. Overview on the pathomechanisms of allergic rhinitis. *Asia Pac. Allergy* **2011**, *1*, 157–167. [CrossRef] [PubMed]

2. Ramirez-Jimenez, F.; Pavon-Romero, G.; Juarez-Martinez, L.L.; Teran, L.M. Allergic rhinitis. *J. Allergy Ther.* **2012**, *S5*, 006. [CrossRef]

3. Jung, D.; Lee, S.; Hong, S. Effects of acupuncture and moxibustion in a mouse model of allergic rhinitis. *Otolaryngol. Head Neck Surg.* **2011**, *146*, 19–25. [CrossRef] [PubMed]

4. Jeong, K.T.; Kim, S.G.; Lee, J.; Park, Y.N.; Park, H.H.; Parl, N.Y.; Kim, K.J.; Lee, H.; Lee, Y.J. Anti-allergic effect of a Korean traditional medicine, Biyeom-Tang on mast cells and allergic rhinitis. *BMC Comp. Altern. Med.* **2014**, *14*, 54. [CrossRef] [PubMed]

5. Van Cauwenberg, P.; Bachert, C.; Passalacua, G. Consensus statement on the treatment of allergic rhinitis. European Academy of Allergology and Clinical Immunology. *Allergy* **2000**, *55*, 116–134. [CrossRef]

6. Ishizawa, K.; Yoshizumi, M.; Kawai, Y.; Terao, J.; Kihira, Y.; Ikeda, Y.; Tomita, S.; Minakuchi, K.; Tsuchiya, K.; Tamaki, T. Pharmacology in health food: Metabolism of quercetin in vivo and its protective effect against arteriosclerosis. *J. Pharmacol. Sci.* **2011**, *115*, 466–470. [CrossRef] [PubMed]

7. Hattori, M.; Mizuguchi, H.; Baba, Y.; Ono, S.; Nakano, T.; Zhang, Q.; Sasaki, Y.; Kobayashi, M.; Kitamura, Y.; Takeda, N.; et al. Quercetin inhibits transcriptional up-regulation of histamine H1 receptor via suppressing protein kinase C-δ/extracellular signal-regulated kinase/poly (ADP-ribose) polymerase-1 signaling pathway in Hela cells. *Int. Immunopharmacol.* **2013**, *15*, 232–239. [CrossRef] [PubMed]

8. Kawada, N.; Seki, S.; Inoue, M.; Kuroki, T. Effect of antioxidants, resveratrol, quercetin, and N-acetylcysteine, on the functions of cultured rat hapatic stellate cells and kupper cells. *Hepatology* **1998**, *27*, 1265–1274. [CrossRef] [PubMed]

9. Amorati, R.; Baschieri, A.; Cowde, A.; Valgimigli, L. The antioxidant activity of quercetin in water solution. *Biomimetics* **2017**, *2*, 9. [CrossRef]

10. Lesjak, M.; Beara, I.; Simin, N.; Pintac, D.; Majkic, T.; Bekvalac, K.; Orcic, D.; Mimica-Dukic, N. Antioxidant and anti-inflammatory activities of quercetin and its derivatives. *J. Funct. Foods* **2018**, *40*, 68–75. [CrossRef]

11. Middleton, E., Jr. Effect of plant flavonoids on immune and inflammatory cell function. *Adv. Exp. Med. Biol.* **1998**, *439*, 175–182. [PubMed]

12. Min, Y.D.; Choi, C.H.; Bark, H.; Son, H.Y.; Park, H.H.; Lee, S.; Park, J.W.; Park, E.K.; Shin, H.I.; Kim, S.H. Quercetin inhibits expression of inflammatory cytokines through attenuation of NF-kB and P38 MAPK in HMC-1 human mast cell line. *Inflamm. Res.* **2007**, *56*, 210–215. [CrossRef] [PubMed]

13. Hirano, T.; Kawai, M.; Arimitsu, J.; Ogawa, M.; Kuwahara, Y.; Hagihara, K.; Shima, Y.; Narazaki, M.; Ogata, A.; Koyanagi, M.; et al. Preventive effect of a flavonoid, enzymatically modified isoquercetin on ocular symptoms of Japanese cedar pollinosis. *Allergol. Int.* **2009**, *58*, 373–382. [CrossRef] [PubMed]

14. Rogerio, A.P.; Kanashiro, A.; Fontanari, C.; de Silva, E.V.; Lucisano-Valim, Y.M.; Soares, E.G.; Faccioli, L.H. Anti-inflammatory activity of quercetin and isoquercetin in experimental murine allergic asthma. *Inflamm. Res.* **2007**, *56*, 402–408. [CrossRef] [PubMed]

15. Dorsch, W.; Bittinger, M.; Kaas, A.; Muller, A.; Kreher, B.; Wagner, H. Antiasthmatic effects of *Galphimia glauca*, gallic acid, and related compounds prevent allergen- and platelet-activating factor-induced bronchial obstruction as well as bronchial hyperreactivity in guinea pigs. *Int. Arch. Allergy Immunol.* **1992**, *97*, 1–7. [CrossRef] [PubMed]

16. Kashiwabara, M.; Asano, K.; Mizuyoshi, T.; Kobayashi, H. Suppression of neuropeptide production by quercetin in allergic rhinitis model rats. *BMC Comp. Altern. Med.* **2016**, *16*, 132. [CrossRef] [PubMed]

17. Min, A.; Lee, Y.A.; Kim, K.; El-Benna, J.; Shin, M.H. Nox2-derived ROS-mediated surface translocation of BLT1 is essential for exocytosis in human eosinophils induced by LBT4. *Int. Arch. Allergy Immunol.* **2014**, *165*, 40–51. [CrossRef] [PubMed]

18. Suojalehto, H.; Vehmas, T.; Lindstrom, I.; Kennedy, D.W.; Kilpelainen, M.; Plosila, T.; Savukoski, S.; Sipilä, J.; Varpula, M.; Wolff, H.; et al. Nasal nitric oxide is dependent on sinus obstruction in allergic rhinitis. *Laryngoscope* **2014**, *124*, E231–E238. [CrossRef] [PubMed]

19. Sen, S.; Chakraborty, R.; Sridhar, C.; Reddy, Y.S.R.; De, B. Free radicals, antioxidants, diseases and phytomedicines: Current status and future prospect. *Int. J. Pharm. Sci. Rev. Res.* **2010**, *3*, 91–100.

20. Burke-Gaffney, A.; Callister, M.E.J.; Nakamura, H. Thioredoxin: Friend or foe in human disease. *Trends Pharmacol. Sci.* **2005**, *26*, 398–404. [CrossRef] [PubMed]

21. Holmgren, A.; Lu, J. Thioredoxin and thioredoxin reductase: Current research with special reference to human disease. *Biochem. Biophys. Res. Commun.* **2010**, *396*, 120–124. [CrossRef] [PubMed]

22. Ichiki, H.; Hoshino, T.; Kinoshita, T.; Imaoka, H.; Kato, S.; Inoue, H.; Nakamura, H.; Yodoi, J.; Young, H.A.; Aizawa, H. Thioredoxin suppresses airway hyperresponsiveness and airway inflammation in asthma. *Biochem. Biophys. Res. Commun.* **2005**, *334*, 1141–1148. [CrossRef] [PubMed]

23. Imaoka, H.; Hoshino, T.; Takei, S.; Sakazaki, Y.; Kinoshita, T.; Okamoto, M.; Kawayama, T.; Yodoi, J.; Kato, S.; Iwanaga, T.; et al. Effects of thioredoxin on established airway remodeling in a chronic antigen exposure asthma model. *Biochem. Biophys. Res. Commun.* **2007**, *360*, 525–530. [CrossRef] [PubMed]

24. Suzaki, I.; Asano, K.; Kanei, A.; Suzaki, H. Enhancement of thioredoxin production from nasal epithelial cells by the macrolide antibiotic, Clarithromycin in vitro. *Vivo* **2013**, *27*, 351–356.

25. Hollman, P.C.; vd Gaag, M.; Mengelers, M.J.; van Trijp, J.M.; de Vries, J.H.; Katan, M.B. Absorption and disposition kinetics of the dietary antioxidant quercetin in man. *Free Radic. Biol. Med.* **1996**, *21*, 703–707. [CrossRef]

26. Wadsworth, T.L.; Koop, D.R. Effects of *Ginkgo biloba* extract (EGb 761) and quercetin on lipopolysaccharide-induced release of nitric oxide. *Biochem. Pharmacol.* **2001**, *137*, 43–58. [CrossRef]

27. Imoto, Y.; Yamada, T.; Tsukahara, H.; Kimura, Y.; Kato, Y.; Sakashita, M.; Fujieda, S. Nitrite/nitrate in nasal lavage fluid reflect nasal symptoms after a single nasal allergen provocation in patients with seasonal allergic rhinitis. *J. Investig. Allergol. Clin. Immunol.* **2015**, *25*, 382–384. [PubMed]

28. Sannohe, S.; Adachi, T.; Hamada, K.; Honda, K.; Yamada, Y.; Saito, N.; Cui, C.H.; Kayaba, H.; Ishikawa, K.; Chihara, J. Upregulated response to chemokines in oxidative metabolism of eosinophils in asthma and allergic rhinitis. *Eur. Respir. J.* **2003**, *21*, 925–931. [CrossRef] [PubMed]

29. Sakai-Kashiwabara, M.; Abe, S.; Asano, K. Suppressive activity of quercetin on the production of eosinophil chemoattractants from eosinophils in vitro. *Vivo* **2014**, *28*, 515–522.

30. Irie, S.; Kashiwabara, M.; Yamada, A.; Asano, K. Suppressive activity of quercetin on periostin functions in vitro. *Vivo* **2016**, *30*, 17–25.

31. Lopez, M.S.; Nieto, A. Glucocorticoids induce the expression of the uteroglobin gene in rabbit fetal lung explants cultured in vitro. *Biochem. J.* **1985**, *225*, 255–258. [CrossRef]

32. Fernandez-Renau, D.; Lombardero, M.; Nieto, A. Glucocorticoid-dependent uteroglobin synthesis and uteroglobin mRNA levels in rabbit lung explants cultured in vitro. *Eur. J. Biochem.* **1984**, *144*, 523–527. [CrossRef] [PubMed]

33. Price, A.; Ramachandran, S.; Ramachandran, S.; Smith, G.P.; Stevenson, M.L.; Pomeranz, M.K.; Cohen, D.E. Oral allergy syndrome (Pollen-food allergy syndrome). *Dermatitis* **2015**, *26*, 78–88. [CrossRef] [PubMed]

34. Lessof, M.H. Pollen-food allergy syndrome. *J. Allergy Clin. Immunol.* **1996**, *98*, 239–240. [CrossRef]

6

Molecular Aspects of Drug-Induced Gingival Overgrowth: An In Vitro Study on Amlodipine and Gingival Fibroblasts

Dorina Lauritano [1,*,†], **Alberta Lucchese** [2,†], **Dario Di Stasio** [2], **Fedora Della Vella** [3], **Francesca Cura** [4], **Annalisa Palmieri** [4] and **Francesco Carinci** [5]

[1] Department of Medicine and Surgery, Centre of Neuroscience of Milan, University of Milano-Bicocca, 20126 Milan, Italy

[2] Multidisciplinary Department of Medical and Dental Specialties, University of Campania- Luigi Vanvitelli, 80138 Naples, Italy; alberta.lucchese@unicampania.it (A.L.); dario.distasio@unicampania.it (D.D.S.)

[3] Interdisciplinary Department of Medicine, University of Bari, 70121 Bari, Italy; fedora.dellavella@uniba.it

[4] Department of Experimental, Diagnostic and Specialty Medicine, University of Bologna, via Belmoro 8, 40126 Bologna, Italy; cura.francesca@tiscali.it (F.C.); annalisa.palmieri@unife.it (A.P.)

[5] Department of Morphology, Surgery and Experimental Medicine, University of Ferrara, 44121 Ferrara, Italy; crc@unife.it

* Correspondence: dorina.lauritano@unimib.it

† Co-first authorship.

Abstract: Gingival overgrowth is a serious side effect that accompanies the use of amlodipine. Several conflicting theories have been proposed to explain the fibroblast's function in gingival overgrowth. To determine whether amlodipine alters the fibrotic response, we investigated its effects on treated gingival fibroblast gene expression as compared with untreated cells. Materials and Methods: Fibroblasts from ATCC® Cell Lines were incubated with amlodipine. The gene expression levels of 12 genes belonging to the "Extracellular Matrix and Adhesion Molecules" pathway was investigated in treated fibroblasts cell culture, as compared with untreated cells, by real time PCR. Results: Most of the significant genes were up-regulated. (*CTNND2, COL4A1, ITGA2, ITGA7, MMP10, MMP11, MMP12, MMP26*) except for *COL7A1, LAMB1, MMP8,* and *MMP16*, which were down-regulated. Conclusion: These results seem to demonstrate that amlodipine has an effect on the extracellular matrix of gingival fibroblast. In the future, it would be interesting to understand the possible effect of the drug on fibroblasts of patients with amlodipine-induced gingival hyperplasia.

Keywords: Gingival overgrowth; gene expression; drugs; amlodipine

1. Introduction

Gingival overgrowth may have multiple causes, however drugs assumption is the most common [1,2]. In addiction, drug-induced gingival overgrowth may be associated with a patient's genetic predisposition [3,4].

The three main classes of drugs inducing gingival overgrowth are anticonvulsants, immunosuppressive, and antihypertensive agents [3,5–7]. The first report regarding gingival overgrowth by the administration of amlodipine was published in 1994 [8]. Subsequently, other authors reported the onset of gingival overgrowth as a side effect in patients who received 10 mg per day of amlodipine within two months [9]. Gingival overgrowth manifests as a side effect within one to three months after amlodipine administration [7,10]. Amlodipine shows a pharmacological profile, as follows: long-acting dihydropyridine; coronary and peripheral arterial vasodilatation; headaches, facial flushing, dizziness, and oedema. The main oral side effect that is induced by amlodipine is gingival overgrowth [11,12].

Gingival overgrowth that is induced by amlodipine (GOIA) must be stimulated by a threshold concentration of amlodipine [13]. However the severity of GOIA is supposed to be related to the concentration of amlodipine in oral fluids [13]. The mean dose of amlodipine reported to cause GOIA in most of the subjects is 5 mg/day. Therefore, it may be suggested that the dosage and duration of amlodipine may have an impact on GOIA [13]. Usually, the gingival manifestations of GOIA appear within the first three months of the drug administration [14]. A longer duration of therapy may increase the exposure of cells to amlodipine, and this may modify the apoptosis of cells, resulting in hyperplasia [14]. Genetic susceptibility is one the factors influencing the severity of GOIA; in fact multidrug resistant (MDR1) gene polymorphisms is supposed to alter the inflammatory response to the amlodipine [15].

Poor plaque control is another risk factor in developing of GOIA. In fact, GOIA hampered routine oral hygiene measures. Additionally, GOIA can favour the accumulation of bacterial plaque, which in turn determines gingival inflammation, causing gingival overgrowth [14]. Amlodipoine, in presence of proinflammatory cytokines (for example TNF-α), may favour the inhibition of apoptosis of human gingival fibroblasts, thus promoting hyperplasia [16].

1.1. Genetic Factors

Evidence suggests that genetic factors, along with patient susceptibility, may play an important role in the pathogenesis of GOIA [15]. A genetic predisposition can influence a number of factors in the drug interactions, cells, and plaque-induced inflammation. These include the functional heterogeneity of gingival fibroblasts, the collagenolytic activity, the drug-receptor binding, the drug metabolism, collagen synthesis, and many other factors.

Since most types of pharmacological agents that are implicated in GOIA can have negative effects on the flow of calcium ions across cell membranes, it has been postulated that these agents can interfere with the synthesis and function of the collagenase [17]. This mechanism of action has been demonstrated for Cyclosporine. In fact, a recent study in vitro have shown that human gingival fibroblasts that were treated with relevant doses of Cyclosporine show significantly reduced levels of secretion of MMP-1 and MMP-3; these reduced levels can contribute to the accumulation of components of the extracellular matrix [18]. An animal study that showed low mRNA levels of collagenase in situ further supported these results, accompanied by a decrease in phagocytosis and degradation of collagen [19]. The genetic predisposition to GOIA has been studied for cyclosporine, while, for what we know, not yet for amlodipine.

1.2. Objective

To determine whether amlodipine can alter the matrix deposition, we investigated its effects on treated gingival fibroblast gene expression as compared with untreated cells.

2. Results

The PrestoBlue™ cell viability test was conducted to determine the optimal concentration of amlodipine to be used for cell treatment that did not significantly affect cell viability. Based on this test, the concentration used for the treatment was 1000 ng/mL.

The gene expression profile of 12 genes belonging to the "Extracellular Matrix and Adhesion Molecules" pathway was analysed using Real time PCR (Figure 1). Table 1 reported the list gene and their fold change.

AMLODIPINE

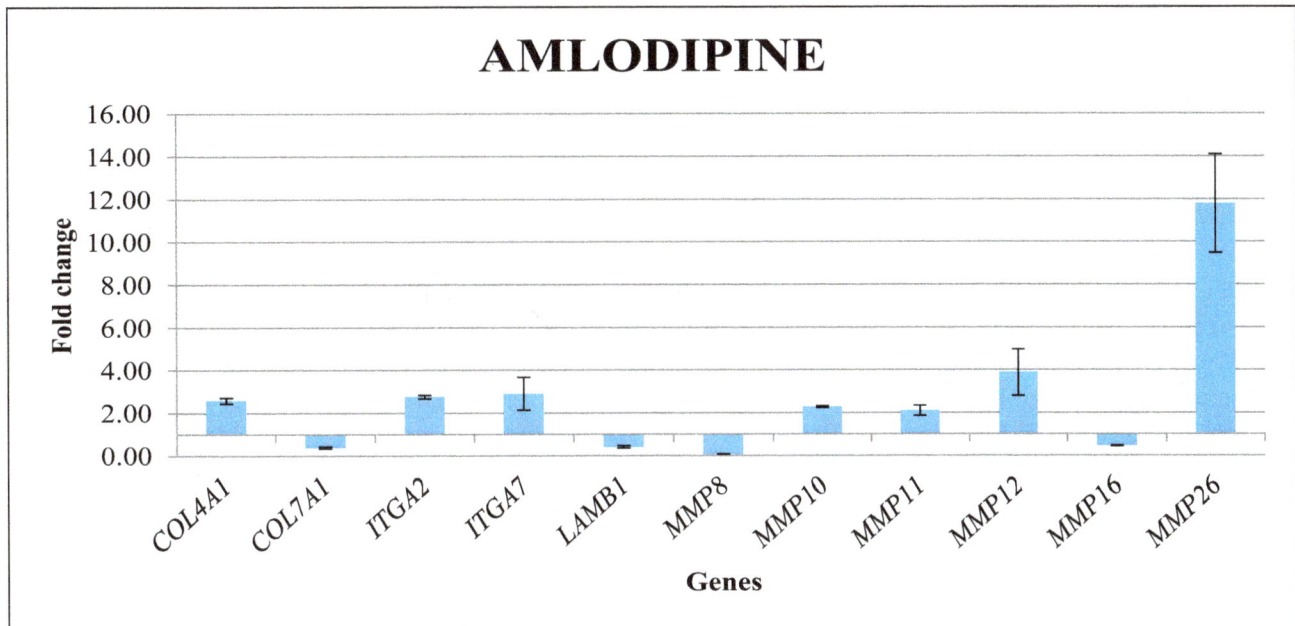

Figure 1. Gene expression profile of fibroblast treated with Amlodipine 1000 ng/mL.

Table 1. Significant gene expression levels after 24 h treatment with Amlodipine, as compared with untreated cells.

Gene	Fold Change	SD (+/−)	Gene Function
CTNND2	2.29	0.03	Cell Adhesion Molecule
COL4A1	2.57	0.13	Collagens & Extracellular Matrix Structural constituent
COL7A1	0.38	0.04	Collagens & Extracellular Matrix Structural constituent
ITGA2	2.75	0.08	Transmembrane Receptor
ITGA7	2.90	0.77	Transmembrane Receptor
LAMB1	0.41	0.05	Basement Membrane Constituent
MMP8	0.06	0.01	Extracellular Matrix Protease
MMP10	2.27	0.03	Extracellular Matrix Protease
MMP11	2.09	0.24	Extracellular Matrix Protease
MMP12	3.88	1.09	Extracellular Matrix Protease
MMP16	0.44	0.02	Extracellular Matrix Protease
MMP26	11.78	2.31	Extracellular Matrix Protease

Bold fonts indicate significant variation of gene expression level: fold change ≥ 2 and p value ≤ 0.05 for up-regulated genes, and fold change ≤ 0.5 and p value ≤ 0.05 for the significantly down-regulated genes.

Among the up-regulated genes, there was *CTNND2*, which code for the cell adhesion protein Catenin Delta 2. Other up-regulated gens were the transmembrane receptor *ITGA2* and *ITGA7* and the basement membrane constituent *LAMB1*. Most of the extracellular matrix proteases were up-regulated (*MMP10, MMP11, MMP12, MMP26*), except for *MMP8* and *MMP16*, which were down-regulated. Other genes that were significantly deregulated genes following the treatment with Amlodipine were *COL7A1*, which was down-regulated and the *COL4A1* that was up-regulated. In Figure 1 the significantly expression levels of the genes up- and down-regulated in fibroblast cells treated with amlodipine were represented.

3. Discussion

The prevalence of GOIA might be as high as 38%, and it is 3.3 times more common in men than in women [20,21]. The pathogenesis may be different for different drugs, even if the oral manifestations of gingival overgrowth are similar. GOIA starts as an enlargement of the interdental papilla of keratinized portions of the gingiva, and it is characterized by an increase in the connective tissue component. Bacteria accumulation appears to be an important uncomfortable effect of GOIA. GOIA may impair oral hygiene and lead to increased oral infections. Oral infection itself is a cause of gingival overgrowth [22]. In addiction, oral infection can potentially impair systemic health and could possibly compromise the general health of patients [22].

The mechanism of action of GOIA is still unknown, however it may be a consequence of the interaction between gingival fibroblasts, cellular and biochemical mediators of inflammation, and drug metabolites [22,23].

Gingival overgrowth is documented more frequently after intake of with phenytoin and rarely with others antihypertensive [24]. Furthermore, poor oral hygiene is indicated as an important risk factor for the expression of GOIA [25,26].

Cross-sectional studies have reported the relationship between bacterial plaque and GOIA. In fact, as previously reported, GOIA can favour the accumulation of bacterial plaque, which in turn determines gingival inflammation, causing gingival overgrowth [26]. The underlying mechanism of GOIA still remains to be fully understood, however two main inflammatory and non-inflammatory pathways have already been suggested [27–29]. One hypothesis may be that amlodipine may induce the alteration of collagenase activity as a consequence of decreased uptake of folic acid, blockage of aldosterone synthesis in adrenal cortex, and consequent feedback increase in the adrenocorticotropic hormone level and the up-regulation of keratinocyte growth factor [30]. Besides, inflammation may be a consequence of the toxic effect of amlodipine in periodontal pocket associated with C pathogens, leading to the up-regulation of several cytokine factors, such as transforming growth factor-beta 1 (TGF-β1) [9]. Another pathogenic mechanism of GOIA is focusing on the effects of amlodipine on gingival fibroblast metabolism and genetic predisposition. In fact, only a subgroup of patients that were treated with this amlodipine will develop GOIA, so it has been hypothesized that these individuals show an abnormal susceptibility to the drug. In fact, elevated levels of protein synthesis, most of which is collagen, characterize the fibroblast of GOIA in these patients. Treatment of GOIA is generally targeted on drug substitution and preventive protocols [12,31]. Surgical intervention is recommended when these measures fail to cause the resolution of GOIA. These treatment modalities, although effective, do not necessarily prevent the recurrence of the lesions [12]. Surgery for treatment of GOIA must be carefully assessed and it is normally performed for cosmetic/aesthetic needs before any functional consequences are present [1,32]. Most reports of GOIA have required surgical intervention [25].

To our knowledge, our study is the first one analysing the effect of amlodipine on genes that belong to the "Extracellular Matrix and Adhesion Molecules" pathway. In this study, gingival fibroblasts were treated for 24 h with 1000 ng/mL of amlodipine. The gene expression profile of 12 genes that belong to the "Extracellular Matrix and Adhesion Molecules" pathway was analysed. Most of the significant genes were up-regulated. (CTNND2, COL4A1, ITGA2, ITGA7, MMP10, MMP11, MMP12, MMP26), except for COL7A1, LAMB1, MMP8, and MMP16, which were down-regulated. These proteins preferentially induce extra cellular matrix deposition. This study demonstrated that, in human gingival fibroblasts that were cultivated in vitro, amlodipine could promote the activities of genes belonging to the "fibroblast matrix and receptors".

It might be part of the underlying reason for the persistent overgrowth of gingiva that was seen when bacterial plaque and local inflammation are present during amlodipine therapy. In fact, GOIA does not allow patient to maintain a good oral hygiene, and this is the reason why GOIA always determines the presence of bacterial plaque and inflammation, which in turn determines gingival overgrowth.

The data presented here suggest that amlodipine may contribute to an extracellular matrix deposition of human gingival fibroblasts inducing gingival overgrowth.

4. Materials and Methods

4.1. Primary Human Fibroblast Cells Culture

We used cells from ATCC® Cell Lines. The cryopreserved cells at the second passage were cultured in 75 cm² culture flasks containing DMEM medium (Sigma Aldrich, Inc., St Louis, Mo, USA) supplemented with 20% fetal calf serum, antibiotics (Penicillin 100U/ml and Streptomycin 100 micrograms/ml-Sigma Aldrich, Inc., St Louis, Mo, USA).

Cell cultures were replicated for subsequent experiments and maintained in a water saturated atmosphere at 37 °C and 5% CO_2.

4.2. Cell Viability Test

A stock solution of amlodipine 1 mg/mL was prepared. Further dilutions were made with the culture medium to the desired concentrations just before use. The cell lines were seeded into 96-well plates at a density of 104 cells per well containing 100 µL of cell culture medium and incubated for 24 h to allow cell adherence. Serial dilution of amlodipine (5000 ng/mL, 2000 ng/mL, 1000 ng/mL, 500 ng/mL, 100 ng/mL) was added (three wells for each concentration). The cell culture medium alone was used negative control.

After 24 h of incubation, cell viability was measured while using PrestoBlue™ Reagent Protocol (Invitrogen, Carlsbad, CA, USA) according to the manufacturer's instructions. Briefly, the PrestoBlue™ solution (10 µL) was added into each well containing 90 µL of treatment solution. The plates were then placed back into the incubator for 1 h, after which absorbance was measured at wavelengths of 570 nm excitation and 620 nm emission by an automated microplate reader (Sunrise™, Tecan Trading AG, Switzerland). Comparing the average absorbance in drug treated wells with average absorbance in control wells exposed to vehicle alone determined the percentage of viable cells.

4.3. Cell Treatment

Gingival fibroblasts were seeded at a density of 1.0×10^5 cells/ml into 9 cm² (3 mL) wells and then subjected to serum starvation for 16 hours at 37 °C. Cells were treated with 1000 ng/mL amlodipine solution for 24 h. This solution was obtained in DMEM that was supplemented with 2% FBS, antibiotics and aminoacids. Cell medium alone was used as control negative. The cells were maintained in a humidified atmosphere of 5% CO_2 at 37 °C. After the end of the exposure time, the cells were trypsinized and processed for RNA extraction.

4.4. RNA Isolation, Reverse Transcription and Quantitative Real-Time RT-PCR

Total RNA was isolated from cultured cells using GenElute mammalian total RNA purification miniprep kit (Sigma-Aldrich, Inc., St Louis, Mo, USA), according to manufacturer's instructions. Pure RNA was quantified at NanoDrop 2000 spectrophotometer (Thermo Scientific, Waltham, Massachusetts, USA).

cDNA synthesis was performed, starting from 500 ng of total RNA, using PrimeScript RT Master Mix (Takara Bio Inc, Kusatsu, Japan). The reaction was incubated at 37 °C for 15 min. and inactivated by heating at 70 °C for 10 s.

cDNA was amplified by Real Time Quantitative PCR using the ViiA™ 7 System (Applied Biosystems, Foster City, CA, USA).

All of the PCR reactions were performed in a 20 µL volume. Each reaction contained 10 µL of 2x qPCRBIO SYGreen Mix Lo-ROX (Pcrbiosystems, London, UK), 400 nM concentration of each primer, and cDNA. Table 2 reported the sequences of the primer that was used in the reaction.

Table 2. Primers sequences of SYBR® Green assay.

Gene Name	Forward Sequence 5′ > 3′	Reverse Sequence 5′ > 3′
CTNND2	AGAGAATTTGGATGGAGAGAC	TTGTTGTCTCCAAAACAGAG
COL4A1	AAAGGGAGATCAAGGGATAG	TCACCTTTTTCTCCAGGTAG
COL7A1	ATGACCTTGGCATTATCTTG	TGAATATGTCACCTCTCAAGG
ITGA2	GGTGGGGTTAATTCAGTATG	ATATTGGGATGTCTGGGATG
ITGA7	CATGAACAATTTGGGTTCTG	GCCCTTCCAATTATAGGTTC
LAMB1	GTGTGTATAGATACTTCGCC	AAAGCACGAAATATCACCTC
MMP8	AAGTTGATGCAGTTTTCCAG	CTGAACTTCCCTTCAACATTC
MMP10	AGCGGACAAATACTGGAG	GTGATGATCCACTGAAGAAG
MMP11	GATAGACACCAATGAGATTGC	TTTGAAGAAAAAGAGCTCGC
MMP12	AGGTATGATGAAAGGAGACAG	AGGTATGATGAAAGGAGAACAG
MMP16	ACCCTCATGACTTGATAACC	TCTGTCTCCCTTGAAGAAATAG
MMP26	AAGGATCCAGCATTTGTATG	CTTTGATCCTCCAATAAACTCC
RPL13	AAAGCGGATGGTGGTTCCT	GCCCCAGATAGGCAAACTTTC

Custom primers belonging to the "Extracellular Matrix and Adhesion Molecules" pathway were purchased from Sigma Aldrich. All of the experiments were performed, including non-template controls to exclude reagents contamination. PCR was performed, including two analytical replicates.

The amplification profile was initiated by 10 min. incubation at 95 °C, followed by two-step amplification of 15 s at 95 °C and 60 s at 60 °C for 40 cycles. As final step, a melt curve dissociation analysis was performed.

4.5. Statistical Analysis

The gene expression levels were normalized to the expression of the reference gene (RPL13) and they were expressed as fold changes relative to the expression of the untreated cells. Quantification was done with the delta/delta Ct calculation method.

5. Conclusions

In this study, most of the significantly genes belonging to the "extracellular matrix proteases" pathway were up-regulated. These results seem to indicate that amlodipine has an effect on the modulation of fibrosis response in gingival fibroblasts, up-regulating extracellular matrix proteases, and favouring the deposition of fibrotic tissue. More explanatory results could probably be obtained by using gingival fibroblasts in which the use of amlodipine seems to aggravate the fibrotic response and the gingival overgrowth.

GOIA is no longer a rare occurrence. From one side, plaque accumulation is an inevitable consequence of GOIA, and from the other, it favours gingival inflammation and overgrowth. The duration of therapy, dosage, and individual genetic susceptibility are considered important risk factors for the development of GOIA. Amlodipine is a widely used drug for the treatment of hypertension and angina, so it is very important that doctors inform patients about side effects, such as GOIA, and about the importance of preventive protocols. Dentists should be able to identify the changes in the oral cavity that are related to the general health of their patients. The patients must be informed of the tendency of certain drugs to cause gingival overgrowth and the associated oral changes and the importance of effective oral hygiene.

Combination therapy consisting of surgical and non-surgical periodontal therapy with drug substitution is the most reliable method in the management of GOIA.

Combination therapy consisting of surgical and non-surgical periodontal therapy with drug substitution is the most reliable method in the management of GOIA.

Author Contributions: Conceptualization, D.L.; Data curation, A.L. and F.C. (Francesca Cura); Investigation, D.D.S.; Supervision, F.C. (Francesco Carinci); Visualization, F.D.V.; Writing—review & editing, A.P.

References

1. Amit, B.; Shalu, B.V. Gingival enlargement induced by anticonvulsants, calcium channel blockers and immunosuppressants: A review. *IRJP* **2012**, *3*, 116–119.
2. Ellis, J.S.; Seymour, R.A.; Steele, J.G.; Roberston, P.; Butler, T.J.; Thomason, J.M. Prevalence of gingival overgrowth induced by calcium channel blockers: A community based study. *J. Periodontol.* **1999**, *70*, 63–67.
3. Bharati, T.; Mukesh Tehmina Veenita Jain, V.V.; Jajoo, U.N. Amlodipine induced gum hypertrophy—A rare case report. *J. Mgims* **2012**, *17*, 63–64.
4. Newman, M.G.; Takei, H.H.; Klokkevold, P.R.; Carranza, F.A. *Carranza's Clinical Periodontology*, 10th ed.; Saunders: St Louis, MO, USA, 2006; pp. 373–377.
5. Drug associated gingival enlargement. *J. Periodontol.* **2004**, *75*, 1424–1431. [CrossRef]
6. Jorgensen, M.G. Prevalence of amlodipine-related gingival hyperplasia. *J. Periodontol.* **1997**, *68*, 676–678.
7. Jose, J.; Santhosh, Y.L.; Naveen, M.R.; Kumar, V. Case report of amlodipine induced gingival hyperplasia—Late onset at a low use. *Asian J. Pharm. Clin. Res.* **2011**, *4*, 65–66.
8. Seymour, R.A.; Ellis, J.S.; Thomason, J.M.; Monkman, S.; Idle, J.R. Amlodipine induced gingival overgrowth. *J. Clin. Periodontal* **1994**, *21*, 281–283.
9. Lafzi, A.; Farahani, R.M.; Shoja, M.A. Amlodipine induced gingival hyperplasia. *Med. Oral Patol. Oral Cir. Bucal.* **2006**, *11*, 480–482.
10. Meraw, S.J.; Sheridan, P.J. Medically induced gingival hyperplasia. *Mayo Clin. Proc.* **1996**, *73*, 1196–1199.
11. Ellis, J.S.; Seymour, R.A.; Monkman, S.C.; Idle, J.R. Gingival sequestration of nifedipine induced gingival overgrowth. *Lancet* **1992**, *39*, 1382–1383.
12. Grover, V.; Kapoor, A.; Marya, C.M. Amlodipine induced gingival hyperplasia. *J. Oral Health Comm. Dent.* **2007**, *1*, 19–22.
13. Daley, T.D.; Wysocki, G.P.; Day, C. Clinical and pharmacologic correlations in cyclosporine-induced gingival hyperplasia. *Oral Surg. Oral Med. Oral Pathol.* **1986**, *62*, 417–421.
14. Pasupuleti, M.K.; Musalaiah, S.V.; Nagasree, M.; Kumar, P.A. Combination of inflammatory and amlodipine induced gingival overgrowth in a patient with cardiovascular disease. *Avicenna J. Med.* **2013**, *3*, 68–72.
15. Meisel, P.; Giebel, J.; Kunert-Keil, C.; Dazert, P.; Kroemer, H.K.; Kocher, T. MDR1 gene polymorphisms and risk of gingival hyperplasia induced by calcium antagonists. *Clin. Pharm. Ther.* **2006**, *79*, 62–71.
16. Takeuchi, R.; Matsumoto, H.; Akimoto, Y.; Fujii, A. The inhibitory action of amlodipine for TNF-α-induced apoptosis in cultured human gingival fibroblasts. *Oral Ther. Pharmacol.* **2012**, *31*, 45–52.
17. Hassell, T.M. Evidence for production of an inactive collagenase by fibroblasts from phenytoin-enlarged human gingiva. *J. Oral Pathol.* **1982**, *11*, 310–317.
18. Bolzani, G.; Della Coletta, R.; Martelli Junior, H.; Martelli Junior, H.; Graner, E. Cyclosporin A inhibits production and activity of matrix metalloproteinases by gingival fibroblasts. *J. Periodontal Res.* **2000**, *35*, 51–58.
19. Kataoka, M.; Shimizu, Y.; Kunikiyo, K.; Asahara, Y.; Yamashita, K.; Ninomiya, M.; Morisaki, I.; Ohsaki, Y.; Kido, J.-I.; Nagata, T. Cyclosporin A decreases the degradation of type I collagen in rat gingival overgrowth. *J. Cell Physiol.* **2000**, *182*, 351–358.
20. Sucu, M.; Yuce, M.; Davatoglu, V. Amlodipine induced massive gingival hypertrophy. *Can. Fam. Phys.* **2011**, *57*, 436–437.
21. Prisant, L.M.; Herman, W. Calcium channel blocker induced gingival overgrowth. *J. Clin. Hypertens.* **2002**, *4*, 310–311.
22. Pradhan, S.; Mishra, P.; Joshi, S. Drug induced gingival enlargement—A review. *PGNM* **2009**, *8*.
23. Amgelpoulous, A.P.; Goaz, P.W. Incidence of diphenylhydantoin gingival hyperplasia. *Oral Surg. Oral Med. Oral Pathol.* **1972**, *34*, 898–906.

24. Hegde, R.; Kale, R.; Jain, A.S. Cyclosporine and amlodipine induced severe gingival overgrowth–etiopathogenesis and management of a case with electrocautery and carbon-dioxide (CO_2) laser. *J. Oral Health. Comm. Dent.* **2012**, *6*, 34–42.

25. Taib, H.; Ali, T.B.T.; Kamin, S. Amlodipine induced gingival overgrowth: A case report. *Arch. Orofac. Sci.* **2007**, *2*, 61–64.

26. Srivastava, A.K.; Kundu, D.; Bandyopadhyay, P.; Pal, A.K. Management of amlodipine induced gingival enlargement: A series of three cases. *J. Indian Soc. Perodontol.* **2010**, *14*, 279.

27. Khan, S.; Mittal, A.; Kanteshwari, I.K. Amlodipine induced gingival overgrowth: A case report. *NJDSR* **2012**, *1*, 65–69.

28. Routray, S.N.; Mishra, T.K.; Pattnaik, U.K.; Satapathy, C.; Mishra, C.K.; Behera, M. Amlodipine induced gingival hyperplasia. *J. Assoc. Phys. India* **2003**, *51*, 818–819.

29. Sharma, S.; Sharma, A. Amlodipine induced gingival enlargement—A clinical report. *Compend. Contin. Educ. Dent.* **2012**, *33*, 78–82.

30. Triveni, M.G.; Rudrakshi, C.; Mehta, D.S. Amlodipine induced gingival overgrowth. *J. Indian Soc. Periodontol.* **2009**, *13*, 160–163.

31. Marshall, R.I.; Bartold, P.M. A clinical review of drug induced gingival overgrowth. *Oral Surg. Oral Med. Oral Pathol.* **1993**, *76*, 543–548.

32. Lombardi, T.; Fiore, D.G.; Belser, U.; Di, F.R. Felodipine induced gingival hyperplasia: A clinical and histologic study. *J. Oral Pathol. Med.* **1991**, *20*, 89–92.

7

Kampo (Traditional Japanese Herbal) Formulae for Treatment of Stomatitis and Oral Mucositis

Masataka Sunagawa[ID]**, Kojiro Yamaguchi**[ID]**, Mana Tsukada, Nachi Ebihara, Hideshi Ikemoto and Tadashi Hisamitsu** *[ID]

Department of physiology, School of medicine, Showa University, Tokyo 142-8555, Japan;
suna@med.showa-u.ac.jp (M.S.); kampo5260@icloud.com (K.Y.); m-tsukada@med.showa-u.ac.jp (M.T.);
BYS00426@nifty.com (N.E.); h_ikemoto@med.showa-u.ac.jp (H.I.)
* Correspondence: tadashi@med.showa-u.ac.jp

Abstract: Stomatitis is occasionally multiple, recurrent, and refractory. Currently, mucositis induced by chemotherapy and radiation therapy in patients with cancer has become a significant clinical problem. Effective treatments have not been established and the treatment of numerous cases remains a challenge for physicians. Traditional Japanese herbal medicines termed Kampo formulae (i.e., Hangeshashinto, Orengedokuto, Inchinkoto, Orento, Byakkokaninjinto, Juzentaihoto, Hochuekkito, and Shosaikoto) are used for treating various types of stomatitis and mucositis. Its use has been based on the Kampo medical theories—empirical rules established over thousands of years. However, recently, clinical and basic research studies investigating these formulae have been conducted to obtain scientific evidence. Clinical studies investigating efficacies of Shosaikoto and Orento for the treatment of cryptogenic stomatitis and acute aphthous stomatitis and those investigating the effects of Hangeshashinto, Orengedokuto, and Juzentaihoto on chemotherapy- or radiotherapy-induced mucositis have been conducted. The Kampo formulae comprise several crude drugs, whose mechanisms of action are gradually being clarified. Most of these drugs that are used for the treatment of stomatitis possess anti-inflammatory, analgesic, and antioxidative properties. In this review, we introduce the clinical applications and summarize the available evidence on the Kampo formulae for the treatment of stomatitis and oral mucositis.

Keywords: kampo formula; traditional Japanese herbal medicine; stomatitis; mucositis; Hangeshashinto

1. Introduction

Stomatitis is a sore and often recurrent inflammatory condition of the oral mucosa, characterized by various symptoms such as the presence of vesicles, erosions, aphthae, and ulcerations. Stomatitis is caused by various factors such as viral, fungal, and bacterial infections, allergic reactions, loose-fitting dental prosthetics, and systemic diseases. Occasionally, stomatitis is multiple, recurrent, and refractory. Currently, mucositis induced by chemotherapy and radiation therapy in patients with cancer has become a significant clinical problem [1]. The pain associated with mucositis often affects a patient's functional status and quality of life.

Kampo formula, a traditional Japanese herbal medicine, has its root in ancient Chinese medicine, and the antecedent form of medicine was introduced to Japan between the 5th and 6th century. It was developed into an individual form of medicine adapting the constitutions of the Japanese people. Kampo formulae have been reported to be effective for the treatment of stomatitis and mucositis [2,3]. The objective of this review was to introduce the clinical applications and summarize the available evidence on the Kampo formulae for the treatment of these two conditions.

2. Clinical Applications

We conducted a questionnaire survey regarding the treatment of stomatitis using the Kampo formulae. According to the results, formulae such as Hangeshashinto (HST), Orengedokuto (OGT), Inchinkoto (ICT), Orento (ORT), Byakkokaninjinto (BKN), Juzentaihoto (JTT), Hochuekkito (HET), and Shosaikoto (SST) were used (Figure 1) [4]. The Kampo formulae are generally composed of at least two kinds of crude drugs and these combinations may suppress the development of infections, inflammation, concomitant oxidative stress, and the underlying causes of stomatitis. The chief ingredient and principal effects of each crude drug included in the formulae frequently used for the treatment of stomatitis are shown in Table 1. Many of these agents possess anti-inflammatory and/or analgesic properties. Of note, *Astragali* Radix, *Scutellariae* Radix, *Phellodendri* Cortex, *Coptidis* Rhizoma, *Glycyrrhizae* Radix, *Bupleuri* Radix, *Paeoniae* Radix, *Artemisiae Lanceae* Rhizoma, *Cimicifugae* Rhizoma, *Cnidii* Rhizoma, *Angelicae* Radix, and *Poria* exert anti-inflammatory effects. Moreover, *Cinnamomi* Cortex, *Cimicifugae* Rhizoma, *Paeoniae* Radix, *Glycyrrhizae* Radix, *Cnidii* Rhizoma, *Angelicae* Radix, *Zingiberis* Rhizoma Processum, and *Magnoliae* Cortex exert analgesic effects [5]. The occurrence of stomatitis is related to the generation of reactive oxygen species (ROS) [6]. Therefore, anti-oxidants contained in these medicinal herbs may effectively mitigate this damaging effect. Dragland et al. [7] assessed the contribution of culinary and medicinal herbs to the total dietary intake of anti-oxidants (Table 1). Notably, *Cinnamomi* Cortex, *Scutellariae* Radix, *Cimicifugae* Rhizoma, *Paeoniae* Radix, *Aurantii Nobilis* Pericarpium, and *Glycyrrhizae* Radix contain high concentrations of anti-oxidants.

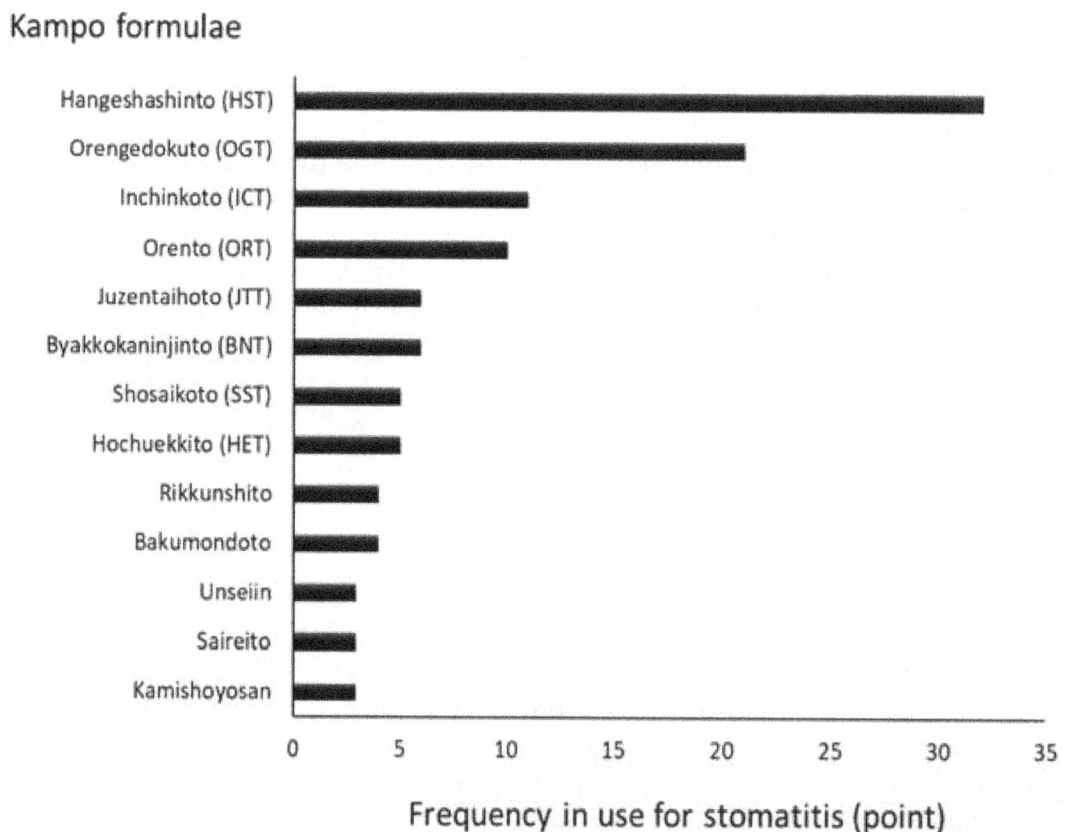

Figure 1. Kampo formulae frequently used for the treatment of stomatitis [4]. The trends in the use of the Kampo formulae at hospitals and faculties of oral surgery of dental/medical universities in Japan were surveyed. A total of 55 hospitals participated in the survey and rated the frequency of Kampo formulae use via a scale from 0 to 3. This graphic summarizes the results of rating.

Table 1. The Kampo formulae frequently used for the treatment of stomatitis and their corresponding crude drugs.

Crude Drug/ Japanese Name	Kampo Formulae									Antioxidant [7] (mmol/100 g)	Chief Ingredient	Principal Effects
	Hangeshashinto (HST)	Orento (ORT)	Orengedokuto (OGT)	Byakkokaninjinto (BKN)	Shosaikoto (SST)	Inchinkoto (ICT)	Heiisan (HIS)	Juzentaihoto (JTT)	Hochuekkito (HET)			
Cinnamomi Cortex Keihi		○						○		120.2	cinnamaldehyde	antipyresis, perspiration, analgesia
Scutellariae Radix Ogon	○		○		○					111.5	baicalin	anti-inflammation, antipyresis, laxative
Cimicifugae Rhizoma Shoma									○	64.3	cimigenol	anti-inflammation, antipyresis, analgesia, antiedema
Paeoniae Radix Shakuyaku								○		55.1	paeoniflorin	analgesia, spasmolysis, anti-inflammation
Aurantii Nobilis Pericarpium Chinpi							○		○	17.5	hesperidin	stomachic, antitussive
Glycyrrhizae Radix Kanzo	○	○		○	○		○	○	○	11.6	glycyrrhizin	anti-inflammation, analgesia, detoxification
Zingiberis Rhizoma Shokyo					○		○		○	7.5	gingerol	stomachic, antinausea
Atractylodis Lanceae Rhizoma Sojutsu							○	○	○	7.4	atractylodin	anti-inflammation, stomachic, diuresis
Cnidii Rhizoma Senkyu								○		6.7	cnidilide	analeptic, nourishing, anti-inflammation, analgesia
Zizyphi Fructus Taiso	○	○			○		○		○	5.9	zizyphus saponin	analeptic, nourishing, stomachic
Bupleuri Radix Saiko					○				○	5.7	saikosaponin	anti-inflammation, antipyresis
Astragali Radix Ogi								○	○	4.9	formononetin	anti-inflammation, analeptic, diuresis, hypotensive
Rhemanniae Radix Jio								○		3.9	catalpol	nourishing, diuresis
Angelicae Radix Toki								○	○	3.0	ligustilide	analeptic, nourishing, anti-inflammation, analgesia
Hoelen Bukuryo								○		2.8	eburicoic acid	antiedema, stomachic
Ginseng Radix Ninjin	○	○		○	○			○	○	1.5	ginsenoside	stomachic, nourishing, antinausea

Table 1. *Cont.*

Crude Drug/ Japanese Name	Kampo Formulae									Antioxidant [7] (mmol/100 g)	Chief Ingredient	Principal Effects
	Hangeshashinto (HST)	Orento (ORT)	Orengedokuto (OGT)	Byakkokaninjinto (BKN)	Shosaikoto (SST)	Inchinkoto (ICT)	Heiisan (HIS)	Juzentaihoto (JTT)	Hochuekkito (HET)			
Pinelliae Tuber Hange	○	○			○					0.3	homogentisic acid	sedation, antinausea, antitussive
Zingiberis Rhizoma Processum Kankyo	○	○									shogaol	warming, analgesia
Coptidis Rhizoma Oren	○	○	○								berberine	anti-inflammation, stomachic, antibacterial, spasmolysis
Phellodendri Cortex Obaku			○								berberine	anti-inflammation, stomachic
Gardeniae Fructus Sanshishi			○			○					geniposide	anti-inflammation, antipyresis, choleresis
Artemisiae Capillaris Flos Inchinko						○					capillarisin	anti-inflammation, antipyresis, choleresis
Rhei Rhizoma Daio						○					sennoside	laxative, blood fluidity improving
Magnoliae Cortex Koboku							○				magnolol	stomachic, analgesia, spasmolysis
Gypsum Sekko				○							calcium sulfate	anti-inflammation, antipyresis, sedation
Oryzae Fructus Kobei				○							starch	stomachic, nourishing
Anemarrhenae Rhizoma Chimo				○							timosaponin AIII	antipyresis, hypoglycemia

Regarding the antioxidative effects of these formulae, only herbs that Dragland, et al. [7] assessed are described.

In addition, *Cinnamomi* Cortex, *Scutellariae* Radix, *Glycyrrhizae* Radix, *Astragali* Radix, *Coptidis* Rhizoma, and *Phellodendri* Cortex inhibit several bacterial infections. Moreover, *Cinnamomi* Cortex, *Scutellariae* Radix, and *Anemarrhenae* Rhizome exert antifungal effects. Furthermore, *Scutellariae* Radix and *Glycyrrhizae* Radix have been shown to inhibit viral infections [8].

In Kampo medicine, the approach to the treatment of stomatitis differs depending on the nature of the symptoms (i.e., acute or chronic). Furthermore, the most appropriate treatment is determined according to the presence of oral and general symptoms. The effectiveness of each Kampo formula according to the pathognomonic symptoms of patients is shown in Table 2. In the acute type, formulae exerting cooling effects (i.e., HST, ORT, OGT, BNT, SST, and ICT) are used. In the chronic type, formulae such as HIS, JTT, and HET are used [3]. The JTT and HET supply energy in patients with symptoms of tiredness, fatigue, or lowered/suppressed immunity [9,10]. The oral cavity is a part of the digestive system; thus, digestive symptoms are important selection criteria for the Kampo formulae. The HST, ORT, OGT, SST, ICT, HIS, JTT, and HET are applied for the treatment of gastrointestinal diseases and symptoms by the national health insurance in Japan.

Table 2. The effectiveness of each Kampo formula according to the pathognomonic symptoms of patients.

Kampo Formulae	Pathognomonic Symptoms
Hangeshashinto (HST)	multiple stomatitis irritation, anxiety, insomnia, rush of blood to the head, anorexia, diarrhea, epigastric discomfort and resistance
Orento (ORT)	multiple stomatitis rush of blood to the head, anorexia, decrease in digestive function, abdominal chill symptom, abdominalgia due to chill, epigastric discomfort and resistance
Orengedokuto (OGT)	multiple stomatitis irritation, insomnia, rush of blood to the head
Byakkokaninjinto (BKN)	thirstiness, dry mouth hyperidrosis, polyuria
Shosaikoto (SST)	bitter in the mouth irritation, depression, anorexia, hypochondriac discomfort and distension, nausea
Inchinkoto (ICT)	multiple stomatitis, dry mouth irritation, insomnia, constipation, oliguria
Heiisan (HIS)	multiple stomatitis anorexia, decrease in digestive function, abdominal distension
Juzentaihoto (JTT)	chronic and repetitive stomatitis, dry mouth depressed, fatigue, dullness, macies, hot sensation, night sweat, anemia, anorexia, decrease in digestive function
Hochuekkito (HET)	chronic and repetitive stomatitis depressed, fatigue, dullness, anorexia, decrease in digestive function

3. Clinical Studies

Use of the Kampo formulae has been based on the Kampo medical theories—empirical rules established over thousands of years. In recent years, clinical and basic research studies investigating the Kampo formulae have been performed to obtain scientific evidence.

For our literature review, PubMed (National Center for Biotechnology Information, Bethesda, MD, USA) and ICHUSHI (Japan Medical Abstracts Society, Tokyo, Japan) were used to identify relevant evidence. Reports of clinical studies (randomized controlled trials, case-control studies, and case series studies) identified through this search are summarized in Table 3.

Ogino, et al. [11] showed that the efficacy of SSK administered to patients with cryptogenic stomatitis accompanied by pain (n = 10) was 80%. SSK was particularly effective against symptoms such as erosion and redness. Oka [12] investigated the effect of ORT in patients with acute aphthous stomatitis (n = 39). The numbers of days until the resolution of pain (2.6 days) and complete cure (6.3 days) were reduced in patients treated with ORT compared with those observed in patients treated with a steroid ointment (pain: 7.5 days; cure: 12.3 days).

Currently, there are effective treatment options for chemotherapy- or radiotherapy-induced stomatitis. HST exerts a preventive effect against these types of stomatitis. Yuki, et al. [13] administered OGT for the treatment of chemotherapy-induced stomatitis and diarrhea in patients with acute myeloblastic or lymphoblastic leukemia (n = 40). The incidence of stomatitis in ORG-treated patients (n = 14) was significantly lower compared with that reported in those who received a gargle consisting of allopurinol, sodium gualenate, and povidone-iodine (n = 25) (27.9% vs. 71.6%, respectively; $p < 0.0001$). Moreover, the incidence of diarrhea was significantly lower (9.3% vs. 31.7%, respectively; $p < 0.005$). HST has been administered for the treatment of chemotherapy-induced mucositis in patients with various types of cancers, such as colorectal [14–17], gastric [16–18], and renal cancers [19]. In all studies, HST extract granules (TJ-14; Tsumura, Tokyo, Japan) were dissolved in drinking water and subjects rinsed their oral cavity with the solution thrice daily. Kono, et al. [14] reported that 92.8% of patients (13/14 patients) with chemotherapy-induced oral mucositis (COM) during treatment with mFOLFOX6 or FOLFIRI for metastasis of advanced colorectal cancer showed significant improvement following a 1-week topical application of HST. Moreover, a significantly decreased mean Common Terminology Criteria for Adverse Events grade was reported in patients treated with HST ($p = 0.0012$). Aoyama, et al. [18] conducted a double-blinded, placebo-controlled, randomized study of HST for the treatment of COM in patients with gastric cancer (n = 91). Although treatment with HST did not reduce the incidence of grade $\geq$ 2 COM, a trend toward the reduction of the risk of grade 1 COM by HST was observed during the screening cycle. Matsuda, et al. [15] also conducted a double-blinded, randomized study investigating the effect of HST against mucositis induced by infusional fluorinated-pyrimidine-based colorectal cancer chemotherapy (n = 93). Although the incidence of grade $\geq$ 2 mucositis was lower in patients treated with HST than in those treated with placebo, the difference was not statistically significant (48.8% vs. 57.4%, respectively; $p = 0.41$). The median duration of grade $\geq$ 2 mucositis was 5.5 days versus 10.5 days, respectively ($p = 0.018$). Nishikawa, et al. [17] demonstrated similar results in patients with gastric and colorectal cancer (n = 181), with a median time to improvement from grade $\geq$ 2 to grade < 1 COM of 8 days versus 15 days in the HST and placebo groups, respectively ($p = 0.072$). Yoshida, et al. [16] and Ohoka, et al. [19] also administered HST to patients with various types of cancer, demonstrating significant decreases in the Common Terminology Criteria for Adverse Events (v4.0) grades. The findings of these studies suggested that HST may be effective for the treatment of chemotherapy- or radiotherapy-induced stomatitis.

A previous study investigated the administration of JTT for the treatment of radiation-induced stomatitis in patients with oral cancer, in whom oral ingestion was not possible (n = 15) [20]. The mean period during which oral ingestion was not possible in these patients showed a reducing trend (i.e., 17.9 $\pm$ 7.1 days vs. 26.0 $\pm$ 11.6 days in the JTT-treated (n = 8) and non-treated (n = 7) groups, respectively ($p < 0.121$)). The clinical use of HST for the treatment of radiation-induced stomatitis has also been reported [21,22].

Table 3. Clinical studies reporting the use of the Kampo formulae for the treatment of stomatitis.

No.	First Author, Year [Reference No.]	Kampo Formula	Study Design	Target Patient	Principal Result
1	Ogino, 1992 [11]	Shosaikoto (SSK)	case series study	cryptogenic stomatitis (n = 10)	Efficacy rate was 80%. (very effective = 2, effective = 4, slightly effective = 2, no change = 2)
2	Oka, 2007 [12]	Orento (ORT)	RCT	acute aphthous stomatitis (n = 39) > non-treated (n = 6), steroid ointment-treated (n = 6) and ORT-treated (n = 27) groups	The administration of Orento reduced the number of days until the disappearance of pain and the complete cure compared to other groups.
3	Yuki, 2003 [13]	Orengedokuto (OGT)	case-control (retrospective) study	chemotherapy-induced stomatitis in patients with acute leukemia (n = 40) > ORG-treated (n = 15) and gargling (n = 25) groups	Incidence of stomatitis was 27.9% in the ORG-treated group, which was significantly lower compared with 71.6% in those who received a gargle consisting of allopurinol, sodium gualenate, and povidone-iodine ($p < 0.0001$).
4	Kono, 2010 [14]		case series study	chemotherapy-induced oral mucositis during mFOLFOX6 or FOLFIRI treatment for metastasis of advanced colorectal cancer (n = 14)	Thirteen patients (92.8%) showed improvements in oral mucositis, with significantly decreased mean CTCAE grades ($p = 0.0012$).
5	Aoyama, 2014 [18]		RCT	gastric cancer chemotherapy-induced oral mucositis (COM) (n = 91) > HST-treated (n = 45) and placebo (n = 46) groups	Although HST treatment did not reduce the incidence of ≥grade 2 COM, a trend was observed in which HST reduced the risk of COM in the patients who developed grade 1 COM.
6	Matsuda, 2015 [15]	Hangeshashinto (HST)	RCT	infusional fluorinated-pyrimidine-based colorectal cancer chemotherapy-induced oral mucositis (n = 93) > HST-treated (n = 46) and placebo (n = 47) groups	Although the incidence of grade ≥2 mucositis was lower for patients treated with HST compared to those treated with placebo, there was no significant difference (48.8 vs. 57.4%; $p = 0.41$). The median duration of grade ≥2 mucositis was 5.5 versus 10.5 days ($p = 0.018$).
7	Yoshida, 2017 [16]		case series study	cancer chemotherapy-induced oral mucositis (grade ≥ 2) (n = 50)	Thirty-seven patients (74%) showed improvements in oral mucositis, with significantly decreased mean NRS and CTC-grade ($p < 0.001$).
8	Nishikawa, 2018 [17]		RCT	chemotherapy-induced oral mucositis (COM) in patients with gastric cancer and colorectal cancer (n = 181) > HST-treated (n = 88) and placebo (n = 93) groups	The incidence of grade ≥2 COM in the HST group was 55.7%, while that in the placebo group was 53.8% ($p = 0.796$). The median time to remission of grade ≥ 2 COM to grade < 1 was 8 days in the HST group and 15 days in the placebo group ($p = 0.072$).
9	Ohoka, 2018 [19]		RCT	sunitinib-induced oral mucositis (OM) in patients with metastatic renal cancer (n = 22) > HST-gargling (n = 12) and non-gargling (n = 10) groups	The gargling with HST significantly improved OM grade and eating status (Global self assessment) ($p = 0.002$).
10	Wada, 2004 [20]	Juzentaihoto (JTT)	RCT	radiation (40 Gy >)-induced stomatitis in patients with oral cancer (n = 15) > JTT-treated (n = 8) and non-treated (n = 7) groups	The mean period that patients could not ingest orally was 17.9 ± 7.1 days in the JTT-treated group, while that in the non-treated group was 26.0 ± 11.6 day ($p = 0.121$).

RCT: randomized controlled trial.

4. Basic Studies of HST

Stomatitis and oral mucositis are induced by various factors, such as infection, inflammation, concomitant oxidative stress, suppressed immunity, depressed function of the digestive tract, malnutrition, psychological stress, and physical stress. Regarding chemotherapy- and radiotherapy-induced mucositis, these treatments induce DNA and non-DNA damage that results in injury of basal epithelial, submucosal, and endothelial cells. In response to this damage, oxidative stress results in the formation of ROS. The presence of ROS damages cell membranes, induces proinflammatory cytokines such as tumor necrosis factor-α, prostaglandin (PG) E_2, interleukin-6, and interleukin-1β, and upregulates cyclooxygenase (COX)-2 in submucosal fibroblasts and endothelial cells leading to mucosal ulceration [23,24]. Furthermore, chemotherapy and radiotherapy reduce immunity, facilitating the development of infectious diseases [25].

Hitomi, et al. [26] conducted in-vivo studies evaluating the analgesic effects of HST using an oral ulcer rat model treated with acetic acid. The topical application of HST in ulcerative oral mucosa suppressed mechanical pain hypersensitivity without exerting effects on healthy mucosa. Moreover, Kamide, et al. [27] assessed the effectiveness of HST for the prevention of radiation-induced mucositis using a hamster model. Administration of HST significantly reduced the severity of mucositis. The percentage of severe mucositis (score $\geq$ 3) was 100% and 16.7% in the untreated and HST groups, respectively. Moreover, HST inhibited the infiltration of neutrophils and expression of COX-2 in irradiated mucosa.

As mentioned earlier in this review, the main characteristic of the Kampo formulae is the combination of several crude drugs (Table 1). These combinations may suppress multiple causes of stomatitis and mucositis. Of note, HST is composed of seven herbs, namely *Scutellariae* Radix, *Glycyrrhizae* Radix, *Zizyphi* Fructus, *Ginseng* Radix, *Pinelliae* Tuber, *Zingiberis* Rhizoma Processum, and *Coptidis* Rhizoma. These constituents, except *Pinelliae* Tuber, exert antioxidative effects [7,28]. Matsumoto, et al. [28] reported that *Glycyrrhizae* Radix, *Ginseng* Radix, and *Zizyphi* Fructus demonstrated scavenging activity for hydroxyl radical, while *Scutellariae* Radix, *Glycyrrhizae* Radix, *Zingiberis* Rhizoma Processum, and *Coptidis* Rhizoma eliminated superoxide. Moreover, *Scutellariae* Radix and *Coptidis* Rhizoma have been shown to eliminate nitroxyl radical.

Regarding its antibacterial action, in vitro studies demonstrated that HST extract inhibited the growth of Gram-negative bacteria including Fusobacterium nucleatum, Porphyromonas gingivalis, Porphyromonas endodontalis, Prevotella intermedia, Prevotella melaninogenica, Tannerella forsythia, Treponema denticola, and Porphyromonas asaccharolytica. However, these inhibitory effects were less pronounced in Gram-positive bacteria and Candida albicans. These effects are thought to be induced by *Scutellariae* Radix (baicalein), *Pinelliae* Tuber (homogentisic acid), *Zingiberis* Rhizoma Processum ([6]-shogaol) and *Coptidis* Rhizoma (berberine, coptisine) [29]. Furthermore, *Glycyrrhizae* Radix [30,31], *Pinelliae* Tuber [31], *Coptidis* Rhizoma [32], and *Ginseng* Radix may enhance immunity. In particular, *Ginseng* Radix was reported to increase the activity of natural killer cells in mice treated orally with it [33,34].

Regarding its anti-inflammatory effect, HST inhibited the production of PGE_2 and suppressed the expression of COX-2 protein. In vitro studies show that *Scutellariae* Radix, *Glycyrrhizae* Radix, *Zingiberis* Rhizoma Processum, and *Coptidis* Rhizoma are involved in these effects [35–38]. As stated earlier in this review, Hitomi, et al. reported the analgesic action of HST [26] and subsequently found through in vitro and in vivo studies that blockage of Na^+ channels by components of *Zingiberis* Rhizoma Processum ([6]-gingerol and ([6]-shogaol) play an essential role in HST-associated analgesia. Moreover, the *Ginseng* Radix extract demonstrated an acceleration of substance permeability into the tissue of the oral ulcer and enhanced the analgesic action of *Zingiberis* Rhizoma Processum [39]. Baicalein—an active constituent of *Scutellariae* Radix—alleviated mechanical allodynia in rats with cancer-induced bone pain [40]. Glycyrrhizin—an active constituent of *Glycyrrhizae* Radix—ameliorated inflammatory pain by inhibiting the microglial activation-mediated inflammatory response in mice with inflammatory pain [41]. HST induces its analgesic effect through the synergistic actions of certain crude drugs.

Therefore, HST exerts a combination of antioxidative, anti-inflammatory, immunostimulatory, and analgesic effects. Moreover, HST is able to control the symptoms and simultaneously eliminate the underlying causes of the condition (Figure 2).

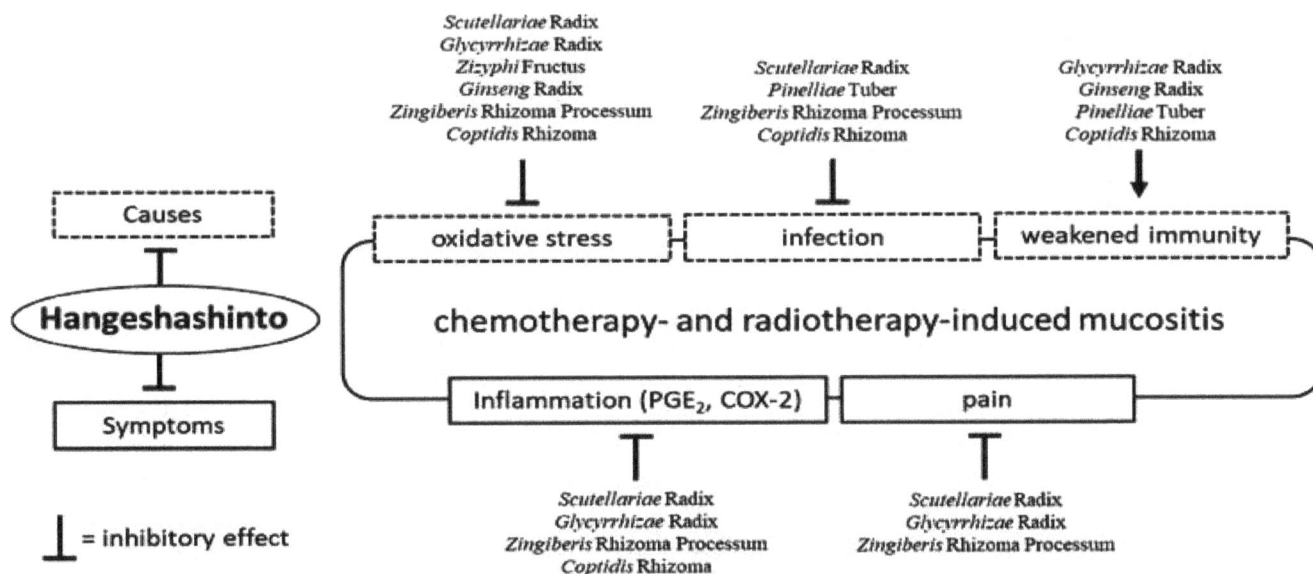

Figure 2. The effects of Hangeshashinto (HST) and the crude drugs on chemotherapy- and radiotherapy-induced mucositis. HST exerts antioxidative, anti-inflammatory, immunostimulatory, and analgesic effects. Moreover, HST is able to control the symptoms and simultaneously eliminate the underlying causes of the condition. PGE$_2$; prostaglandin E$_2$. COX-2; cyclooxygenase-2.

5. Conclusions

In general, western medicines such as steroid ointments, nonsteroidal anti-inflammatory drugs, and antiviral and antifungal drugs are applied for stomatitis and oral mucositis according to the causes and symptoms. In contrast to western medicines which generally include a single component, the Kampo formulae contain multiple components and their effects are exerted through complex mechanisms of action. Use of the Kampo formulae may be an alternative treatment option for patients who failed to respond to conventional therapies. In addition, the concomitant use of Kampo formulae with western medicines may be useful. Kobayashi [42] reported effective cases in which the concomitant use of HST with steroid ointment was applied. In this review, we introduced the clinical applications and summarized the available evidence of the Kampo formulae for the treatment of stomatitis and oral mucositis. Despite the availability of clinical reports, the evidence (except for that related to treatment with HST) is limited. Future clinical and basic research studies are warranted to further investigate the effectiveness on the Kampo formulae against these conditions.

Author Contributions: T.H. designed and supervised the work. M.S. wrote the initial draft with support from M.T., N.E. and H.I., and K.Y. edited the manuscript. All authors approved the final version of the manuscript.

Acknowledgments: The authors would like to thank Shigemasa Kubo for his valuable assistance during the preparation of this manuscript and Enago (www.enago.jp) for English language review.

Abbreviations

BKN	Byakkokaninjinto
COM	chemotherapy-induced oral mucositis
COX	cyclooxygenase
HET	Hochuekkito

HST   Hangeshashinto
ICT   Inchinkoto
IL   interleukin
JTT   Juzentaihoto
OGT   Orengedokuto
ORT   Orento
PG   prostaglandin
RCT   randomized controlled trial
ROS   reactive oxygen species
SST   Shosaikoto

References

1.   Curra, M.; Junior, S.; Valente, L.A.; Martins, M.D.; Santos, P.S.D.S. Chemotherapy protocols and incidence of oral mucositis. An integrative review. *Einstein* **2018**, *16*, eRW4007. [CrossRef] [PubMed]
2.   Zheng, L.W.; Hua, H.; Cheung, L.K. Traditional Chinese medicine and oral diseases: Today and tomorrow. *Oral Dis.* **2011**, *17*, 7–12. [CrossRef] [PubMed]
3.   Yamaguchi, K. Traditional Japanese herbal medicines for treatment of odontopathy. *Front. Pharmacol.* **2015**, *6*, 176. [CrossRef] [PubMed]
4.   Sunagawa, M.; Wang, P.L.; Yohkoh, N.; Kameyama, A.; Mukunashi, K.; Mori, S.; Makiishi, T.; Takahashi, S. Survey on trends in the use of Kampo medicines in dentistry and oral surgery among the hospitals of universities. *J. Jpn. Dent. Soc. Orient. Med.* **2011**, *30*, 8–17. (In Japanese)
5.   Kenkyukai, K.C. *Clinical Research of Chinese Traditional Medicine—Pharmacognosy*, 1st ed.; Ishiyaku Publishers, Inc.: Tokyo, Japan, 1992; pp. 36–553. ISBN 4-263-73065-8. (In Japanese)
6.   Tugrul, S.; Koçyiğit, A.; Doğan, R.; Eren, S.B.; Senturk, E.; Ozturan, O.; Ozar, O.F. Total antioxidant status and oxidative stress in recurrent aphthous stomatitis. *Int. J. Dermatol.* **2016**, *55*, e130–e135. [CrossRef] [PubMed]
7.   Dragland, S.; Senoo, H.; Wake, K.; Holte, K.; Blomhoff, R. Several culinary and medicinal herbs are important sources of dietary antioxidants. *J. Nutr.* **2003**, *133*, 1286–1290. [CrossRef] [PubMed]
8.   Toriizuka, K. *Monographs of Pharmacological Research on Traditional Herbal Medicine*; Ishiyaku Publishers, Inc.: Tokyo, Japan, 2003; pp. 9–379. ISBN 978-4-263-20188-6. (In Japanese)
9.   Ikemoto, T.; Shimada, M.; Iwahashi, S.; Saito, Y.; Kanamoto, M.; Mori, H.; Morine, Y.; Imura, S.; Utsunomiya, T. Changes of immunological parameters with administration of Japanese Kampo medicine (Juzen-Taihoto/TJ-48) in patients with advanced pancreatic cancer. *Int. J. Clin. Oncol.* **2014**, *19*, 81–86. [CrossRef]
10.   Kuroiwa, A.; Liou, S.; Yan, H.; Eshita, A.; Naitoh, S.; Nagayama, A. Effect of a traditional Japanese herbal medicine, hochu-ekki-to (Bu-Zhong-Yi-Qi Tang), on immunity in elderly persons. *Int. Immunopharmacol.* **2004**, *4*, 317–324. [CrossRef]
11.   Ogino, S.; Harada, T. The effects of Tsumura Shosaikoto on stomatitis. *J. New Rem. Clin.* **1992**, *41*, 592–595. (In Japanese)
12.   Oka, S. The effects of Oren-to on Stomatitis. *Pharm. Med.* **2007**, *25*, 35–38. (In Japanese)
13.   Yuki, F.; Kawaguchi, T.; Hazemoto, K.; Asou, N. Preventive effects of oren-gedoku-to on mucositis caused by anticancer agents in patients with acute leukemia. *Jpn. Cancer Chemother.* **2003**, *30*, 1303–1307. (In Japanese)
14.   Kono, T.; Satomi, M.; Chisato, N.; Ebisawa, Y.; Suno, M.; Asama, T.; Karasaki, H.; Matsubara, K.; Furukawa, H. Topical Application of Hangeshashinto (TJ-14) in the Treatment of Chemotherapy-Induced Oral Mucositis. *World J. Oncol.* **2010**, *1*, 232–235. [PubMed]
15.   Matsuda, C.; Munemoto, Y.; Mishima, H.; Nagata, N.; Oshiro, M.; Kataoka, M.; Sakamoto, J.; Aoyama, T.; Morita, S.; Kono, T. Double-blind, placebo-controlled, randomized phase II study of TJ-14 (Hangeshashinto) for infusional fluorinated-pyrimidine-based colorectal cancer chemotherapy-induced oral mucositis. *Cancer Chemother. Pharmacol.* **2015**, *76*, 97–103. [CrossRef] [PubMed]
16.   Yoshida, N.; Taguchi, T.; Okayama, T.; Ishikawa, T.; Naito, Y.; Kanazawa, M.; Kanbayashi, Y.; Hosokawa, T.; Kohno, R.; Ito, Y. The effects of Hangeshashinto infiltration method for cancer chemotherapy-induced oral mucositis. *Prog. Med.* **2017**, *37*, 1339–1343. (In Japanese)

17. Nishikawa, K.; Aoyama, T.; Oba, M.S.; Yoshikawa, T.; Matsuda, C.; Munemoto, Y.; Takiguchi, N.; Tanabe, K.; Nagata, N.; Imano, M.; et al. The clinical impact of Hangeshashinto (TJ-14) in the treatment of chemotherapy-induced oral mucositis in gastric cancer and colorectal cancer: Analyses of pooled data from two phase II randomized clinical trials (HANGESHA-G and HANGESHA-C). *J. Cancer* **2018**, *9*, 1725–1730. [CrossRef]

18. Aoyama, T.; Nishikawa, K.; Takiguchi, N.; Tanabe, K.; Imano, M.; Fukushima, R.; Sakamoto, J.; Oba, M.S.; Morita, S.; Kono, T.; et al. Double-blind, placebo-controlled, randomized phase II study of TJ-14 (hangeshashinto) for gastric cancer chemotherapy-induced oral mucositis. *Cancer Chemother. Pharmacol.* **2014**, *73*, 1047–1054. [CrossRef] [PubMed]

19. Ohoka, H. The Clinical Usefulness of Gargling with Hangeshashinto for Treatment of Oral Mucositis Caused by Sunitinib in Patients with Metastatic Renal Cancer. *Kampo Med.* **2018**, *69*, 1–6. (In Japanese) [CrossRef]

20. Wada, S.; Furuta, I. The preventive effects of Juzentaihoto on side effects of radiation therapy for oral cancer. *Sci. Kampo Med.* **2004**, *28*, 76–78. (In Japanese)

21. Nagai, A.; Ogawa, K.; Miura, J.; Kobayashi, K. Therapeutic effects of Hangeshashinto, a Japanese Kampo medicine, on radiation-induced enteritis and oral mucositis: Case series. *Kampo Med.* **2014**, *65*, 108–114. (In Japanese) [CrossRef]

22. Tanaka, Y.; Yamashita, T.; Matsunobu, T.; Shiotani, A. Two Cases of Radiotherapy-induced Oral Mucositis Alleviated with Hange-shashin-to. *Pract. Oto-Rhino-Laryngol.* **2012**, *105*, 1199–1203. (In Japanese) [CrossRef]

23. Logan, R.M.; Gibson, R.J.; Sonis, S.T.; Keefe, D.M. Nuclear factor-kappaB (NF-kappaB) and cyclooxygenase-2 (COX-2) expression in the oral mucosa following cancer chemotherapy. *Oral Oncol.* **2007**, *43*, 395–401. [CrossRef] [PubMed]

24. Al-Dasooqi, N.; Gibson, R.J.; Bowen, J.M.; Logan, R.M.; Stringer, A.M.; Keefe, D.M. Matrix metalloproteinases are possible mediators for the development of alimentary tract mucositis in the dark agouti rat. *Exp. Biol. Med.* **2010**, *235*, 1244–1256. [CrossRef] [PubMed]

25. Al-Ansari, S.; Zecha, J.A.; Barasch, A.; de Lange, J.; Rozema, F.R.; Raber-Durlacher, J.E. Oral Mucositis Induced by Anticancer Therapies. *Curr. Oral Health Rep.* **2015**, *2*, 202–211. [CrossRef] [PubMed]

26. Hitomi, S.; Ono, K.; Yamaguchi, K.; Terawaki, K.; Imai, R.; Kubota, K.; Omiya, Y.; Hattori, T.; Kase, Y.; Inenaga, K. The traditional Japanese medicine hangeshashinto alleviates oral ulcer-induced pain in a rat model. *Arch. Oral Biol.* **2016**, *66*, 30–37. [CrossRef] [PubMed]

27. Kamide, D.; Yamashita, T.; Araki, K.; Tomifuji, M.; Shiotani, A. Hangeshashinto (TJ-14) prevents radiation-induced mucositis by suppressing cyclooxygenase-2 expression and chemotaxis of inflammatory cells. *Clin. Transl. Oncol.* **2017**, *19*, 1329–1336. [CrossRef]

28. Matsumoto, C.; Sekine-Suzuki, E.; Nyui, M.; Ueno, M.; Nakanishi, I.; Omiya, Y.; Fukutake, M.; Kase, Y.; Matsumoto, K. Analysis of the antioxidative function of the radioprotective Japanese traditional (Kampo) medicine, hangeshashinto, in an aqueous phase. *J. Radiat. Res.* **2015**, *56*, 669–677. [CrossRef]

29. Fukamachi, H.; Matsumoto, C.; Omiya, Y.; Arimoto, T.; Morisaki, H.; Kataoka, H.; Kadena, M.; Funatsu, T.; Fukutake, M.; Kase, Y.; et al. Effects of Hangeshashinto on Growth of Oral Microorganisms. *Evid. Based Complement. Alternat. Med.* **2015**, *2015*, 512947. [CrossRef]

30. Chan, A.; Pang, H.; Yip, E.C.; Tam, Y.K.; Wong, Y.H. The aqueous extract of Radix Glycyrrhizae stimulates mitogen-activated protein kinases and nuclear factor-kappaB in Jurkat T-cells and THP-1 monocytic cells. *Am. J. Chin. Med.* **2006**, *34*, 263–278. [CrossRef]

31. Matsuura, K.; Kawakita, T.; Nakai, S.; Saito, Y.; Suzuki, A.; Nomoto, K. Role of B-lymphocytes in the immunopharmacological effects of a traditional Chinese medicine, xiao-chai-hu-tang (shosaiko-to). *Int. J. Immunopharmacol.* **1993**, *15*, 237–243. [CrossRef]

32. Zhou, X.; Peng, Y.; Li, L.; He, K.; Huang, T.; Mou, S.; Feng, M.; Han, B.; Ye, X.; Li, X. Effects of dietary supplementations with the fibrous root of *Rhizoma Coptidis* and its main alkaloids on non-specific immunity and disease resistance of common carp. *Vet. Immunol. Immunopathol.* **2016**, *173*, 34–38. [CrossRef]

33. Jang, A.Y.; Song, E.J.; Shin, S.H.; Hwang, P.H.; Kim, S.Y.; Jin, Y.W.; Lee, E.K.; Lim, M.J.; Oh, I.S.; Ahn, J.Y.; et al. Potentiation of natural killer (NK) cell activity by methanol extract of cultured cambial meristematic cells of wild ginseng and its mechanism. *Life Sci.* **2015**, *135*, 138–146. [CrossRef] [PubMed]

34. Liou, C.J.; Huang, W.C.; Tseng, J. Short-term oral administration of ginseng extract induces type-1 cytokine production. *Immunopharmacol. Immunotoxicol.* **2006**, *28*, 227–240. [CrossRef] [PubMed]

35. Kato, T.; Segami, N.; Sakagami, H. Anti-inflammatory Activity of Hangeshashinto in IL-1β-stimulated Gingival and Periodontal Ligament Fibroblasts. *In Vivo* **2016**, *30*, 257–263. [PubMed]

36. Kaneko, T.; Chiba, H.; Horie, N.; Kato, T.; Kobayashi, M.; Hashimoto, K.; Kusama, K.; Sakagami, H. Effect of Scutellariae radix ingredients on prostaglandin E(2) production and COX-2 expression by LPS-activated macrophage. *In Vivo* **2009**, *23*, 577–581. [PubMed]

37. Kase, Y.; Saitoh, K.; Ishige, A.; Komatsu, Y. Mechanisms by which Hange-shashin-to reduces prostaglandin E2 levels. *Biol. Pharm. Bull.* **1998**, *21*, 1277–1281. [CrossRef] [PubMed]

38. Kono, T.; Kaneko, A.; Matsumoto, C.; Miyagi, C.; Ohbuchi, K.; Mizuhara, Y.; Miyano, K.; Uezono, Y. Multitargeted effects of hangeshashinto for treatment of chemotherapy-induced oral mucositis on inducible prostaglandin E2 production in human oral keratinocytes. *Integr. Cancer Ther.* **2014**, *13*, 435–445. [CrossRef] [PubMed]

39. Hitomi, S.; Ono, K.; Terawaki, K.; Matsumoto, C.; Mizuno, K.; Yamaguchi, K.; Imai, R.; Omiya, Y.; Hattori, T.; Kase, Y.; et al. [6]-gingerol and [6]-shogaol, active ingredients of the traditional Japanese medicine hangeshashinto, relief oral ulcerative mucositis-induced pain via action on Na$^+$ channels. *Pharmacol. Res.* **2017**, *117*, 288–302. [CrossRef] [PubMed]

40. Hu, S.; Chen, Y.; Wang, Z.F.; Mao-Ying, Q.L.; Mi, W.L.; Jiang, J.W.; Wu, G.C.; Wang, Y.Q. The Analgesic and Antineuroinflammatory Effect of Baicalein in Cancer-Induced Bone Pain. *Evid. Based Complement. Altern. Med.* **2015**, *2015*, 973524. [CrossRef]

41. Sun, X.; Zeng, H.; Wang, Q.; Yu, Q.; Wu, J.; Feng, Y.; Deng, P.; Zhang, H. Glycyrrhizin ameliorates inflammatory pain by inhibiting microglial activation-mediated inflammatory response via blockage of the HMGB1-TLR4-NF-kB pathway. *Exp. Cell Res.* **2018**, *369*, 112–119. [CrossRef]

42. Kobayashi, E. Clinical study on 184 cases of stomatitis. *J. Kampo Med.* **2007**, *54*, 108–115. (In Japanese)

8

Pathogenic Viruses Commonly Present in the Oral Cavity and Relevant Antiviral Compounds Derived from Natural Products

Daisuke Asai⦿ and Hideki Nakashima *

Department of Microbiology, St. Marianna University School of Medicine, Kawasaki 216-8511, Japan
* Correspondence: nakahide@marianna-u.ac.jp

Abstract: Many viruses, such as human herpesviruses, may be present in the human oral cavity, but most are usually asymptomatic. However, if individuals become immunocompromised by age, illness, or as a side effect of therapy, these dormant viruses can be activated and produce a variety of pathological changes in the oral mucosa. Unfortunately, available treatments for viral infectious diseases are limited, because (1) there are diseases for which no treatment is available; (2) drug-resistant strains of virus may appear; (3) incomplete eradication of virus may lead to recurrence. Rational design strategies are widely used to optimize the potency and selectivity of drug candidates, but discovery of leads for new antiviral agents, especially leads with novel structures, still relies mostly on large-scale screening programs, and many hits are found among natural products, such as extracts of marine sponges, sea algae, plants, and arthropods. Here, we review representative viruses found in the human oral cavity and their effects, together with relevant antiviral compounds derived from natural products. We also highlight some recent emerging pharmaceutical technologies with potential to deliver antivirals more effectively for disease prevention and therapy.

Keywords: anti-human immunodeficiency virus (HIV); antiviral; natural product; human virus

1. Introduction

The human oral cavity is home to a rich microbial flora, including bacteria, fungi, and viruses. Oral tissues are constantly exposed to these microbes, which form a complex ecological community that influences oral and systemic health [1]. Discussion of the microbiological aspects of oral disease traditionally focuses on bacteria and fungi, but viruses are attracting increasing attention as pathogens. Viruses are generally more difficult to detect among pathogenic microbes, at least with traditional methods such as in vitro cultivation; however, the development of sophisticated molecular tools, including monoclonal antibodies and viral genome sequencing, have greatly advanced the field of virology over the past decade or so. A number of viruses have been found in the oral cavity, of which many are thought to be involved in the development of various types of oral ulcers, oral tumors, classical oral infectious diseases, and periodontitis. For example, herpes simplex virus 1 (HSV-1) causes gingivostomatitis, and the virus can subsequently enter a dormant state in the trigeminal ganglion. Blood-borne viruses such as human immunodeficiency virus (HIV) can enter the mouth via gingival crevicular fluid, and viruses causing upper respiratory tract infections are also found in the mouth [2]. Similarly, the mumps virus is known to infect the salivary glands and can be found in saliva of affected individuals. Human papillomavirus (HPV) is responsible for several oral conditions, including papilloma, condylomas, and focal epithelial hyperplasia, and has also been implicated in head and neck squamous cell carcinoma.

The field of antiviral research acquired new urgency since the 1980s, owing to the global spread of HIV, which causes acquired immune deficiency syndrome (AIDS). HIV is a member of the RNA retroviruses, which contain a reverse transcriptase (RT) enzyme that transcribes RNA into DNA in infected cells, leading to integration of the retroviral genomic information into chromosomal DNA of the host cell. Antiretroviral drugs (ARVs) often target RT, but are always given in combination with other ARVs for antiretroviral therapy (ART) in order to increase efficacy and reduce the development of resistance. The anti-HIV agent zidovudine (AZT) is a representative ARV, and was the first to be approved in the United States in 1986; however, recently, many new classes of drugs have been introduced [3], together with new formulations such as long-acting depot-type anti-HIV drugs and easy-to-use gel formulations for preventing rectal HIV infection [4].

The enormous research effort directed at the treatment of HIV has led to important advances in basic science and many therapeutic breakthroughs, including the development of inhibitors targeting a range of human viruses. Nevertheless, large-scale screening of natural products, such as extracts of marine sponges, sea algae, plants, and arthropods, remains an important source of leads for new antiviral agents, whose potency and selectivity can then be optimized with the aid of rational design strategies, including computational approaches. Thus, the aim of this review is to provide a personal viewpoint on natural-product-derived antiviral agents that are available for the treatment of pathogenic viruses, especially HIV, that may cause symptoms in the oral cavity, considered from a historic perspective. As major candidates for viruses involved in oral diseases, we focus on (1) HSV-1 and HSV-2; (2) Epstein–Barr virus (EBV); (3) Kaposi sarcoma-associated herpesvirus (KSHV); (4) human papilloma virus (HPV); and (5) HIV.

2. Viruses Associated with Oral Diseases of Humans

Members of the human herpesvirus (HHV) family cause common primary viral infections of the oral mucous membrane, and may also play a role in periodontitis. There are eight members of the HHV family, which are among the largest and most complex human viruses. We focus here on HSV-1, HSV-2, EBV, and KSHV; the others are varicella-zoster virus (VZV), human cytomegalovirus (HCMV), HHV-6, and HHV-7 (Table 1). HPV is a diverse family of viruses, which can cause a variety of pathologies, including oral squamous cell carcinoma, and chronic infection of the skin or mucosal epithelium. Furthermore, the retrovirus HIV causes a decline in immunocompetence, which can lead to various cutaneous manifestations [5]. In this section, we present a brief overview of these viruses.

Table 1. Human herpesviruses (HHVs) and their associated diseases.

Type	Target	Oral Manifestations	Other Pathology
1. HSV-1	Mucoepithelial	Herpes ulcers	Genital ulcers
2. HSV-2	Mucoepithelial	Herpes ulcers	Genital ulcers
3. VZV	Mucoepithelial	Possible oral manifestations of chicken pox and herpes zoster	Chicken pox and herpes zoster
4. EVB	B cells and epithelial cells	Hairy leukoplakia, Periodontitis (nasopharyngeal carcinoma)	Mononucleosis and lymphoma
5. HCMV	Monocytes, lymphocytes, and epithelial cells	Periodontitis	
6. HHV-6	Monocytes and macrophages		Roseola in infants
7. HHV-7	T cells and possibly others		Roseola in infants
8. KSHV	B cells and possibly others		Kaposi sarcoma (in AIDS patients)

HSV-1, herpes simplex virus 1; HSV-2, herpes simplex virus 2; VZV, varicella-zoster virus; EBV, Epstein–Barr virus; HCMV, human cytomegalovirus; HHV-6, human herpesvirus 6; HHV-7, human herpesvirus 7; KSHV, Kaposi sarcoma-associated herpesvirus; AIDS, acquired immune deficiency syndrome.

2.1. HSV-1 and HSV-2

HSVs are relatively large, enveloped, double-stranded DNA viruses with icosahedral symmetry. Infections by HSV-1 are referred to as upper body infections to distinguish them from the genital infection caused by HSV-2. The formal designations of these viruses are human herpesvirus 1 (HHV-1) and 2 (HHV-2). Oral herpes is a viral infection mainly around the mouth and lips caused by herpes simplex viruses. HSV-1 causes painful sores on the upper and lower lips, gums, tongue, roof of the mouth, inside the cheeks or nose, and sometimes on the face, chin, and neck. In addition, HSV-1 can cause symptoms such as swollen lymph nodes, fever, and muscle aches. HSV-2 is primarily associated with the genitals and most often causes genital herpes. However, it may spread to the mouth during oral sex, causing oral herpes. HSVs characteristically establish latent infection in sensory nerve ganglia, and, in this case, signs appear only when the virus is reactivated. Following recovery from primary oropharyngeal infection, the individual retains HSV DNA in the trigeminal ganglion, but the virus becomes dormant. Infected individuals have at least a 50% chance of suffering sporadic recurrent attacks of herpes labialis (otherwise known as facial herpes, herpes simplex, fever blisters, or cold sores) from time to time throughout the remainder of their life.

At present, the drug of choice for the treatment of HSV infections is acyclovir (ACV; 9-(2-hydroxyethoxymethyl)guanine). Its unique advantage over earlier nucleoside derivatives is that HSV-encoded thymidine kinase (TK), which has broader specificity than cellular TK, phosphorylates ACV to ACV-monophosphate (ACV-P). A cellular guanosine monophosphate (GMP) kinase then completes the phosphorylation to generate the active agent, ACV-triphosphate (ACV-PPP). ACV-PPP acts as both an inhibitor and a substrate of the viral enzyme, competing with guanosine triphosphate (GTP) for incorporation into DNA; this results in chain termination, because ACV lacks the 3'-hydroxyl group required for chain elongation. Before ACV was introduced, vidarabine (Ara-A) which was the first nucleoside analog antiviral to be systemically administered, was used. Ara-A is also sequentially phosphorylated by kinases to afford the triphosphate ara-ATP, which competitively inhibits deoxyATP (dATP). However, the mechanism of Ara-A is different in that all three phosphorylations are mediated by host adenosine kinases, resulting in a lack of specificity. Indeed, Ara-A is more toxic and less metabolically stable than ACV, although it is still employed against ACV-resistant strains. In addition, valaciclovir (VACV), an ester of ACV, is a prodrug that has greater oral bioavailability than ACV. VACV provides high plasma levels of the parent compound and offers greater efficacy, as well as decreased dosing frequency. Additionally, guanosine analog famciclovir (FCV) is another choice for the treatment of HSV infections.

2.2. EBV

EBV, formally human herpesvirus 4 (HHV-4), has a small DNA genome, and its main host cells are B lymphocytes and epithelial cells. EBV replicates in epithelial cells of the nasopharynx and salivary glands, especially the parotid, lysing them and releasing infectious virions into saliva. EBV attaches to B lymphocytes via binding of the viral glycoprotein gp350/EBV to CD21 receptors on the lymphocyte. The major characteristic of infected B lymphocytes is transformation. When this occurs, only a small amount of the viral DNA integrates into the host chromosome, and most of the viral DNA stays in a separate circular episome form. The B lymphocytes infiltrating the lymphatic tissue of the infected oropharyngeal mucosa may, in turn, become infected, but are generally not permissive for virus production. EBV is transmitted only after repeated contact with infected individuals. It can manifest in the oral cavity and/or head and neck region, e.g., as Burkitt's lymphoma (BL), mononucleosis, or oral hairy leukoplakia (OHL), and the prevalence and disease severity are increased in individuals co-infected with HIV. Mononucleosis is common, irrespective of HIV infection status, and is associated with a primary EBV infection during adolescence and young adulthood. OHL is an oral mucosal lesion that is associated with EBV infection and is often asymptomatic, commonly presenting as non-removable white patches on the lateral borders of the tongue. OHL is now an established phenomenon in a range of conditions affecting immune competence, e.g., in immunosuppressed patients with HIV infection or bone marrow transplant recipients [6]. EBV-positive Hodgkin's and non-Hodgkin's lymphomas may manifest in the head and neck. Nasopharyngeal carcinoma (NPC) is also a head and neck cancer associated with EBV infection. No effective anti-EBV drugs have yet been developed. EBV is sensitive to ACV in vitro, but systemic administration of this drug has little effect on clinical illness.

2.3. KSHV

The formal designation of human herpesvirus 8 (HHV-8) was proposed for KSHV, in keeping with the systematic nomenclature adopted for all human herpesviruses. KSHV is the causative virus of Kaposi sarcoma (KS), multicentric Castleman's disease, and primary effusion lymphoma. Humans are thought to be the natural host for KSHV, which is primarily transmitted via saliva. Infection occurs during childhood and increases with age. KSHV is detected in endothelial and spindle cells of Kaposi sarcoma lesions, as well as in circulating endothelial cells, primary effusion lymphoma cells, B lymphocytes, macrophages, dendritic cells, oropharynx and prostatic glandular epithelium, and keratinocytes. Epidemiological studies indicate that there are four clinical variants of KS: (1) classic; (2) endemic (African); (3) iatrogenic (transplant-associated); and (4) HIV/AIDS-associated (epidemic) (HIV-KS). It is well known that KS is an AIDS-defining illness and the most frequent AIDS-associated neoplasm. HIV-KS commonly affects the oral cavity, with the oral mucosa being the initial site of clinical disease in 20% of patients [7]. ART has successfully decreased the prevalence and incidence of HIV-KS. A liposome-encapsulated form of doxorubicin (Doxil) is often used primarily for the treatment of AIDS-related KS.

2.4. HPV

HPV is a small, non-enveloped, double-stranded DNA virus with icosahedral symmetry. There is wide genetic diversity among HPVs, and more than 70 genotypes of HPVs have been identified so far. Some of them are associated with a variety of benign papillomatous lesions of the skin and squamous mucosa. The mechanism of malignant transformation is not fully understood and is difficult to study because HPV is difficult to grow in culture. It is thought that the viral DNA remains episomal in benign lesions, whereas it is integrated into host chromosomal DNA in malignant cells, e.g., cervical carcinoma. Oral papillomas of the conventional kind can be caused by sexually transmitted HPV types 6, 11, and 16. Common warts are most frequently caused by type 2 [8].

HPVs induce benign tumors of the epithelium in their natural host. The discovery of the role of HPV in cervical cancer has led to the widespread use of HPV vaccines for young women, but it is still uncertain whether HPV actually plays an essential role [9]. Based on their putative role in cervical carcinoma, the viruses are classified as having either high (primarily 16 and 18) or low (primarily 6 and 11) oncogenic potential. HPVs are often found in oral samples from healthy mouths, such as brush samples of mucosa, but their prevalence is typically reported to be higher in biopsies from oral lesions, including leukoplakia and/or cancers. The association with oncogenic HPVs is less obvious in the case of leukoplakia, while there are many reports of HPVs in malignant cancers. The observed prevalence in oral cancers is considerably lower than that in cervical cancers, but the case for a role of HPVs is still reasonably strong [2]. When generations who have received papillomavirus vaccines grow up, we should find out whether the prevalence of oral carcinomas declines along with the expected decline in cervical cancer. Imiquimod is used as a patient-applied cream to treat genital warts. Imiquimod is a Toll-like receptor 7 (TLR7) agonist, promoting the secretion of inflammatory cytokines. Traditional treatments consist of locally destructive techniques, such as cautery, surgical excision, and cryotherapy using liquid nitrogen.

2.5. HIV

HIV is an enveloped retrovirus that is transmitted through sexual contact or by contact with infected body fluids. Retroviral RT allows the virus to integrate its genetic information into the host chromosome. HIV targets CD4-positive T-helper cells, and the resulting development of immunodeficiency leads to AIDS. Viral infections are a significant cause of morbidity and mortality in immunosuppressed patients. In general, diseases or medical treatments that have cytostatic or cytotoxic effects on lymphocytes increase the risk of viral infections, and the viral infection rate depends on the nature and degree of immunosuppression. The reactivation of latent virus is the most important determinant of the type of viral infection, and this occurs most commonly in immunosuppressed patients. Skin and mucous membrane manifestations of HIV infection may result from opportunistic disorders secondary to the decline in immunocompetence caused by the infection. HIV-related oral conditions occur in a large proportion of patients, and frequently are misdiagnosed or inadequately treated. Dental expertise is necessary for appropriate management of oral manifestations of HIV infection; however, in practice, many patients do not receive adequate dental care. Common or notable HIV-related oral conditions include the following symptoms: xerostomia (dry mouth), candidiasis, OHL, periodontal diseases such as linear gingival erythema and necrotizing ulcerative periodontitis, KS, HPV-associated warts, ulcerative conditions including HSV lesions, recurrent aphthous ulcers, and neutropenic ulcers. In 1993, consensus was reached on the classification of the oral manifestations of HIV, so-called the 1993 EC-Clearinghouse classification. It classifies oral lesions associated with HIV (HIV-OLs) into three groups: (1) lesions strongly associated with HIV infection; (2) those less commonly associated with HIV infection; and (3) lesions seen in HIV infection [10]. The sequence of events associated with HIV infection, from the cellular level of infection to oral manifestations in HIV-infected patients, is illustrated in Figure 1, together with the classification of HIV-OLs.

HIV is one of the best-studied viruses and, thus, anti-HIV agents show the widest range of structural variation among antiviral agents. Since the introduction of combination therapy (ART) for patients, HIV infection has been transformed into a long-term and manageable disorder; indeed, ART can reduce plasma virus titers to below detectable levels for more than one year and slow the disease progression. The major classes of drugs used in ART regimens include entry inhibitors (EI), nucleoside reverse-transcriptase inhibitors (NRTI), non-nucleoside reverse-transcriptase inhibitors (NNRTI), protease inhibitors (PI), and integrase strand-transfer inhibitors (INSTI).

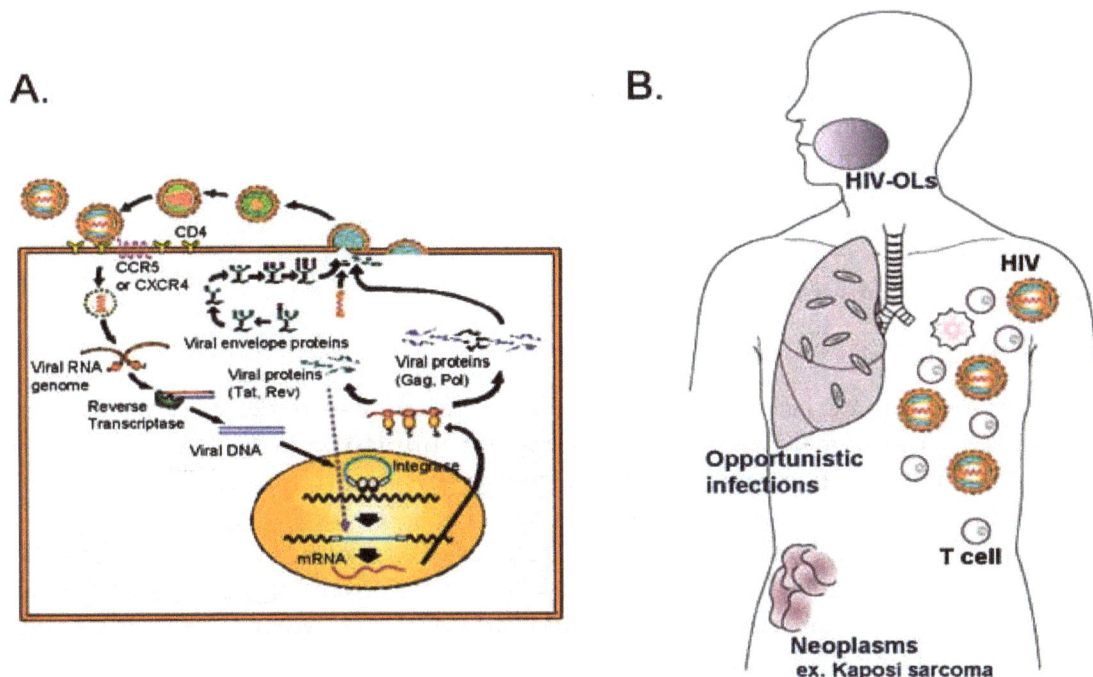

Figure 1. *Cont.*

C.

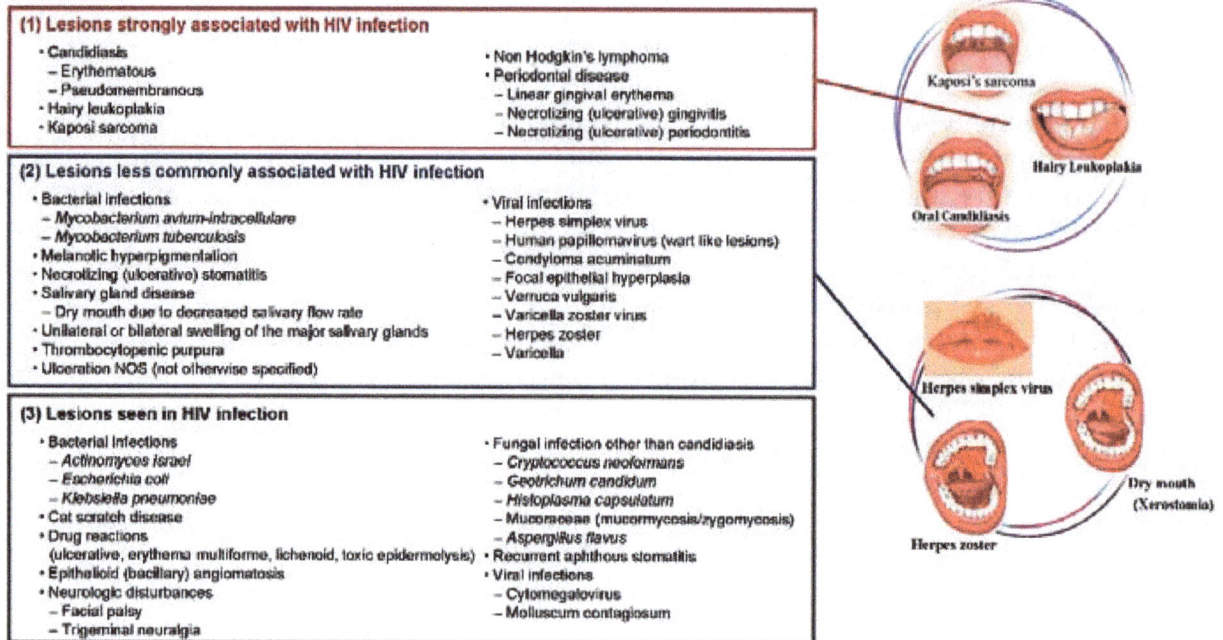

Figure 1. Life cycle and effects of human immunodeficiency virus (HIV). (**A**) The HIV infection of cells begins when the envelope glycoprotein of a viral particle binds to both cluster of differentiation 4 (CD4) and a co-receptor that is a member of the chemokine receptor family. Once inside the cells, the viral genome is reverse-transcribed into DNA and incorporated into the cellular genome. Viral gene transcription and viral reproduction are stimulated by signals that normally activate the host cell. Production of the virus is accompanied by cell death. (**B**) Infection with HIV induces immunosuppression, which in turn enables many kinds of bacteria, fungi, and viruses to grow in the oral cavity. HIV-infected individuals usually exhibit immune dysfunction prior to depletion of their CD4-positive T-helper cells. The progressive immune deficiency is accompanied by a wide range of opportunistic infections and neoplasms, such as candidiasis, Kaposi sarcoma, and hairy leukoplakia, in the oral cavity. (**C**) The 1993 EC-Clearinghouse classification for oral lesions associated with HIV (HIV-OLs) is still globally used, despite some controversy as to its current relevance to periodontal diseases.

3. Natural Products as Antiviral Agents

3.1. Early History of Antivirals

Extracts of natural materials, such as herbs, spices, roots, tree barks, leaves, etc., have a long anecdotal, as well as proven history of use in treating human ailments. Indeed, many drugs now in clinical use have their origins in plants, marine organisms, bacteria, and fungi that were traditionally believed to have desirable pharmacological activities. However, it is difficult to isolate pure active compounds from a complex array of substances, some of which may be cytotoxic, present in natural materials. Nevertheless, the discoveries of antiviral-active nucleosides, spongothymidine and spongouridine, more than half a century ago made scientists aware of the potential value of antivirals from natural sources (Figure 2) [11].

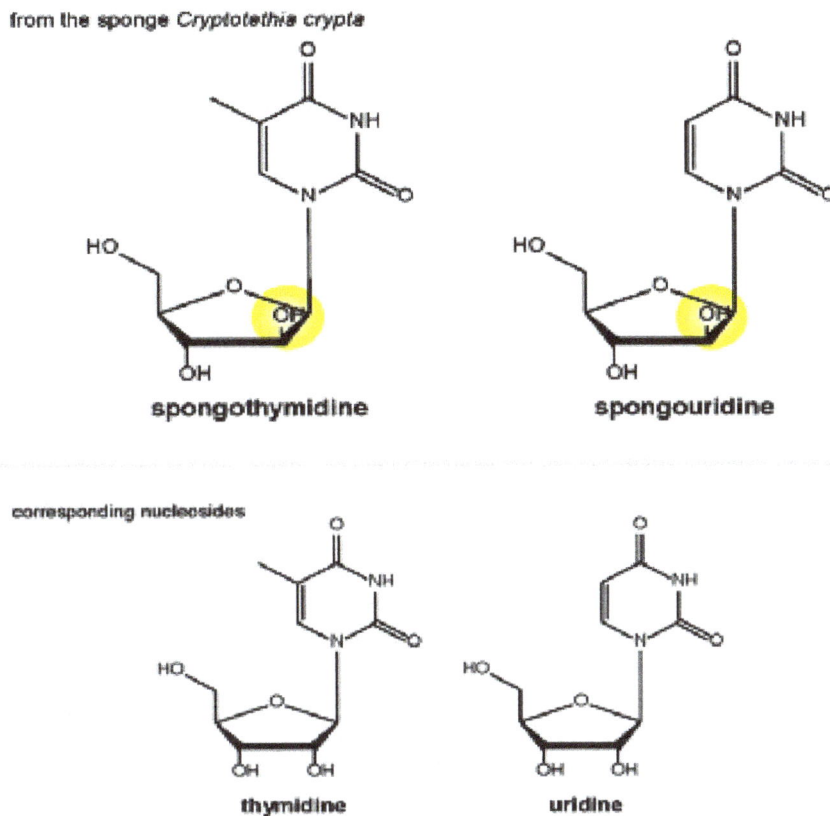

Figure 2. Chemical structures of arabinosyl nucleosides from the sponge *Cryptotethia crypta*, together with the corresponding human nucleosides. The key structural features are highlighted in yellow. Arabinosyl nucleosides contain arabinofuranose instead of β-D-ribofuranose.

3.2. Antivirals in the Latter Half of the 20th Century

Since the early work on marine-derived antivirals, thousands of novel compounds with antiviral activities have been isolated from natural sources, and some have been successfully developed for clinical use. Perhaps the most important contribution was the isolation and characterization of arabinosyl nucleosides from a Caribbean sponge (phylum Porifera) called *Tethya cripta* (Tethylidae), which provided the basis for drug design of nucleoside analogs used in medicine today. In this context, the most important antivirals that have come onto the market so far are acyclovir (ACV) [12], vidarabine (Ara-A) [13], and azidothymidine (zidovudine) (AZT) [14] (Figure 3). ACV and Ara-A are nucleic acid analogs that competitively inhibit herpes viral DNA polymerases, preventing further viral DNA synthesis. As for AZT, the active intracellular metabolite, AZT-triphosphate, is an HIV RT inhibitor, and is a key constituent of standard ART regimens. Our group investigated the inhibition of HIV replication by AZT and its cytopathic effect by means of time-of-addition experiments using HIV-bearing MT-4 cells [15], confirming and extending previous work [16].

Given the history of marine organism-based drug discovery, attention subsequently turned to marine sponges, which proved to be a rich source of compounds with antiviral properties (Table 2). Cytarabine (Ara-C) is a structural analog of cytosine arabinoside and is currently used in the routine treatment of patients with leukemia and lymphoma [13]. Avarol blocks the synthesis of glutamine transfer RNA (tRNA), which is crucial for a viral protein synthesis [17]. Manzamine A is an alkaloid with a diverse range of bioactivity, including anti-HIV activity [18]. Mycalamide A was found to inhibit HSV-1 replication by blocking viral protein synthesis [19]. Papuamide A inhibits viral entry into host cells independently of the CD4-gp120/HIV and C–C chemokine receptor type 5 (CCR5)-gp41/HIV interactions [20].

Synthetic derivatives of arabinosyl nucleosides from sponge, *Tethya cripta*

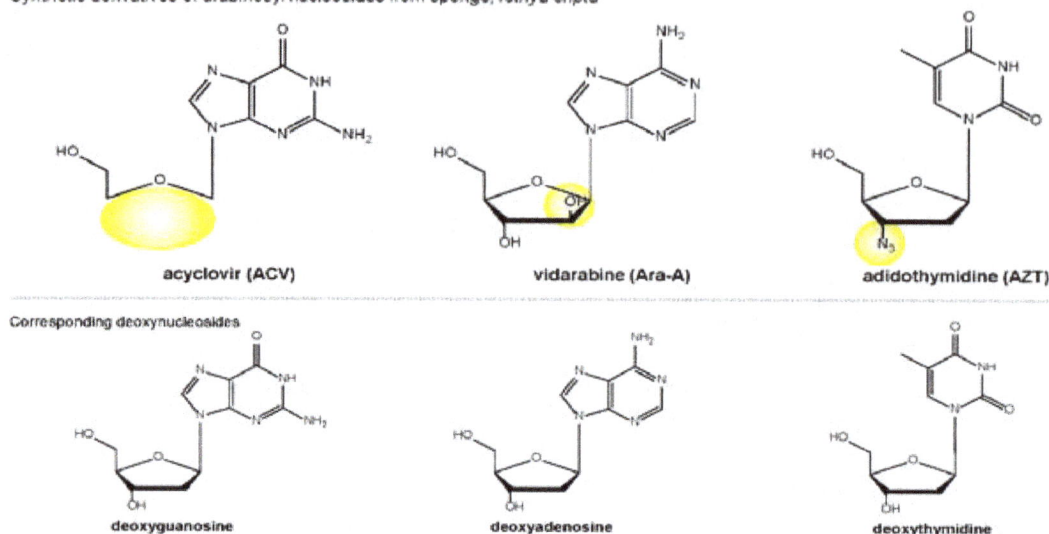

acyclovir (ACV)   vidarabine (Ara-A)   adidothymidine (AZT)

Corresponding deoxynucleosides

deoxyguanosine   deoxyadenosine   deoxythymidine

Figure 3. Chemical structures of nucleic acid analogs clinically used as key antivirals today, together with those of analogous competitors. Acyclovir (ACV) is used for the treatment of herpes simplex virus infections, chickenpox, and shingles. ACV inhibits viral DNA polymerase activity in a deoxyguanosine triphosphate (dGTP)-competitive manner. Vidarabine (Ara-A) is active against herpes simplex and varicella zoster viruses. Ara-A inhibits viral DNA polymerase activity in a deoxyadenosine triphosphate (dATP)-competitive manner. Azidothymidine, also called zidovudine (AZT), is the most common drug prescribed for individuals who have acquired immune deficiency syndrome (AIDS). AZT inhibits viral reverse transcriptase (RT) activity in a deoxythymidine triphosphate (dTTP)-competitive manner. The key structural features are highlighted in yellow.

Table 2. Sponge-derived antivirals reported in the latter part of the twentieth century. Compounds below the horizontal dotted line are more recent medicines. HIV—human immunodeficiency virus.

Compound	Organism	Target Virus	Reference
Acyclovir	*Tethya cripta*	HSV, VZV	Elion et al., 1977 [12]
Cytarabine	*Tethya cripta*	HSV [*1]	Privat and de Rudder, 1964 [13]
Vidarabine	*Tethya cripta*	HSV	Privat and de Rudder, 1964 [13]
Zidovudine	*Tethya cripta*	HIV	Horwitz et al., 1964 [14]
Avarol	*Disidea avara*	HIV	Muller et al., 1987 [17]
Manzamine A	*Haliclona* sp.	HIV	Sakai et al., 1986 [18]
Mycalamide A	*Mycale*	HSV	Perry et al., 1988 [19]
Papuamide A	*Theonella mirabilis*		Ford et al., 1999 [20]

[*1]: presently used as an anti-tumor agent.

Compounds extracted from algae have activity against a wide range of viruses, including HIV and HSV [21]. For example, galactan sulfate, which is a polysaccharide isolated from the red seaweed *Agardhiella tenera*, shows potent HIV replication-inhibitory activity [22]. A citrate buffer extract of the marine red alga *Schizymenia pacifca* inhibited RT of avian myeloblastosis virus and Rauscher murine leukemia virus [23], and the main component of this "sea algal extract" (SAE) was characterized as a member of the λ-carrageenan family, being a sulfated polysaccharide composed of galactose (73%), sulfonate (20%), and 3,6-anhydrogalactose (0.65%) with a molecular weight of approximately 2000 kDa [24]. SAE was demonstrated to be a specific inhibitor of HIV RT and HIV replication in vitro, and its sulfate residues were hypothesized to play a key role in the inhibition. Various types of sulfated polysaccharides such as dextran sulfate have been reported as potent inhibitors of HIV infection by researchers from around the world, including our group [25–34]. However, these observations did not generate much interest because the antiviral actions of these compounds were considered to be largely nonspecific [35]. Subsequent studies revealed that the target of sulfated polysaccharides is the binding of gp120/HIV to the cell-surface protein CD4 on naive cells [36–38].

Various plant-derived natural products have also been reported as potential lead compounds for anti-HIV agents. Lignin extracted from pine cones is a natural polyphenolic material generated by oxidative polymerization of phenylpropanoid monomers. Sakagami and co-workers have reported on the anti-HIV activity of lignin toward cultured cells [39,40]. Lignin was suggested to suppress the absorption of HIV onto the surface of cultured cells, although the details are unclear. Mitsuhashi et al. proposed that low-molecular-weight lignin inhibits HIV replication through suppression of HIV transcription from long terminal repeats (LTRs), including activation via nuclear factor kappa B (NF-κB) [41]. Betulinic acid (triterpenoid), isolated from the leaves of *Syzigium claviflorum*, inhibited HIV replication in a mechanism-blind screening [42]. The activity-directed derivatization of betulinic acid contributed to the creation of bevirimat, which disrupts core condensation by targeting a late step in Gag/HIV processing [43–45].

Cationic host-defense peptides, tachyplesins and polyphemusins, which were isolated from the hemocytes of horseshoe crabs (*Tachypleus tridentatus* and *Limulus polyphemus*), were reported to possess anti-HIV activity by Iwanaga's group [46,47]. These peptides consist of 17 or 18 amino-acid residues with two intramolecular disulfide bridges. We investigated the structure–anti-HIV activity relationship (SAR) of these peptides and found that [Tyr-5,12, Lys-7]polyphemusin II (named T22) showed strong anti-HIV activity and low cytotoxicity [48,49]. Our continuing studies led to shortened polyphemusin analogs comprising 14 amino-acid residues, T134 [50] and T140 [51], as potent anti-HIV peptides. Moreover, FC131, which has a lower molecular weight than T134/T140, was found in a library of cyclic pentapeptides designed by means of a pharmacophore-guided approach based on SAR studies [52]. These peptides include a potent C–X–C chemokine receptor type 4 (CXCR4; HIV co-receptor) antagonist that strongly blocks X4-HIV-1 entry through competitive binding to CXCR4 [53–55]. Development of polyphemusin-derived CXCR4 antagonists from natural sources is a good example of a success story from natural product screening supported by fine synthetic technology using peptide chemistry (Figure 4). Currently, the biostable T140 analog BKT-140 (BioLineRx Ltd.) is a phase II drug candidate for the treatment of acute myeloid leukemia (AML) [56].

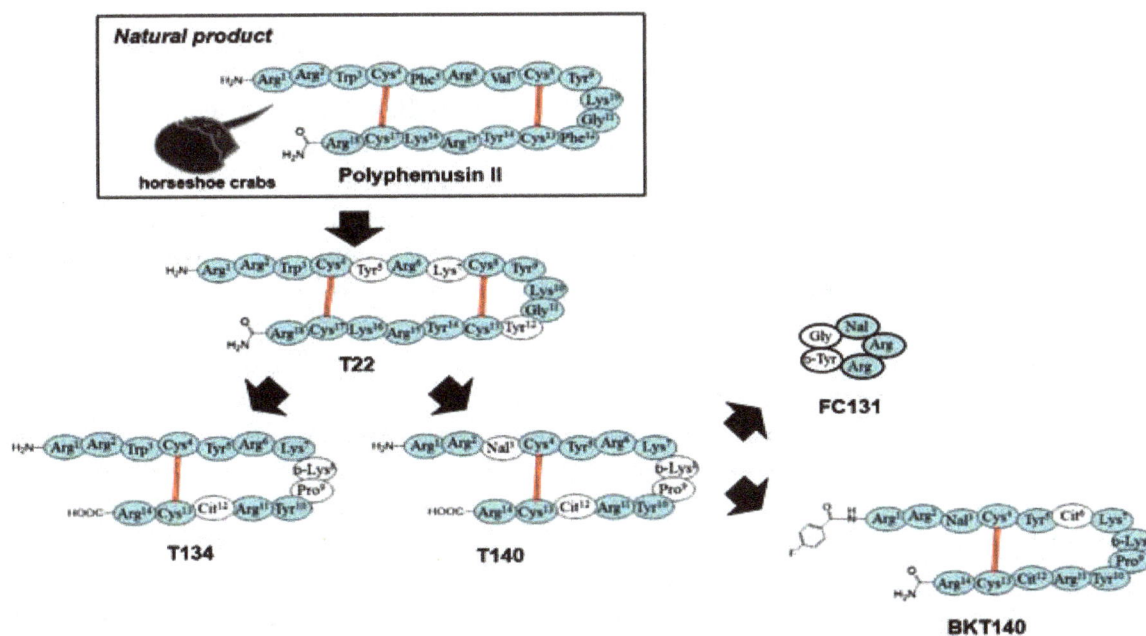

Figure 4. Discovery and development of C–X–C chemokine receptor type 4 (CXCR4) antagonists with potent anti-HIV activity from host-defense peptide of horseshoe crabs. Substitutions are highlighted in white. Red lines indicate intramolecular disulfide bond formation. Cit, L-citrulline; Nal, L-3-(2-naphthyl)alanine.

3.3. Antivirals in the 21st century

3.3.1. Status of Anti-HIV Natural Products

The mainstream of antiviral discovery from natural sources continues to be directed against HIV and HSV. In the past decade, some unique compounds with anti-HIV activity have been reported from sponges, algae, and also from natural product libraries. Ma et al. reported the isolation of phenylspirodrimane, named stachybotrin D, from the marine sponge-associated fungus *Stachybotrys chartarum* MXH-X73, as a novel NNRTI [57]. Vidal et al. reported that daphnane diterpenes (daphnetoxin) extracted from the aerial parts of *Daphne gnidium* L. (Thymelaeaceae) with dichloromethane possessed anti-HIV inhibitory activity, interfering directly with the expression of the two main HIV co-receptors, CCR5 and CXCR4 [58]. Ixoratannin A-2 (doubly linked, A-type proanthrocyanidin trimer) and boldine (aporphine alkaloid) were identified as novel viral protein U (Vpu)/HIV-interacting anti-HIV inhibitors from the pan-African Natural Product Library (p-ANAPL), which is the largest collection of medicinal plant-derived pure compounds on the African continent [59]. The activities of these compounds require further characterization. The red algal protein griffithsin (GRFT) comprising 121 amino-acid residues shows promising potent anti-HIV inhibitory activity without cellular toxicity [60]. The potent HIV entry inhibitor GRFT was found to be a lectin that targets high-mannose *N*-linked glycans displayed on the surface of HIV envelope glycoproteins, and is of interest because unique technology has been developed for its large-scale production by genetic engineering using *Nicotiana benthamiana* plants transduced with a tobacco mosaic virus (TMV)-based vector expressing GRFT [61]. Recently, gnidimacrin, a daphnane-type diterpenoid extracted from the roots of *Stellera chamaejasme* (Thymelaeaceae), was reported to reduce latent HIV-1 DNA and the frequency of HIV-1-infected cells through activation of protein kinase C beta 1 and 2 (PKCβI and βII) in peripheral blood mononuclear cells (PBMC) from patients [62]. Persistent HIV infection is currently incurable owing to the presence of latent viral reservoirs of long-lived memory T cells, so targeting of latent viruses is an attractive strategy for complete HIV eradication, especially for ART-interrupted patients.

3.3.2. Status of Anti-HSV Natural Products

The second most advanced antiviral development program after anti-HIV is anti-HSV. Anti-herpes drugs were the first antivirals targeting human pathogenic viruses and, thus, HSV infections are considered to be manageable, even though the available drugs have only limited therapeutic efficacy. It should be noted that chronic HSV infections of HIV-positive individuals, or solid organ transplant recipients, or patients with cancer may require prolonged antiviral treatment. In particular, HSV encephalitis is highly lethal. Unfortunately, prolonged therapies with available anti-herpes drugs may result in undesirable side effects, and can also induce the emergence of drug-resistant strains. Therefore, the discovery of novel anti-herpesvirus agents is still necessary.

There are many reports of compounds derived from various plant species as potential antiherpetic agents. Hassan et al. recently published a comprehensive review about bioactive natural products with anti-HSV properties, including nucleosides, polysaccharides, proteins, peptides, terpenes, phenolic compounds, and alkaloids [63]. Here, we focus on some of the materials currently considered most promising. Based on the successful development of ACV and Ara-A, marine organisms are anticipated to be a key source of novel anti-HSV drugs [64]. Mandal et al. showed that the polysaccharide xylan isolated from red algae *Scinaia hatei* exhibits activity against HSVs [65]. In addition, some sulfated polysaccharides, such as sulfated galactan, were reported to have antiviral activity for HSV [66,67], as well as HIV. These compounds may inhibit virus adsorption on cells. In 2005, a methanol extract of algae *Sargassum latiuscula* (Rhodomelaceae) collected in Korea was reported to display antiviral activities against not only wild-type HSV-1, but also ACV-resistant and/or thymidine kinase-deficient HSV-1 strains in vitro without apparent cytotoxicity, and it was also effective in a mouse HSV-1 infection model without noticeable toxic effects [68]. Fractionation of this extract afforded the active components 2,3,6-tribromo-4,5-dihydroxybenzyl methyl ether (TDB) and TDB alcohol. Meliacine isolated from *Melia azedarach* is a plant-derived glycopeptide exhibiting a therapeutic effect on HSV-induced ocular disease and genital herpetic infection in mice, possibly by inhibiting viral protein synthesis [69,70]. Various other natural products have yielded candidate anti-HSVs, including diterpenes from *Scoparia dulcis* L. (a medicinal plant) [71], a sulfated polysaccharide called calcium spirulan (Ca-SP) from *Spirulina platensis* (cyanobacteria) [72], fucoidan from *Undaria pinnatifida* (edible seaweed) [73], and nostoflan from *Nostoc flagelliforme* (terrestrial cyanobacterium) [74].

3.3.3. Status of Natural Products with Activity against Other Viruses

Although HIV and HSVs have been the mainstream of attention, screening for and testing of natural compounds for activity against other viruses has also been progressing. For example, resveratrol (trans-3,4′,5 trihydroxystilbene) has in vitro antiviral activities against several members of the HHV family, including varicella-zoster virus (VZV) [75], EBV [76], human cytomegalovirus (HCMV) [77], and KSHV [78]. The compound appears to act on cellular pathways that affect viral replication, though the details are unclear. Anti-EBV peptide, an N-myristoylated peptide containing six amino acids, was isolated from hemolymph (blood) of larvae of tobacco budworm, *Heliothis virescens* [79]. This peptide has antiviral activity against several viruses, and Ourth proposed that the "myristate plus basic" motif in this peptide may prevent assembly and/or budding of viruses from the host cell. These two compounds are of interest, because there are no effective antiviral drugs or vaccines in clinical use for diseases caused by EBV and KSHV. Curcumin, a natural polyphenol derived from the rhizome of the medical plant *Curcuma longa Linn*, was reported to have anti-HPV activity due to downregulation of HPV18 transcription via inhibition of activator protein 1 (AP-1) [80]. This seems noteworthy, because curcumin is readily available and inexpensive. Slater et al. reported that indolocarbazoles derived from the natural product arcyriafavin A (an alkaloid) are potent and selective inhibitors of replication of HCMV [81]. Arcyriafavin A is a potent cyclin-dependent kinase 4 (CDK4)/cyclin D1 and Ca^{2+}/calmodulin-dependent (CaM) kinase II inhibitor, and seems to be a promising candidate for further development.

At present, the most promising next-generation antiviral agents from natural sources may be the red algal protein GRFT and the algae-derived polysaccharide carrageenan (CG). GRFT is a potent anti-HIV agent, and also inhibits infection with other sexually transmitted infectious viruses, including HSV by targeting viral entry and cell-to-cell transmission [82], HPV by mediating receptor internalization [83], and HCV by targeting cell entry [84]. CG blocks the binding of HPV to cells [85,86], and is well established as a thickening agent in various foods and cosmetic products, including some brands of sexual lubricant [87]. It has, therefore, the advantage of being recognized as safe by the Food and Drug Administration (FDA), and a microbicide gel formulation for vaginal application has been developed, taking advantage of its gel-forming property. Recently, the combination of GRFT and CG was reported to show broad antiviral activity against HSV-2 and HPV in murine models [83]. The combination of GRFT and CG seems promising, and we discuss it further below in connection with new pharmaceutical formulation technologies.

4. Formulation of Natural-Product-Derived Antivirals Using New Pharmaceutical Technologies

Recently, innovations in drug formulation technology have attracted great interest as a means of improving clinical outcomes. Drug delivery systems (DDS) such as nano- and microparticles, targeted carriers, prodrugs, polyethylene glycol (PEG)ylation, hydrogel depots, and so on are attractive technologies to enable a drug to act at the right time, at the right site, and at the required concentration. The objectives of these systems include controlled drug release, prolongation of drug lifetime, acceleration of drug permeation and absorption, and drug targeting. For example, a prodrug modification of ACV is the L-valyl ester (VACV), which shows increased cell-membrane permeability, enabling a reduction in the frequency of administration and reduced side effects. Some formulations of natural products themselves have been reported to serve as topical microbicides. Cellulose sulfate, an HIV entry inhibitor in vitro, was investigated for use as a sulfated polysaccharide vaginal gel formulation [88,89]. Unfortunately, however, no significant effect of cellulose sulfate on the risk of HIV acquisition was found, compared with the placebo [90]. In an alternative approach, sodium carboxymethylcellulose (Na CMC) has been used as a gelling agent together with maraviroc and tenofovir (both of which are in clinical use) for prevention of rectal acquisition of HIV [4]. In a macaque model, these drugs were detectable in plasma at 30 minutes after gel application and remained in rectal fluids at more than 95%-inhibitory concentrations for 24 h. The algae-derived anti-HPV polysaccharide CG (see Section 3.3.3) is a macromolecular gel, and the CG-based gel formulation Carraguard is now a phase III drug candidate as a sexual lubricant with anti-HPV properties. More recently, the combination of the red algal protein GRFT and CG in a novel formulation called a freeze-dried fast-dissolving insert (FDI) was reported to protect rhesus macaques from vaginal simian–human immunodeficiency virus (SHIV) challenge, as well as mice from vaginal HSV-2 and HPV pseudovirus challenge, and current phase I trials are looking at the anti-HPV properties of a GRFT/CG combination gel as a sexual lubricant [91]. Thus, formulations with good retention at invasion sites using natural products acting outside infected cells, e.g., entry and/or budding inhibitors for host cells, seem promising, especially for pre-exposure prophylaxis (PrEP).

Some drug formulation studies of curcumin, an anti-HPV natural product from medical plants, were recently reported. Curcumin inspired considerable interest based on its extensive physiological activities; however, poor bioavailability restricts its clinical translation. Treatment of cervical cancer with a curcumin nanoparticle formulation in poly(lactic-co-glycolic acid) (PGLA) was investigated in an orthotopic mouse model [92,93]. Various hydrogel formulations for curcumin have also been proposed [94,95]. The results of these pre-clinical experiments suggested that suitably formulated curcumin could be an effective therapeutic modality for HPV-induced cervical cancer.

5. Prospects

Most viral infections of the oral cavity involve HHVs, especially in HIV-infected individuals. As described in Section 2, HSV type 1 (HHV-1) and 2 (HHV-2) produce shallow, small, painful ulcers which may coalesce. The development of antiviral agents with their delivery systems that successfully stop the recurrence of oral ulceration (recurrent aphthous stomatitis (RAS)) is anticipated [96]. VZV (HHV-3) is responsible for chickenpox upon primary infection, and shingles in its reactivated form. EBV (HHV-4) causes infectious mononucleosis and/or glandular fever. HCMV (HHV-5) can cause large, painful ulceration on any oral surface. EBV and HCMV were also reported to associate with periodontitis [97]; therefore, the discovery of new antiviral agents is necessary, especially for chronic periodontitis. HHV-6 and -7 are associated with facial rashes in babies and oral ulceration. Also, reactivated HHV-6 can cause encephalitis in patients after transplantation [98]. KSHV (HHV-8) is associated with KS in AIDS patients. In HIV-infected individuals, herpes infections often persist for long period of time. In addition, HPV infections are also found in AIDS patients, and may give rise to exophytic warts, often at the corners of the mouth. In patients with AIDS, there is a danger that viremias may spread to life-threatening sites, and early treatment of oral herpetic infections is essential.

Recent developments in anti-HIV drugs has mainly been focused on creating novel formulations to improve medication compliance, such as mixed formulations including drugs with different mechanisms of action in a single tablet. For example, Complera® is a once-a-day medication, consisting of a single tablet containing rilpivirine (NNRTI), emtricitabine (NRTI), and tenofovir (NRTI). Prezcobix® utilizes a pharmacokinetic (PK) booster strategy, with a single tablet containing darunavir (PI) and a cytochrome P450 3A (CYP3A) inhibitor to prolong the blood half-life of darunavir. We have reported a depot strategy for the peptide drug Fuzeon®, which is used for the treatment of HIV-infected individuals and AIDS patients with multidrug-resistant HIV infections [99]. Natural-product-derived peptides with anti-viral activity may be candidates for PrEP and post-exposure therapy if appropriate pharmaceutical technology is employed. Also, there is still an enormous range of natural resources (plants, etc.) that remain to be explored for new antiviral candidates. Thus, discovery and development of new drugs in combination with improved pharmaceutical formulation technologies offers great promise for the future treatment of viral infections.

Author Contributions: D.A. wrote the first draft of the manuscript and reviewed it under research supervision by H.N. H.N. reviewed and edited the manuscript.

Acknowledgments: We thank the members of the Department of Microbiology, St. Marianna University School of Medicine, and the Department of Microbiology and Immunology, Kagoshima University Dental School, for much helpful discussion and technical support. We also thank Dr. Nobutaka Fujii (Kyoto University), Dr. Hiroshi Sakagami (Meikai University), and Dr. Naoki Yamamoto (Tokyo Medical and Dental University) for collaboration in our research on anti-HIV compounds.

References

1. Aas, J.A.; Paster, B.J.; Stokes, L.N.; Olsen, I.; Dewhirst, F.E. Defining the normal bacterial flora of the oral cavity. *J. Clin. Microbiol.* **2005**, *43*, 5721–5732. [CrossRef] [PubMed]

2. Grinde, B.; Olsen, I. The role of viruses in oral disease. *J. Oral Microbiol.* **2010**, *2*. [CrossRef] [PubMed]

3. Caplan, M.R.; Daar, E.S.; Corado, K.C. Next generation fixed dose combination pharmacotherapies for treating HIV. *Expert Opin. Pharmacother.* **2018**, *19*, 589–596. [CrossRef] [PubMed]

4. Dobard, C.W.; Taylor, A.; Sharma, S.; Anderson, P.L.; Bushman, L.R.; Chuong, D.; Pau, C.P.; Hanson, D.; Wang, L.; Garcia-Lerma, J.G.; et al. Protection Against Rectal Chimeric Simian/Human Immunodeficiency Virus Transmission in Macaques by Rectal-Specific Gel Formulations of Maraviroc and Tenofovir. *J. Infect. Dis.* **2015**, *212*, 1988–1995. [CrossRef] [PubMed]

5. Cedeno-Laurent, F.; Gomez-Flores, M.; Mendez, N.; Ancer-Rodriguez, J.; Bryant, J.L.; Gaspari, A.A.; Trujillo, J.R. New insights into HIV-1-primary skin disorders. *J. Int. AIDS Soc.* **2011**, *14*, 5. [CrossRef] [PubMed]

6. Khammissa, R.A.; Fourie, J.; Chandran, R.; Lemmer, J.; Feller, L. Epstein-Barr Virus and Its Association with Oral Hairy Leukoplakia: A Short Review. *Int. J. Dent.* **2016**, *2016*, 4941783. [CrossRef] [PubMed]

7. Khammissa, R.A.; Pantanowitz, L.; Feller, L. Oral HIV-Associated Kaposi Sarcoma: A Clinical Study from the Ga-Rankuwa Area, South Africa. *AIDS Res. Treat.* **2012**, *2012*, 873171. [CrossRef] [PubMed]

8. Cubie, H.A. Diseases associated with human papillomavirus infection. *Virology* **2013**, *445*, 21–34. [CrossRef] [PubMed]

9. Giuliano, A.R.; Tortolero-Luna, G.; Ferrer, E.; Burchell, A.N.; de Sanjose, S.; Kjaer, S.K.; Munoz, N.; Schiffman, M.; Bosch, F.X. Epidemiology of human papillomavirus infection in men, cancers other than cervical and benign conditions. *Vaccine* **2008**, *26* (Suppl. 10), K17–K28. [CrossRef] [PubMed]

10. Classification and Diagnostic Criteria for Oral Lesions in HIV Infection. EC-Clearinghouse on Oral Problems Related to HIV Infection and WHO Collaborating Centre on Oral Manifestations of the Immunodeficiency Virus. *J. Oral Pathol. Med.* **1993**, *22*, 289–291. [CrossRef]

11. Bergmann, W.; Feeney, R.J. Contributions to the study of marine products. XXXII. The nucleosides of sponges. I. *J. Org. Chem.* **1951**, *16*, 981–987. [CrossRef]

12. Elion, G.B.; Furman, P.A.; Fyfe, J.A.; de Miranda, P.; Beauchamp, L.; Schaeffer, H.J. Selectivity of action of an antiherpetic agent, 9-(2-hydroxyethoxymethyl) guanine. *Proc. Natl. Acad. Sci. USA* **1977**, *74*, 5716–5720. [CrossRef] [PubMed]

13. Privat de Garilhe, M.; de Rudder, J. Effect of 2 arabinose nucleosides on the multiplication of herpes virus and vaccine in cell culture. *C. R. Hebd. Seances Acad. Sci.* **1964**, *259*, 2725–2728.

14. Horwitz, J.P.; Chua, J.; Noel, M. Nucleosides. V. The Monomesylates of 1-(2′-Deoxy-β-D-lyxofuranosyl)thymine[1,2]. *J. Org. Chem.* **1964**, *29*, 2076–2078. [CrossRef]

15. Nakashima, H.; Matsui, T.; Harada, S.; Kobayashi, N.; Matsuda, A.; Ueda, T.; Yamamoto, N. Inhibition of replication and cytopathic effect of human T cell lymphotropic virus type III/lymphadenopathy-associated virus by 3′-azido-3′-deoxythymidine in vitro. *Antimicrob. Agents Chemother.* **1986**, *30*, 933–937. [CrossRef] [PubMed]

16. Mitsuya, H.; Weinhold, K.J.; Furman, P.A.; St Clair, M.H.; Lehrman, S.N.; Gallo, R.C.; Bolognesi, D.; Barry, D.W.; Broder, S. 3'-Azido-3'-deoxythymidine (BW A509U): An antiviral agent that inhibits the infectivity and cytopathic effect of human T-lymphotropic virus type III/lymphadenopathy-associated virus in vitro. *Proc. Natl. Acad. Sci. USA* **1985**, *82*, 7096–7100. [CrossRef] [PubMed]

17. Muller, W.E.; Sobel, C.; Diehl-Seifert, B.; Maidhof, A.; Schroder, H.C. Influence of the antileukemic and anti-human immunodeficiency virus agent avarol on selected immune responses in vitro and in vivo. *Biochem. Pharmacol.* **1987**, *36*, 1489–1494. [CrossRef]

18. Sakai, R.; Higa, T.; Jefford, C.W.; Bernardinelli, G. Manzamine A, a novel antitumor alkaloid from a sponge. *J. Am. Chem. Soc.* **1986**, *108*, 6404–6405. [CrossRef]

19. Perry, N.B.; Blunt, J.W.; Munro, M.H.G.; Pannell, L.K. Mycalamide A, an antiviral compound from a New Zealand sponge of the genus Mycale. *J. Am. Chem. Soc.* **1988**, *110*, 4850–4851. [CrossRef]

20. Ford, P.W.; Gustafson, K.R.; McKee, T.C.; Shigematsu, N.; Maurizi, L.K.; Pannell, L.K.; Williams, D.E.; de Silva, E.D.; Lassota, P.; Allen, T.M.; et al. Papuamides A–D, HIV-inhibitory and cytotoxic depsipeptides from the sponges *Theonella mirabilis* and *Theonella swinhoei* collected in Papua New Guinea. *J. Am. Chem. Soc.* **1999**, *121*, 5899–5909. [CrossRef]

21. Yasuhara-Bell, J.; Lu, Y. Marine compounds and their antiviral activities. *Antivir. Res.* **2010**, *86*, 231–240. [CrossRef] [PubMed]

22. Witvrouw, M.; Este, J.A.; Mateu, M.Q.; Reymen, D.; Andrei, G.; Snoeck, R.; Ikeda, S.; Pauwels, R.; Bianchini, N.V.; Desmyter, J.; et al. Activity of a sulfated polysaccharide extracted from the red seaweed *Aghardhiella tenera* against human immunodeficiency virus and other enveloped viruses. *Antivir. Chem. Chemother.* **1994**, *5*, 297–303. [CrossRef]

23. Nakashima, H.; Kido, Y.; Kobayashi, N.; Motoki, Y.; Neushul, M.; Yamamoto, N. Antiretroviral activity in a marine red alga: Reverse transcriptase inhibition by an aqueous extract of *Schizymenia pacifica*. *J. Cancer Res. Clin. Oncol.* **1987**, *113*, 413–416. [CrossRef] [PubMed]

24. Nakashima, H.; Kido, Y.; Kobayashi, N.; Motoki, Y.; Neushul, M.; Yamamoto, N. Purification and characterization of an avian myeloblastosis and human immunodeficiency virus reverse transcriptase inhibitor, sulfated polysaccharides extracted from sea algae. *Antivir. Chem. Chemother.* **1987**, *31*, 1524–1528. [CrossRef]

25. Mitsuya, H.; Looney, D.J.; Kuno, S.; Ueno, R.; Wong-Staal, F.; Broder, S. Dextran sulfate suppression of viruses in the HIV family: Inhibition of virion binding to CD4+ cells. *Science* **1988**, *240*, 646–649. [CrossRef] [PubMed]

26. Nakashima, H.; Yoshida, O.; Baba, M.; De Clercq, E.; Yamamoto, N. Anti-HIV activity of dextran sulphate as determined under different experimental conditions. *Antivir. Res.* **1989**, *11*, 233–246. [CrossRef]

27. Busso, M.E.; Resnick, L. Anti-human immunodeficiency virus effects of dextran sulfate are strain dependent and synergistic or antagonistic when dextran sulfate is given in combination with dideoxynucleosides. *Antimicrob. Agents Chemother.* **1990**, *34*, 1991–1995. [CrossRef] [PubMed]

28. Yoshida, T.; Nakashima, H.; Yamamoto, N.; Uryu, T. Anti-AIDS virus activity in vitro of dextran sulfates obtained by sulfation of synthetic and natural dextrans. *Polym. J.* **1993**, *25*, 1069–1077. [CrossRef]

29. Yoshida, O.; Nakashima, H.; Yoshida, T.; Kaneko, Y.; Yamamoto, I.; Matsuzaki, K.; Uryu, T.; Yamamoto, N. Sulfation of the immunomodulating polysaccharide lentinan: A novel strategy for antivirals to human immunodeficiency virus (HIV). *Biochem. Pharmacol.* **1988**, *37*, 2887–2891. [CrossRef]

30. Kaneko, Y.; Yoshida, O.; Nakagawa, R.; Yoshida, T.; Date, M.; Ogihara, S.; Shioya, S.; Matsuzawa, Y.; Nagashima, N.; Irie, Y.; et al. Inhibition of HIV-1 infectivity with curdlan sulfate in vitro. *Biochem. Pharmacol.* **1990**, *39*, 793–797. [CrossRef] [PubMed]

31. Gao, Y.; Fukuda, A.; Katsuraya, K.; Kaneko, Y.; Mimura, T.; Nakashima, H.; Uryu, T. Synthesis of regioselective substituted curdlan sulfates with medium molecular weights and their specific anti-HIV-1 activities. *Macromolecules* **1997**, *30*, 3224–3228. [CrossRef]

32. Yamamoto, I.; Takayama, K.; Gonda, T.; Matsuzaki, K.; Hatanaka, K.; Yoshida, T.; Uryu, T.; Yoshida, O.; Nakashima, H.; Yamamoto, N.; et al. Synthesis, structure and antiviral activity of sulfates of curdlan and its branched derivatives. *Br. Polym. J.* **1990**, *23*, 245–250. [CrossRef]

33. Koizumi, N.; Sakagami, H.; Utsumi, A.; Fujinaga, S.; Takeda, M.; Asano, K.; Sugawara, I.; Ichikawa, S.; Kondo, H.; Mori, S.; et al. Anti-HIV (human immunodeficiency virus) activity of sulfated paramylon. *Antivir. Res.* **1993**, *21*, 1–14. [CrossRef]

34. Nakashima, H.; Inazawa, K.; Ichiyama, K.; Ito, M.; Ikushima, N.; Shoji, T.; Katsuraya, K.; Uryu, T.; Yamamoto, N.; Juodawlkis, A.S.; et al. Sulfated alkyl oligosaccharides inhibit human immunodeficiency virus in vitro and provide sustained drug levels in mammals. *Antivir. Chem. Chemother.* **1995**, *6*, 271–280. [CrossRef]

35. Witvrouw, M.; De Clercq, E. Sulfated polysaccharides extracted from sea algae as potential antiviral drugs. *Gen. Pharmacol.* **1997**, *29*, 497–511. [CrossRef]

36. Batinic, D.; Robey, F.A. The V3 region of the envelope glycoprotein of human immunodeficiency virus type 1 binds sulfated polysaccharides and CD4-derived synthetic peptides. *J. Biol. Chem.* **1992**, *267*, 6664–6671. [PubMed]

37. Callahan, L.N.; Phelan, M.; Mallinson, M.; Norcross, M.A. Dextran sulfate blocks antibody binding to the principal neutralizing domain of human immunodeficiency virus type 1 without interfering with gp120-CD4 interactions. *J. Virol.* **1991**, *65*, 1543–1550. [PubMed]

38. Mbemba, E.; Chams, V.; Gluckman, J.C.; Klatzmann, D.; Gattegno, L. Molecular interaction between HIV-1 major envelope glycoprotein and dextran sulfate. *Biochim. Biophys. Acta* **1992**, *1138*, 62–67. [CrossRef]

39. Lai, P.K.; Donovan, J.; Takayama, H.; Sakagami, H.; Tanaka, A.; Konno, K.; Nonoyama, M. Modification of human immunodeficiency viral replication by pine cone extracts. *AIDS Res. Hum. Retrovir.* **1990**, *6*, 205–217. [CrossRef] [PubMed]

40. Nakashima, H.; Murakami, T.; Yamamoto, N.; Naoe, T.; Kawazoe, Y.; Konno, K.; Sakagami, H. Lignified materials as medicinal resources. V. Anti-HIV (human immunodeficiency virus) activity of some synthetic lignins. *Chem. Pharm. Bull.* **1992**, *40*, 2102–2105. [CrossRef] [PubMed]

41. Mitsuhashi, S.; Kishimoto, T.; Uraki, Y.; Okamoto, T.; Ubukata, M. Low molecular weight lignin suppresses activation of NF-κB and HIV-1 promoter. *Bioorg. Med. Chem.* **2008**, *16*, 2645–2650. [CrossRef] [PubMed]

42. Fujioka, T.; Kashiwada, Y.; Kilkuskie, R.E.; Cosentino, L.M.; Ballas, L.M.; Jiang, J.B.; Janzen, W.P.; Chen, I.S.; Lee, K.H. Anti-AIDS agents, 11. Betulinic acid and platanic acid as anti-HIV principles from *Syzigium claviflorum*, and the anti-HIV activity of structurally related triterpenoids. *J. Nat. Prod.* **1994**, *57*, 243–247. [CrossRef] [PubMed]

43. Kashiwada, Y.; Hashimoto, F.; Cosentino, L.M.; Chen, C.H.; Garrett, P.E.; Lee, K.H. Betulinic acid and dihydrobetulinic acid derivatives as potent anti-HIV agents. *J. Med. Chem.* **1996**, *39*, 1016–1017. [CrossRef] [PubMed]

44. Kanamoto, T.; Kashiwada, Y.; Kanbara, K.; Gotoh, K.; Yoshimori, M.; Goto, T.; Sano, K.; Nakashima, H. Anti-human immunodeficiency virus activity of YK-FH312 (a betulinic acid derivative), a novel compound blocking viral maturation. *Antimicrob. Agents Chemother.* **2001**, *45*, 1225–1230. [CrossRef] [PubMed]

45. Li, F.; Goila-Gaur, R.; Salzwedel, K.; Kilgore, N.R.; Reddick, M.; Matallana, C.; Castillo, A.; Zoumplis, D.; Martin, D.E.; Orenstein, J.M.; et al. PA-457: A potent HIV inhibitor that disrupts core condensation by targeting a late step in Gag processing. *Proc. Natl. Acad. Sci. USA* **2003**, *100*, 13555–13560. [CrossRef] [PubMed]

46. Morimoto, M.; Mori, H.; Otake, T.; Ueba, N.; Kunita, N.; Niwa, M.; Murakami, T.; Iwanaga, S. Inhibitory effect of tachyplesin I on the proliferation of human immunodeficiency virus in vitro. *Chemotherapy* **1991**, *37*, 206–211. [CrossRef] [PubMed]

47. Murakami, T.; Niwa, M.; Tokunaga, F.; Miyata, T.; Iwanaga, S. Direct virus inactivation of tachyplesin I and its isopeptides from horseshoe crab hemocytes. *Chemotherapy* **1991**, *37*, 327–334. [CrossRef] [PubMed]

48. Nakashima, H.; Masuda, M.; Murakami, T.; Koyanagi, Y.; Matsumoto, A.; Fujii, N.; Yamamoto, N. Anti-human immunodeficiency virus activity of a novel synthetic peptide, T22 ([Tyr-5,12, Lys-7]polyphemusin II): A possible inhibitor of virus-cell fusion. *Antimicrob. Agents Chemother.* **1992**, *36*, 1249–1255. [CrossRef] [PubMed]

49. Masuda, M.; Nakashima, H.; Ueda, T.; Naba, H.; Ikoma, R.; Otaka, A.; Terakawa, Y.; Tamamura, H.; Ibuka, T.; Murakami, T.; et al. A novel anti-HIV synthetic peptide, T-22 ([Tyr5,12,Lys7]-polyphemusin II). *Biochem. Biophys. Res. Commun.* **1992**, *189*, 845–850. [CrossRef]

50. Arakaki, R.; Tamamura, H.; Premanathan, M.; Kanbara, K.; Ramanan, S.; Mochizuki, K.; Baba, M.; Fujii, N.; Nakashima, H. T134, a small-molecule CXCR4 inhibitor, has no cross-drug resistance with AMD3100, a CXCR4 antagonist with a different structure. *J. Virol.* **1999**, *73*, 1719–1723. [PubMed]

51. Tamamura, H.; Xu, Y.; Hattori, T.; Zhang, X.; Arakaki, R.; Kanbara, K.; Omagari, A.; Otaka, A.; Ibuka, T.; Yamamoto, N.; et al. A low-molecular-weight inhibitor against the chemokine receptor CXCR4: A strong anti-HIV peptide T140. *Biochem. Biophys. Res. Commun.* **1998**, *253*, 877–882. [CrossRef] [PubMed]

52. Fujii, N.; Oishi, S.; Hiramatsu, K.; Araki, T.; Ueda, S.; Tamamura, H.; Otaka, A.; Kusano, S.; Terakubo, S.; Nakashima, H.; et al. Molecular-size reduction of a potent CXCR4-chemokine antagonist using orthogonal combination of conformation- and sequence-based libraries. *Angew. Chem. Int. Ed. Engl.* **2003**, *42*, 3251–3253. [CrossRef] [PubMed]

53. Murakami, T.; Nakajima, T.; Koyanagi, Y.; Tachibana, K.; Fujii, N.; Tamamura, H.; Yoshida, N.; Waki, M.; Matsumoto, A.; Yoshie, O.; et al. A small molecule CXCR4 inhibitor that blocks T cell line-tropic HIV-1 infection. *J. Exp. Med.* **1997**, *186*, 1389–1393. [CrossRef] [PubMed]

54. Xu, Y.; Tamamura, H.; Arakaki, R.; Nakashima, H.; Zhang, X.; Fujii, N.; Uchiyama, T.; Hattori, T. Marked increase in anti-HIV activity, as well as inhibitory activity against HIV entry mediated by CXCR4, linked to enhancement of the binding ability of tachyplesin analogs to CXCR4. *AIDS Res. Hum. Retrovir.* **1999**, *15*, 419–427. [CrossRef] [PubMed]

55. Murakami, T.; Zhang, T.Y.; Koyanagi, Y.; Tanaka, Y.; Kim, J.; Suzuki, Y.; Minoguchi, S.; Tamamura, H.; Waki, M.; Matsumoto, A.; et al. Inhibitory mechanism of the CXCR4 antagonist T22 against human immunodeficiency virus type 1 infection. *J. Virol.* **1999**, *73*, 7489–7496. [CrossRef] [PubMed]

56. Ohashi, N.; Tamamura, H. Peptide-derived mid-sized anti-HIV agents. *Amino Acids Pept. Proteins* **2017**, *41*, 1–29. [CrossRef]

57. Ma, X.; Li, L.; Zhu, T.; Ba, M.; Li, G.; Gu, Q.; Guo, Y.; Li, D. Phenylspirodrimanes with anti-HIV activity from the sponge-derived fungus *Stachybotrys chartarum* MXH-X73. *J. Nat. Prod.* **2013**, *76*, 2298–2306. [CrossRef] [PubMed]

58. Vidal, V.; Potterat, O.; Louvel, S.; Hamy, F.; Mojarrab, M.; Sanglier, J.J.; Klimkait, T.; Hamburger, M. Library-based discovery and characterization of daphnane diterpenes as potent and selective HIV inhibitors in *Daphne gnidium*. *J. Nat. Prod.* **2012**, *75*, 414–419. [CrossRef] [PubMed]

59. Tietjen, I.; Ntie-Kang, F.; Mwimanzi, P.; Onguene, P.A.; Scull, M.A.; Idowu, T.O.; Ogundaini, A.O.; Meva'a, L.M.; Abegaz, B.M.; Rice, C.M.; et al. Screening of the Pan-African natural product library identifies ixoratannin A-2 and boldine as novel HIV-1 inhibitors. *PLoS ONE* **2015**, *10*, e0121099. [CrossRef] [PubMed]

60. Mori, T.; O'Keefe, B.R.; Sowder, R.C., 2nd; Bringans, S.; Gardella, R.; Berg, S.; Cochran, P.; Turpin, J.A.; Buckheit, R.W., Jr.; McMahon, J.B.; et al. Isolation and characterization of griffithsin, a novel HIV-inactivating protein, from the red alga *Griffithsia* sp. *J. Biol. Chem.* **2005**, *280*, 9345–9353. [CrossRef] [PubMed]

61. O'Keefe, B.R.; Vojdani, F.; Buffa, V.; Shattock, R.J.; Montefiori, D.C.; Bakke, J.; Mirsalis, J.; d'Andrea, A.L.; Hume, S.D.; Bratcher, B.; et al. Scaleable manufacture of HIV-1 entry inhibitor griffithsin and validation of its safety and efficacy as a topical microbicide component. *Proc. Natl. Acad. Sci. USA* **2009**, *106*, 6099–6104. [CrossRef] [PubMed]

62. Lai, W.; Huang, L.; Zhu, L.; Ferrari, G.; Chan, C.; Li, W.; Lee, K.H.; Chen, C.H. Gnidimacrin, a Potent Anti-HIV Diterpene, Can Eliminate Latent HIV-1 Ex Vivo by Activation of Protein Kinase C beta. *J. Med. Chem.* **2015**, *58*, 8638–8646. [CrossRef] [PubMed]

63. Hassan, S.T.; Masarcikova, R.; Berchova, K. Bioactive natural products with anti-herpes simplex virus properties. *J. Pharm. Pharmacol.* **2015**, *67*, 1325–1336. [CrossRef] [PubMed]

64. Vo, T.S.; Ngo, D.H.; Ta, Q.V.; Kim, S.K. Marine organisms as a therapeutic source against herpes simplex virus infection. *Eur. J. Pharm. Sci.* **2011**, *44*, 11–20. [CrossRef] [PubMed]

65. Mandal, P.; Pujol, C.A.; Damonte, E.B.; Ghosh, T.; Ray, B. Xylans from *Scinaia hatei*: Structural features, sulfation and anti-HSV activity. *Int. J. Biol. Macromol.* **2010**, *46*, 173–178. [CrossRef] [PubMed]

66. Duarte, M.E.; Noseda, D.G.; Noseda, M.D.; Tulio, S.; Pujol, C.A.; Damonte, E.B. Inhibitory effect of sulfated galactans from the marine alga *Bostrychia montagnei* on herpes simplex virus replication in vitro. *Phytomedicine* **2001**, *8*, 53–58. [CrossRef] [PubMed]

67. Talarico, L.B.; Zibetti, R.G.; Faria, P.C.; Scolaro, L.A.; Duarte, M.E.; Noseda, M.D.; Pujol, C.A.; Damonte, E.B. Anti-herpes simplex virus activity of sulfated galactans from the red seaweeds *Gymnogongrus griffithsiae* and *Cryptonemia crenulata*. *Int. J. Biol. Macromol.* **2004**, *34*, 63–71. [CrossRef] [PubMed]

68. Park, H.J.; Kurokawa, M.; Shiraki, K.; Nakamura, N.; Choi, J.S.; Hattori, M. Antiviral activity of the marine alga *Symphyocladia latiuscula* against herpes simplex virus (HSV-1) in vitro and its therapeutic efficacy against HSV-1 infection in mice. *Biol. Pharm. Bull.* **2005**, *28*, 2258–2262. [CrossRef] [PubMed]

69. Pifarre, M.P.; Berra, A.; Coto, C.E.; Alche, L.E. Therapeutic action of meliacine, a plant-derived antiviral, on HSV-induced ocular disease in mice. *Exp. Eye Res.* **2002**, *75*, 327–334. [CrossRef] [PubMed]

70. Petrera, E.; Coto, C.E. Therapeutic effect of meliacine, an antiviral derived from *Melia azedarach* L., in mice genital herpetic infection. *Phytother. Res.* **2009**, *23*, 1771–1777. [CrossRef] [PubMed]

71. Hayashi, T.; Kawasaki, M.; Miwa, Y.; Taga, T.; Morita, N. Antiviral agents of plant origin. III. Scopadulin, a novel tetracyclic diterpene from *Scoparia dulcis* L. *Chem. Pharm. Bull.* **1990**, *38*, 945–947. [CrossRef] [PubMed]

72. Hayashi, T.; Hayashi, K.; Maeda, M.; Kojima, I. Calcium spirulan, an inhibitor of enveloped virus replication, from a blue-green alga *Spirulina platensis*. *J. Nat. Prod.* **1996**, *59*, 83–87. [CrossRef] [PubMed]

73. Lee, J.B.; Hayashi, K.; Hashimoto, M.; Nakano, T.; Hayashi, T. Novel antiviral fucoidan from sporophyll of *Undaria pinnatifida* (Mekabu). *Chem. Pharm. Bull.* **2004**, *52*, 1091–1094. [CrossRef] [PubMed]

74. Kanekiyo, K.; Lee, J.B.; Hayashi, K.; Takenaka, H.; Hayakawa, Y.; Endo, S.; Hayashi, T. Isolation of an antiviral polysaccharide, nostoflan, from a terrestrial cyanobacterium, *Nostoc flagelliforme*. *J. Nat. Prod.* **2005**, *68*, 1037–1041. [CrossRef] [PubMed]

75. Docherty, J.J.; Sweet, T.J.; Bailey, E.; Faith, S.A.; Booth, T. Resveratrol inhibition of varicella-zoster virus replication in vitro. *Antivir. Res.* **2006**, *72*, 171–177. [CrossRef] [PubMed]

76. De Leo, A.; Arena, G.; Lacanna, E.; Oliviero, G.; Colavita, F.; Mattia, E. Resveratrol inhibits Epstein Barr Virus lytic cycle in Burkitt's lymphoma cells by affecting multiple molecular targets. *Antivir. Res.* **2012**, *96*, 196–202. [CrossRef] [PubMed]

77. Evers, D.L.; Wang, X.; Huong, S.M.; Huang, D.Y.; Huang, E.S. 3,4′,5-Trihydroxy-trans-stilbene (resveratrol) inhibits human cytomegalovirus replication and virus-induced cellular signaling. *Antivir. Res.* **2004**, *63*, 85–95. [CrossRef] [PubMed]

78. Dyson, O.F.; Walker, L.R.; Whitehouse, A.; Cook, P.P.; Akula, S.M. Resveratrol inhibits KSHV reactivation by lowering the levels of cellular EGR-1. *PLoS ONE* **2012**, *7*, e33364. [CrossRef] [PubMed]

79. Ourth, D.D. Susceptibility in vitro of Epstein-Barr Virus to myristoylated-peptide. *Peptides* **2010**, *31*, 1409–1411. [CrossRef] [PubMed]

80. Prusty, B.K.; Das, B.C. Constitutive activation of transcription factor AP-1 in cervical cancer and suppression of human papillomavirus (HPV) transcription and AP-1 activity in HeLa cells by curcumin. *Int. J. Cancer* **2005**, *113*, 951–960. [CrossRef] [PubMed]

81. Slater, M.J.; Cockerill, S.; Baxter, R.; Bonser, R.W.; Gohil, K.; Gowrie, C.; Robinson, J.E.; Littler, E.; Parry, N.; Randall, R.; et al. Indolocarbazoles: Potent, selective inhibitors of human cytomegalovirus replication. *Bioorg. Med. Chem.* **1999**, *7*, 1067–1074. [CrossRef]

82. Nixon, B.; Stefanidou, M.; Mesquita, P.M.; Fakioglu, E.; Segarra, T.; Rohan, L.; Halford, W.; Palmer, K.E.; Herold, B.C. Griffithsin protects mice from genital herpes by preventing cell-to-cell spread. *J. Virol.* **2013**, *87*, 6257–6269. [CrossRef] [PubMed]

83. Levendosky, K.; Mizenina, O.; Martinelli, E.; Jean-Pierre, N.; Kizima, L.; Rodriguez, A.; Kleinbeck, K.; Bonnaire, T.; Robbiani, M.; Zydowsky, T.M.; et al. Griffithsin and Carrageenan Combination To Target Herpes Simplex Virus 2 and Human Papillomavirus. *Antimicrob. Agents Chemother.* **2015**, *59*, 7290–7298. [CrossRef] [PubMed]

84. Takebe, Y.; Saucedo, C.J.; Lund, G.; Uenishi, R.; Hase, S.; Tsuchiura, T.; Kneteman, N.; Ramessar, K.; Tyrrell, D.L.; Shirakura, M.; et al. Antiviral lectins from red and blue-green algae show potent in vitro and in vivo activity against hepatitis C virus. *PLoS ONE* **2013**, *8*, e64449. [CrossRef] [PubMed]

85. Buck, C.B.; Thompson, C.D.; Roberts, J.N.; Muller, M.; Lowy, D.R.; Schiller, J.T. Carrageenan is a potent inhibitor of papillomavirus infection. *PLoS Pathog.* **2006**, *2*, e69. [CrossRef] [PubMed]

86. Roberts, J.N.; Buck, C.B.; Thompson, C.D.; Kines, R.; Bernardo, M.; Choyke, P.L.; Lowy, D.R.; Schiller, J.T. Genital transmission of HPV in a mouse model is potentiated by nonoxynol-9 and inhibited by carrageenan. *Nat. Med.* **2007**, *13*, 857–861. [CrossRef] [PubMed]

87. Marais, D.; Gawarecki, D.; Allan, B.; Ahmed, K.; Altini, L.; Cassim, N.; Gopolang, F.; Hoffman, M.; Ramjee, G.; Williamson, A.L. The effectiveness of Carraguard, a vaginal microbicide, in protecting women against high-risk human papillomavirus infection. *Antivir. Ther.* **2011**, *16*, 1219–1226. [CrossRef] [PubMed]

88. Malonza, I.M.; Mirembe, F.; Nakabiito, C.; Odusoga, L.O.; Osinupebi, O.A.; Hazari, K.; Chitlange, S.; Ali, M.M.; Callahan, M.; Van Damme, L. Expanded Phase I safety and acceptability study of 6% cellulose sulfate vaginal gel. *AIDS* **2005**, *19*, 2157–2163. [CrossRef] [PubMed]

89. El-Sadr, W.M.; Mayer, K.H.; Maslankowski, L.; Hoesley, C.; Justman, J.; Gai, F.; Mauck, C.; Absalon, J.; Morrow, K.; Masse, B.; et al. Safety and acceptability of cellulose sulfate as a vaginal microbicide in HIV-infected women. *AIDS* **2006**, *20*, 1109–1116. [CrossRef] [PubMed]

90. Van Damme, L.; Govinden, R.; Mirembe, F.M.; Guedou, F.; Solomon, S.; Becker, M.L.; Pradeep, B.S.; Krishnan, A.K.; Alary, M.; Pande, B.; et al. Lack of effectiveness of cellulose sulfate gel for the prevention of vaginal HIV transmission. *N. Engl. J. Med.* **2008**, *359*, 463–472. [CrossRef] [PubMed]

91. Derby, N.; Lal, M.; Aravantinou, M.; Kizima, L.; Barnable, P.; Rodriguez, A.; Lai, M.; Wesenberg, A.; Ugaonkar, S.; Levendosky, K.; et al. Griffithsin carrageenan fast dissolving inserts prevent SHIV HSV-2 and HPV infections in vivo. *Nat. Commun.* **2018**, *9*, 3881. [CrossRef] [PubMed]

92. Punfa, W.; Yodkeeree, S.; Pitchakarn, P.; Ampasavate, C.; Limtrakul, P. Enhancement of cellular uptake and cytotoxicity of curcumin-loaded PLGA nanoparticles by conjugation with anti-P-glycoprotein in drug resistance cancer cells. *Acta Pharmacol. Sin.* **2012**, *33*, 823–831. [CrossRef] [PubMed]

93. Zaman, M.S.; Chauhan, N.; Yallapu, M.M.; Gara, R.K.; Maher, D.M.; Kumari, S.; Sikander, M.; Khan, S.; Zafar, N.; Jaggi, M.; et al. Curcumin Nanoformulation for Cervical Cancer Treatment. *Sci. Rep.* **2016**, *6*, 20051. [CrossRef] [PubMed]

94. Gong, C.; Wu, Q.; Wang, Y.; Zhang, D.; Luo, F.; Zhao, X.; Wei, Y.; Qian, Z. A biodegradable hydrogel system containing curcumin encapsulated in micelles for cutaneous wound healing. *Biomaterials* **2013**, *34*, 6377–6387. [CrossRef] [PubMed]

95. Chen, G.; Li, J.; Cai, Y.; Zhan, J.; Gao, J.; Song, M.; Shi, Y.; Yang, Z. A Glycyrrhetinic Acid-Modified Curcumin Supramolecular Hydrogel for liver tumor targeting therapy. *Sci. Rep.* **2017**, *7*, 44210. [CrossRef] [PubMed]

96. Porter, S.R.; Al-Johani, K.; Fedele, S.; Moles, D.R. Randomised controlled trial of the efficacy of HybenX in the symptomatic treatment of recurrent aphthous stomatitis. *Oral Dis.* **2009**, *15*, 155–161. [CrossRef] [PubMed]

97. Nibali, L.; Atkinson, C.; Griffiths, P.; Darbar, U.; Rakmanee, T.; Suvan, J.; Donos, N. Low prevalence of subgingival viruses in periodontitis patients. *J. Clin. Periodontol.* **2009**, *36*, 928–932. [CrossRef] [PubMed]

98. Agut, H.; Bonnafous, P.; Gautheret-Dejean, A. Laboratory and clinical aspects of human herpesvirus 6 infections. *Clin. Microbiol. Rev.* **2015**, *28*, 313–335. [CrossRef] [PubMed]

99. Asai, D.; Kanamoto, T.; Takenaga, M.; Nakashima, H. In situ depot formation of anti-HIV fusion-inhibitor peptide in recombinant protein polymer hydrogel. *Acta Biomater.* **2017**, *64*, 116–125. [CrossRef] [PubMed]

9

Antimicrobial Susceptibilities of Oral Isolates of *Abiotrophia* and *Granulicatella* According to the Consensus Guidelines for Fastidious Bacteria

Taisei Kanamoto [1,2,*], Shigemi Terakubo [2] and Hideki Nakashima [2]

[1]   Laboratory of Microbiology, Showa Pharmaceutical University, Machida, Tokyo 194-8543, Japan
[2]   Department of Microbiology, St. Marianna University School of Medicine, Kawasaki,
     Kanagawa 216-8511, Japan; biseibutsu-001@marianna-u.ac.jp (S.T.); nakahide@marianna-u.ac.jp (H.N.)
[*]   Correspondence: kanamoto@ac.shoyaku.ac.jp

Abstract: Background: The genera *Abiotrophia* and *Granulicatella*, previously known as nutritionally variant streptococci (NVS), are fastidious bacteria requiring vitamin B_6 analogs for growth. They are members of human normal oral microbiota, and are supposed to be one of the important pathogens for so-called "culture-negative" endocarditis. **Methods:** The type strains and oral isolates identified, by using both phenotypic profiles and the DNA–DNA hybridization method, were examined for susceptibilities to 15 antimicrobial agents including penicillin (benzylpenicillin, ampicillin, amoxicillin, and piperacillin), cephem (cefazolin, ceftazidime, ceftriaxone, and cefaclor), carbapenem (imipenem), aminoglycoside (gentamicin), macrolide (erythromycin), quinolone (ciprofloxacin), tetracycline (minocycline), glycopeptide (vancomycin), and trimethoprim-sulfamethoxazole complex. The minimum inhibitory concentration and susceptibility criterion were determined, according to the consensus guideline from the Clinical and Laboratory Standards Institute. **Results:** Isolates of *Abiotrophia defectiva* were susceptible to ampicillin, amoxicillin ceftriaxone, cefaclor, imipenem, ciprofloxacin, and vancomycin. Isolates of *Granulicatella adiacens* were mostly susceptible to benzylpenicillin, ampicillin, amoxicillin, cefazolin, ceftriaxone, imipenem, minocycline, and vancomycin. The susceptibility profile of *Granulicatella elegans* was similar to that of *G. adiacens*, and the susceptibility rate was higher than that of *G. adiacens*. **Conclusions:** Although *Abiotrophia* and *Granulicatella* strains are hardly distinguishable by their phenotypic characteristics, their susceptibility profiles to the antimicrobial agents were different among the species. Species-related differences in susceptibility of antibiotics should be considered in the clinical treatment for NVS related infections.

Keywords: nutritionally variant streptococci; antimicrobial susceptibilities; oral microbiota; infective endocarditis

1. Introduction

The bacteria formerly known as nutritionally variant streptococci (NVS) are characterized by their growth as small satellite colonies supported by helper bacteria such as *Staphylococcus aureus* The NVS strains require vitamin B_6 analogs for growth and produce bacteriolytic enzymes, pyrrolidonyl arylamidase and chromophore in common and were supposed to be auxotrophic variants of viridans group streptococci [2]. After several taxonomic alterations, they were finally transferred into two new genera, *Abiotrophia* and *Granulicatella*, on the basis of 16S rRNA gene sequence homology analysis [3,4]. They have been estimated as one of the important pathogens of so-called 'culture-negative endocarditis' [2,5,6]; however, because of their fastidiousness in growth, difficulty in identification, and complication in taxonomic position, the clinical importance of these bacteria has been underestimated by clinicians [7].

Although there have been several studies on the antimicrobial susceptibility of NVS, most of the previous studies dealt with a small number of strains, and methods and results were variable [2]. Furthermore, the taxonomic backgrounds of the tested isolates were uncertain. Commercial identification systems, based on the phenotypic characteristics of cultured bacteria, have often misidentified the clinical isolates of *Granulicatella* as *Gemella morbillorum*, and cannot distinguish *Granulicatella adiacens* and *Granulicatella elegans* [8–10]. To distinguish the two species of *Granulicatella*, molecular genetic analysis is required [11]. We previously isolated 91 strains of NVS from the human oral microbiota and classified them based on the phenotypic characteristics [9]. Among the oral isolates, 37 isolates confirmed their taxonomic identification by using DNA–DNA hybridization homology analysis, and we reported genetic heterogeneities in genus *Granulicatella* [10].

The Clinical and Laboratory Standards Institute (CLSI) published a laboratory guideline of antimicrobial susceptibility testing of infrequently encountered or fastidious bacteria, not covered in previous CLSI publications [12]. In this study, we determined the minimum inhibitory concentrations (MICs) of the taxonomically confirmed strains of *Abiotrophia* and *Granulicatella*, according to the consensus guideline provided by CLSI.

2. Materials and Methods

2.1. Bacterial Strains

Seven *Abiotrophia defectiva*, 17 *Granulicatella adiacens*, and six *Granulicatella elegans* (including type strains and oral isolates) were examined (see Tables 1 and 2). All isolates were identified using the rapid ID32 STREP system (Bio Mérieux SA, Marcy-l'Etoile, France) and DNA-DNA hybridization homology analysis [10]. The reference strains, *A. defectiva* ATCC 49176^T, NVS-47, and PE7, *G. adiacens* ATCC 49175^T, and *G. elegans* DSM11693^T, were from patients with endocarditis or bacteremia [13–15], and the other 25 isolates were derived from the oral cavity of healthy volunteers [9]. The strain *Streptococcus pneumoniae* ATCC 49619 was included in the assay to monitor accuracy of the MIC tests. The ATCC strains were obtained from American Type Culture Collection (Manassas, VA, USA), the DSM strain was obtained from Deutsche Sammlung von Mikroorganismen und Zellkulturen GmbH (Braunschweig, Germany), and the other strains were from the stock culture collection in our laboratory.

Table 1. MICs (μg/mL) of 15 antibiotics against *Abiotrophia* isolates.

Strains	PEN	AMP	AMX	PIP	CFZ	CAZ	CRO	CEC	IPM	GEN	ERY	CIP	MIN	VAN	SXT
A. defectiva															
ATCC49176[T]	0.125	0.016	0.016	1	1	16	1	0.125	0.125	32	0.5	1	0.063	0.25	256/4864
NVS-47	0.125	0.032	0.016	1	2	16	1	0.125	0.125	32	0.5	1	0.032	0.25	256/4864
PE7	0.032	0.016	0.016	4	1	8	1	0.125	0.125	32	0.5	1	0.063	0.25	256/4864
YTS2	0.063	0.016	0.063	1	4	8	0.5	0.5	0.125	32	0.5	1	0.063	0.25	256/4864
C8-3	0.25	0.125	0.063	1	2	8	0.5	0.5	0.125	16	0.25	0.5	4	0.25	0.016/0.3
C1-2	2	0.5	0.25	4	16	16	1	32	0.25	16	128	1	8	0.25	128/2432
YK-3	0.25	0.125	0.125	2	16	16	1	1	0.25	64	4	1	16	0.25	128/2432
range	0.032	0.016	0.016	1	1	8	0.5	0.125	0.125	16	0.25	0.5	0.032	—	0.016/0.3
	—	—	—	—	—	—	—	—	—	—	—	—	—	0.25	—
	2	0.5	0.25	4	16	16	1	32	0.25	64	128	1	16		256/4864

Type strain and strains NVS-47 and PE7 were derived from blood cultures with endocarditis and the others were oral isolates from healthy volunteers. MIC: minimum inhibitory concentration, PEN: benzylpenicillin, AMP: ampicillin, AMX: amoxicillin, PIP: piperacillin, CFZ: cefazolin, CAZ: ceftazidime, CRO: ceftriaxone, CEC: cefaclor, IPM: imipenem, GEN: gentamicin, ERY: erythromycin, CIP: ciprofloxacin, MIN: minocycline, VAN: vancomycin, SXT: sulfamethoxazole-trimethoprim complex.

Table 2. MICs (μg/mL) of 15 antibiotics against *Granulicatella* isolates.

Strains	PEN	AMP	AMX	PIP	CFZ	CAZ	CRO	CEC	IPM	GEN	ERY	CIP	MIN	VAN	SXT
G. adiacens															
ATCC49175[T]	0.032	0.032	0.016	0.5	0.125	16	0.25	0.5	0.016	32	0.5	2	0.063	0.5	128/2432
HHC3	0.125	0.063	0.032	1	2	32	0.5	2	0.032	32	0.25	4	8	0.5	64/1216
HHP1	0.063	0.032	0.016	0.25	0.25	4	0.25	1	0.016	32	0.5	2	0.063	0.5	256/4864
P6-1	0.063	0.032	0.016	0.25	0.25	4	0.25	2	0.016	64	0.25	1	0.063	0.5	64/1216
YTC1	0.125	0.063	0.032	0.5	1	32	0.5	2	0.016	16	0.5	2	0.032	0.5	256/4864
S961-2	0.032	0.032	0.016	0.25	0.25	4	2	0.25	0.016	32	0.5	2	0.016	0.5	32/608
S1058-2	0.125	0.032	0.032	0.25	0.25	2	0.25	1	0.016	32	0.25	1	0.032	0.5	32/608
TK-T1	0.032	0.032	0.032	0.25	0.25	4	1	0.5	0.016	32	0.5	2	0.125	0.5	64/1216
HKT1-4	0.25	0.125	0.063	0.5	1	8	1	4	0.032	32	0.5	2	0.125	0.5	32/608
HKT2-2	0.125	0.125	0.063	0.5	1	8	0.25	4	0.032	32	0.125	2	0.016	0.25	32/608
C4-3	0.016	0.008	0.008	0.063	0.125	4	1	0.5	0.016	16	0.25	4	0.016	0.5	256/4864

Table 2. *Cont.*

Strains	PEN	AMP	AMX	PIP	CFZ	CAZ	CRO	CEC	IPM	GEN	ERY	CIP	MIN	VAN	SXT
HKT1-1	0.25	0.125	0.063	0.5	1	16	2	4	0.032	32	0.125	1	0.016	0.25	64/1216
NMP2	0.125	0.125	0.063	0.5	1	4	1	2	0.032	32	0.25	2	0.032	0.5	64/1216
P7-4	0.5	0.25	0.125	0.5	2	4	4	4	0.016	32	0.25	2	0.016	0.5	16/304
S49-2	0.032	0.032	0.032	0.25	0.25	4	8	0.5	0.016	32	0.25	2	0.063	0.5	128/2432
YTT3	0.063	0.032	0.032	0.25	0.25	64	0.25	1	0.032	16	0.25	2	0.125	0.5	64/1216
TK-T2	0.063	0.063	0.063	0.25	0.5	16	1	1	0.016	32	0.5	2	0.125	0.5	256/4864
range	0.016 – 0.5	0.008 – 0.25	0.008 – 0.125	0.063 – 1	0.125 – 2	2 – 64	0.25 – 8	0.25 – 4	0.016 – 0.032	16 – 64	0.125 – 0.5	1 – 4	0.016 – 8	0.25 – 0.5	16/304 – 256/4864
G. elegans															
DSM11693[T]	0.016	0.063	0.125	0.125	0.125	2	0.5	0.5	0.016	16	8	1	0.25	4	0.5/9.5
NMP3	0.032	0.032	0.016	0.125	0.25	1	0.008	0.5	0.016	16	0.5	2	0.032	0.5	1/19
S1052-1	0.016	0.016	0.016	0.25	0.5	2	0.008	0.5	0.032	16	1	2	0.063	0.5	2/38
YTM1	0.032	0.032	0.016	0.25	0.25	1	0.016	0.5	0.016	16	0.5	4	0.063	0.5	512/9728
HHC5	0.032	0.032	0.016	0.25	0.5	2	0.032	0.5	0.032	8	0.5	2	0.016	0.5	2/38
C9-2	0.063	0.063	0.063	0.25	0.5	1	0.032	2	0.063	16	32	4	2	0.5	1/19
range	0.016 – 0.063	0.016 – 0.63	0.016 – 0.125	0.125 – 0.25	0.125 – 0.5	1 – 2	0.08 – 0.5	0.5 – 2	0.016 – 0.63	8 – 16	0.5 – 32	1 – 4	0.016 – 2	0.5 – 4	0.5/9.5 – 512/9728

Type strains were derived from blood cultures with endocarditis and the others were oral isolates from healthy volunteers. MIC: minimum inhibitory concentration, PEN: benzylpenicillin, AMP: ampicillin, AMX: amoxicillin, PIP: piperacillin, CFZ: cefazolin, CAZ: ceftazidime, CRO: ceftriaxone, CEC: cefaclor, IPM: imipenem, GEN: gentamicin, ERY: erythromycin, CIP: ciprofloxacin, MIN: minocycline, VAN: vancomycin, SXT: sulfamethoxazole-trimethoprim complex.

2.2. Antimicrobial Agents

Fifteen antimicrobial agents including penicillin, cephem, carbapenem, aminoglycoside, macrolide, tetracycline, quinolone, glycopeptide, and sulfonamide were used for this study (see Table 3). The following agents were purchased from Wako Pure Chemical Industries, Ltd. (Osaka, Japan): benzylpenicillin, cefazolin, piperacillin, ciprofloxacin, minocycline, and trimethoprim-sulfamethoxazole complex. Ampicillin, ceftazidime, ceftriaxone, cefaclor, gentamicin, erythromycin, and vancomycin were obtained from Sigma Chemical Co. (St. Louis, MO, USA). Amoxicillin was purchased from Fluka Biochemika (Bucks, Switzerland). Imipenem was kindly supplied by the Banyu Pharmaceutical Co., Ltd. (Tokyo, Japan).

Table 3. Percentage of susceptible isolates of *Abiotrophia* and *Granulicatella* against antimicrobial agents.

Antimicrobial Agent	% of Susceptible Isolates		
	A. defectiva (n = 7)	G. adiacens (n = 17)	G. elegans (n = 6)
Penicillin			
Benzylpenicillin	57.1	82.4	100
Ampicillin	85.7	100	100
Amoxicillin [a]	100	100	100
Piperacillin [a]	0	52.9	100
Cephem			
Cefazolin [b]	28.6	88.2	100
Ceftazidime [b]	0	0	50
Ceftriaxone	100	76.4	100
Cefaclor [b]	85.7	52.9	83.3
Carbapenem			
Imipenem	100	100	100
Aminoglycoside			
Gentamicin [c]	0	0	0
Macrolide			
Erythromycin	14.3	58.8	0
Quinolone			
Ciprofloxacin	100	17.6	16.7
Tetracycline			
Minocycline [d]	57.1	94.1	100
Glycopeptide			
Vancomycin	100	100	83.3
Other			
Sulfamethoxazole-trimethoprim [e]	14.3	0	16.7

Susceptibilities of the strains to the antimicrobial agents were determined according to the CLSI guideline M45-A2 for *Abiotrophia* spp. and *Granulicatella* spp. Susceptibilities to the antimicrobial agents unlisted in the guideline were determined as below; [a,b] Determined according to the guideline for ampicillin and cephems, respectively; [c] Determined according to the CLSI guideline M100-S18 for *S. aureus*; [d] Determined according to the CLSI guideline M100-S18 for tetracycline for *Streptococcus* spp. Viridans group; [e] Determined by the MIC values under 2/38 µg/mL.

2.3. MIC Testing

For preparation of inoculum, tested isolates were cultured anaerobically at 37 °C for 20 to 24 h with Mueller-Hinton broth (MHB; Difco Becton Dickinson and company, Sparks, MD, USA) containing 0.001% pyridoxal hydrochloride (Wako) and the bacterial cell suspensions were adjusted to yield about 5×10^5 CFU/mL. MICs for the *Abiotrophia* and *Granulicatella* strains were determined using the microdilution broth method with MHB containing 2.5% lysed horse blood (Strepto hemo supplement 'Eiken', Eiken Chemical Co., Ltd., Tokyo, Japan) and 0.001% pyridoxal hydrochloride, according to the consensus guideline from the CLSI for fastidious bacteria [12]. Briefly, the antimicrobial agents (100 µL/well) were diluted on 96-well round bottom plates (Sumilon, Sumitomo Bakelite Co., Ltd.,

Tokyo, Japan) in serial two-fold with the supplemented MHB, and 5 μL of the bacterial inoculum was added to each well. The plates were incubated at 35 °C in anaerobic condition for 20 h. The MIC values were defined as the lowest concentrations of antimicrobial agents that completely inhibited the bacterial growth in the microdilution wells, detected by unaided eyes. The strain of *S. pneumoniae* ATCC 49619 was used for quality control testing, and all MIC values for the strain were within the acceptable limits.

2.4. Susceptibility Criteria

The MIC values for bacterial isolates to the antimicrobial agents benzylpenicillin, ampicillin, ceftriaxone imipenem, erythromycin, ciprofloxacin, and vancomycin were interpreted into 3 categories: Susceptible, intermediate, and resistant, according to the CLSI guideline for *Abiotrophia* spp. and *Granulicatella* spp.

The MIC values for amoxicillin and piperacillin, and those for cefazolin, ceftazidime, and cefaclor were interpreted using criteria for ampicillin and cephems in the guideline for *Abiotrophia* and *Granulicatella*, respectively [16]. The MIC values for gentamicin and minocycline were interpreted using criteria in the CLSI guideline for *S. aureus* and for *Streptococcus* spp. Viridans group, respectively. The MIC values under 2/38 μg/mL for trimethoprim-sulfamethoxazole were interpreted as susceptible [17].

3. Results

The susceptibility percentage of the NVS isolates for 15 antimicrobial agents was summarized in Table 3. Although the phenotypic characteristics of the NVS isolates were similar, the profiles of susceptibility were unique among the species. The NVS isolates were susceptible to ampicillin (96.7%), amoxicillin (100%), imipenem (100%), and vancomycin (96.7%). In addition, *A. defectiva* strains were susceptible to ceftriaxone (100%), cefaclor (85.7%), and ciprofloxacin (100%); and *G. adiacens* strains were susceptible to benzylpenicillin (82.7%), cefazolin (88.2%), ceftriaxone (76.4%), and minocycline (94.1%). The susceptibility profile of *G. elegans* was similar to that of *G. adiacens*, and the susceptibility percentages of *G. elegans* to beta-lactams were higher than that of *G. adiacens*. On the other hand, no NVS strains were susceptible to gentamicin, and 93.3% of the strains were not susceptible to trimethoprim/sulfamethoxazole. Piperacillin susceptibility rate of *A. defectiva* was 0%, while that of *G. adiacens* and *G. elegans* were 52.9% and 100%, respectively. All *A. defectiva* strains were susceptible to ciprofloxacin, but only 17.4% of *Granulicatella* strains were susceptible to it.

Individual MIC values of *A. defectiva* and *Granulicatella* isolates to the antimicrobial agents were shown in Tables 1 and 2, respectively. Benzylpenicillin-nonsusceptible oral isolates of *A. defectiva* C1-2 and YK-3 were highly resistant to cefazolin and ceftazidime (both MICs = 16 μg/mL) and C1-2 showed additional resistance to cefaclor (MIC = 32 μg/mL), but were susceptible to ceftriaxone (MIC ≤ 1 μg/mL). Oral isolate of *G. adiacens* HHC3 was highly multi-drug resistant to ceftazidime, gentamycin, ciprofloxacin, and minocycline. The benzylpenicillin-nonsusceptible oral isolate of *G. adiacens* P7-4 was resistant to cephems, including ceftazidime, ceftriaxone, and cefaclor (all MICs = 4 μg/mL). Among the NVS isolates, only *G. elegans* DSM11693[T] was resistant to vancomycin (MIC = 4 μg/mL).

4. Discussion

Abiotrophia and *Granulicatella* species are very common inhabitants in human normal oral microbiota, in spite of their fastidiousness in growth [9,11,18–20], and are significant causative pathogens of endocarditis, bacteremia, and other systemic infections [21–24]. They often cannot grow on commercial blood agar plates used for the usual clinical examination, and even if they could grow on supplemented culture plates, their colonies are sometimes small, 0.2 to 0.5 mm in diameter [1,25]. Therefore, these fastidious microorganisms have been overlooked in clinical specimens from foci of infective diseases, especially when they are concomitant with easily recovered bacteria (such as *S. aureus*). Based on their phenotypic characteristics, *Abiotrophia* and *Granulicatella* spp. were initially classified as members of genus *Streptococcus*. Although genera *Abiotrophia* and *Granulicatella* were transferred and divided into two groups, based on the 16S rRNA sequence homology analysis, they have been treated as a same bacterial group of NVS in the field of clinical infectious diseases because they have common phenotypic characteristics, such as requiring vitamin B_6 analogs in growth and producing bacteriolytic enzymes. The human oral cavity is assumed to be a reservoir for the pathogens of many systemic infective diseases, so it is important to examine the antimicrobial susceptibilities of oral bacteria. In this study, we determined MICs of genetically identified seven *Abiotrophia* and 23 *Granulicatella* isolates (including oral isolates), according to the guideline from CLSI. Although NVS species have biochemical and phenotypic properties in common, and are difficult to distinguish without molecular genetical identification methods, the susceptibility profiles to antimicrobial agents were different among the species (Table 3).

Because of their fastidiousness, NVS species often were not recovered from the specimen in the usual clinical examination for infectious diseases caused by these bacteria. When no bacteria are recovered from the specimen of infective diseases, and that happens often, the empiric therapy with broad-spectrum antimicrobial agents (such as carbapenem, macrolide, quinolone, and tetracycline) is selected by the clinicians. As with the antimicrobials tested, all NVS isolates were susceptible to imipenem, and species-related differences were observed with respect to susceptibilities to ciprofloxacin and minocycline. The ciprofloxacin susceptibility rate for *A. defectiva* isolates was 100%, and that for *Granulicatella* isolates was 17.4%. In contrast, the susceptibility rate of minocycline for *Abiotrophia* isolates was 57.1%, and that for *Granulicatella* isolates was 95.7%. Species-related differences in susceptibility of antibiotics should be considered in the empiric therapy for NVS related infections.

In case of infective endocarditis (IE) caused by NVS, a combination of benzylpenicillin and gentamycin has been used for the antibiotic therapy [26–29]. However, 42.9% of *A. defectiva* isolates were not susceptible to benzylpenicillin and no strains of NVS isolates were susceptible to gentamycin in this study. Aminopenicillins, ampicillin, and amoxicillin showed better susceptible rates than benzylpenicillin and piperacillin. Ceftriaxone and ceftazidime are both third generation cephem, but the susceptible rates were contrary: Only three isolates of *G. elegans* (10.0% of the NVS isolates) were susceptible to ceftazidime. In contrast, 86.6% of the NVS isolates were susceptible to ceftriaxone (Table 3). According to the guidelines for endocarditis treatment by the British Society for Antimicrobial Chemotherapy, vancomycin can be used alone for the NVS IE patients with penicillin allergy [29]. The susceptibility rate of vancomycin for NVS isolates in our study was 96.7%. In the antimicrobial treatment of NVS IE, the recommended initial drugs (the combination of benzylpenicillin and gentamycin) may not be effective, and the regimen of initial drugs should be reconsidered.

Some isolates showed unique susceptibility profiles, for example, *A. defectiva* C1-2 showed multi-drug resistance to piperacillin, cefazolin, ceftazidime, cefaclor, gentamicin, erythromycin, and minocycline, but was susceptible to amoxicillin and ceftriaxone. Some *G. adiacens* isolates, such as HHC3, YTC1, and YTT3, were highly resistant to ceftazidime but susceptible to ceftriaxone, ampicillin, and amoxicillin. *G. adiacens* P7-4 was not susceptible to benzylpenicillin, piperacillin, and cefazolin, and was resistant to ceftriaxone, ceftazidime, and cefaclor, but was susceptible to ampicillin and amoxicillin. In the antimicrobial process, beta-lactams are bound to the penicillin binding protein (PBP) of the bacteria and inhibit their cell wall synthesis. The minor variations of PBP(s) may affect the antimicrobial susceptibilities of these isolates. Further molecular genetic research is needed to determine the mechanism of resistance in the NVS isolates with unique susceptibility profiles.

Author Contributions: T.K. and H.N. conceived the study. T.K. and S.T. performed the laboratory work. T.K. wrote the manuscript. All authors read and approved the final manuscript.

Acknowledgments: We thank Hiromu Takemura, for advice and stimulating discussions.

References

1. Frenkel, A.; Hirsch, W. Spontaneous development of L forms of streptococci requiring secretions of other bacteria or sulphydryl compounds for normal growth. *Nature* **1961**, *191*, 728–730. [CrossRef] [PubMed]
2. Ruoff, K.L. Nutritionally variant streptococci. *Clin. Microbiol. Rev.* **1991**, *4*, 184–190. [CrossRef] [PubMed]
3. Kawamura, Y.; Hou, X.G.; Sultana, F.; Liu, S.; Yamamoto, H.; Ezaki, T. Transfer of *Streptococcus adjacens* and *Streptococcus defectivus* to *Abiotrophia* gen. nov. as *Abiotrophia adiacens* comb. nov. and *Abiotrophia defectiva* comb. nov., respectively. *Int. J. Syst. Bacteriol.* **1995**, *45*, 798–803. [CrossRef] [PubMed]
4. Collins, M.D.; Lawson, P.A. The genus *Abiotrophia* (Kawamura et al.) is not monophyletic: Proposal of *Granulicatella* gen. nov., *Granulicatella adiacens* comb. nov., *Granulicatella elegans* comb. nov. and *Granulicatella balaenopterae* comb. nov. *Int. J. Syst. Evol. Microbiol.* **2000**, *50 Pt 1*, 365–369. [CrossRef] [PubMed]
5. Casalta, J.P.; Habib, G.; La Scola, B.; Drancourt, M.; Caus, T.; Raoult, D. Molecular diagnosis of *Granulicatella elegans* on the cardiac valve of a patient with culture-negative endocarditis. *J. Clin. Microbiol.* **2002**, *40*, 1845–1847. [CrossRef] [PubMed]
6. Tattevin, P.; Watt, G.; Revest, M.; Arvieux, C.; Fournier, P.E. Update on blood culture-negative endocarditis. *Med. Mal. Infect.* **2015**, *45*, 1–8. [CrossRef] [PubMed]
7. Tellez, A.; Ambrosioni, J.; Llopis, J.; Pericas, J.M.; Falces, C.; Almela, M.; Garcia de la Maria, C.; Hernandez-Meneses, M.; Vidal, B.; Sandoval, E.; et al. Epidemiology, Clinical Features, and Outcome of Infective Endocarditis due to *Abiotrophia* Species and *Granulicatella* Species: Report of 76 Cases, 2000–2015. *Clin. Infect. Dis.* **2018**, *66*, 104–111. [CrossRef]
8. Coto, H.; Berk, S.L. Endocarditis caused by *Streptococcus morbillorum*. *Am. J. Med. Sci.* **1984**, *287*, 54–58. [CrossRef]
9. Kanamoto, T.; Eifuku-Koreeda, H.; Inoue, M. Isolation and properties of bacteriolytic enzyme-producing cocci from the human mouth. *FEMS Microbiol. Lett.* **1996**, *144*, 135–140. [CrossRef]
10. Kanamoto, T.; Sato, S.; Inoue, M. Genetic heterogeneities and phenotypic characteristics of strains of the genus *Abiotrophia* and proposal of *Abiotrophia para-adiacens* sp. nov. *J. Clin. Microbiol.* **2000**, *38*, 492–498.
11. Sato, S.; Kanamoto, T.; Inoue, M. *Abiotrophia elegans* strains comprise 8% of the nutritionally variant streptococci isolated from the human mouth. *J. Clin. Microbiol.* **1999**, *37*, 2553–2556. [PubMed]
12. Jorgensen, J.H.; Hindler, J.F. New consensus guidelines from the Clinical and Laboratory Standards Institute for antimicrobial susceptibility testing of infrequently isolated or fastidious bacteria. *Clin. Infect. Dis.* **2007**, *44*, 280–286. [CrossRef] [PubMed]
13. Bouvet, A.; Grimont, F.; Grimont, P.A.D. *Streptococcus defectivus* sp. nov. and *Streptococcus adjacens* sp. nov., nutritionally variant streptococci from human clinical specimens. *Int. J. Syst. Bacteriol.* **1989**, *39*, 290–294. [CrossRef]
14. van de Rijn, I.; George, M. Immunochemical study of nutritionally variant streptococci. *J. Immunol.* **1984**, *133*, 2220–2225. [PubMed]
15. Roggenkamp, A.; Abele-Horn, M.; Trebesius, K.H.; Tretter, U.; Autenrieth, I.B.; Heesemann, J. *Abiotrophia elegans* sp. nov., a possible pathogen in patients with culture-negative endocarditis. *J. Clin. Microbiol.* **1998**, *36*, 100–104. [PubMed]
16. CLSI. *Methods for Antimicrobial Dilution and Disk Susceptibility Testing of Infrequently Isolated or Fastidious Bacteria*; Approved Guideline M45-A; Clinical and Laboratory Standards Institute: Wayne, PA, USA, 2006; Volume 26, pp. 10–11.
17. CLSI. Methods for Dilution Antimicirobial Susceptibility Tests for Bacteria That Grow Aerobically; Approved Standard-Seventh Edition M7-A7. In *Performance Standards for Antimicrobial Susceptibility Testing*; Eighteenth Informational Supplement M100-S18; Wikler, M.A., Ed.; Clinical and Laboratory Standards Institute: Wayne, PA, USA, 2008; Volume 27, pp. 86–161.
18. Aas, J.A.; Paster, B.J.; Stokes, L.N.; Olsen, I.; Dewhirst, F.E. Defining the normal bacterial flora of the oral cavity. *J. Clin. Microbiol.* **2005**, *43*, 5721–5732. [CrossRef]
19. Diaz, P.I.; Chalmers, N.I.; Rickard, A.H.; Kong, C.; Milburn, C.L.; Palmer, R.J., Jr.; Kolenbrander, P.E. Molecular characterization of subject-specific oral microflora during initial colonization of enamel. *Appl. Environ. Microbiol.* **2006**, *72*, 2837–2848. [CrossRef]
20. Zaura, E.; Keijser, B.J.; Huse, S.M.; Crielaard, W. Defining the healthy "core microbiome" of oral microbial communities. *BMC Microbiol.* **2009**, *9*, 259. [CrossRef]

21. Brouqui, P.; Raoult, D. Endocarditis due to rare and fastidious bacteria. *Clin. Microbiol. Rev.* **2001**, *14*, 177–207. [CrossRef]

22. Woo, P.C.; To, A.P.; Lau, S.K.; Fung, A.M.; Yuen, K.Y. Phenotypic and molecular characterization of erythromycin resistance in four isolates of *Streptococcus*-like gram-positive cocci causing bacteremia. *J. Clin. Microbiol.* **2004**, *42*, 3303–3305. [CrossRef]

23. Senn, L.; Entenza, J.M.; Greub, G.; Jaton, K.; Wenger, A.; Bille, J.; Calandra, T.; Prod'hom, G. Bloodstream and endovascular infections due to *Abiotrophia defectiva* and *Granulicatella* species. *BMC Infect. Dis.* **2006**, *6*, 9. [CrossRef] [PubMed]

24. De Luca, M.; Amodio, D.; Chiurchiu, S.; Castelluzzo, M.A.; Rinelli, G.; Bernaschi, P.; Calo Carducci, F.I.; D'Argenio, P. *Granulicatella* bacteraemia in children: Two cases and review of the literature. *BMC Pediatr.* **2013**, *13*, 61. [CrossRef] [PubMed]

25. Reimer, L.G.; Reller, L.B. Growth of nutritionally variant streptococci on laboratory media supplemented with blood of eight animal species. *Med. Lab. Sci.* **1982**, *39*, 79–81. [PubMed]

26. Cargill, J.S.; Scott, K.S.; Gascoyne-Binzi, D.; Sandoe, J.A. *Granulicatella* infection: Diagnosis and management. *J. Med. Microbiol.* **2012**, *61*, 755–761. [CrossRef] [PubMed]

27. Ohara-Nemoto, Y.; Kishi, K.; Satho, M.; Tajika, S.; Sasaki, M.; Namioka, A.; Kimura, S. Infective endocarditis caused by *Granulicatella elegans* originating in the oral cavity. *J. Clin. Microbiol.* **2005**, *43*, 1405–1407. [CrossRef] [PubMed]

28. Lin, C.H.; Hsu, R.B. Infective endocarditis caused by nutritionally variant streptococci. *Am. J. Med. Sci.* **2007**, *334*, 235–239. [CrossRef] [PubMed]

29. Gould, F.K.; Denning, D.W.; Elliott, T.S.; Foweraker, J.; Perry, J.D.; Prendergast, B.D.; Sandoe, J.A.; Spry, M.J.; Watkin, R.W.; Working Party of the British Society for Antimicrobial Chemotherapy. Guidelines for the diagnosis and antibiotic treatment of endocarditis in adults: A report of the Working Party of the British Society for Antimicrobial Chemotherapy. *J. Antimicrob. Chemother.* **2012**, *67*, 269–289. [CrossRef] [PubMed]

10

Search for Drugs Used in Hospitals to Treat Stomatitis

Yaeko Hara [1],*, Hiroshi Shiratuchi [2], Tadayoshi Kaneko [2] and Hiroshi Sakagami [3]

[1]   Second Division of Oral and Maxillofacial Surgery, Department of Diagnostic and Therapeutic Sciences, Meikai University School of Dentistry, 1-1 Keyakidai, Sakado, Saitama 350-0283, Japan

[2]   Department of Oral Maxillofacial Surgery, Nihon University School of Dentistry; 1-8-13 Kanda Surugadai, Chiyoda-ku, Tokyo 101-8310, Japan; shiratsuchi.hiroshi@nihon-u.ac.jp (H.S.); kaneko.tadayoshi@nihon-u.ac.jp (T.K.)

[3]   Meikai University Research Institute of Odontology (M-RIO), 1-1 Keyakidai, Sakado, Saitama 350-0283, Japan; sakagami@dent.meikai.ac.jp

*   Correspondence: hara.yaeko@dent.meikai.ac.jp

Abstract: Stomatitis is an inflammatory disease of the oral mucosa, often accompanied by pain. Usually it is represented by aphthous stomatitis, for which treatment steroid ointment is commonly used. However, in the cases of refractory or recurrent stomatitis, traditional herbal medicines have been used with favorable therapeutic effects. Chemotherapy, especially in the head and neck region, induces stomatitis at higher frequency, which directly affects the patient's quality of life and treatment schedule. However, effective treatment for stomatitis has yet to be established. This article presents the clinical report of Kampo medicines on the stomatitis patients in the Nihon university, and then reviews the literature of traditional medicines for the treatment of stomatitis. Among eighteen Kampo medicines, Hangeshashinto has been the most popular for the treatment of stomatitis, due to its prominent anti-inflammatory activity. It was unexpected that clinical data of Hangeshashinto on stomatitis from Chinese hospital are not available. Kampo medicines have been most exclusively administered to elder person, as compared to pediatric population. Supplementation of alkaline plant extracts rich in lignin-carbohydrate complex may further extend the applicability of Kampo medicines to viral diseases.

Keywords: Chinese herbal remedies; stomatitis

1. Introduction

Stomatitis is an inflammation induced by various factors such as trauma, viruses and bacterial infections, genetic factors, stress and vitamin deficiency [1–3]. Chemotherapy and radiotherapy may produce active oxygen species and free radicals, that cause oxidative injury, inflammation of the oral mucosa and pain [4,5]. Like the digestive tract, oral mucosa membrane is susceptible to stress, and prone to be deteriorated by contact with teeth and unsanitary oral hygiene. Therefore, anti-stomatitis therapy with herbal medicines should be based on their anti-stress, anti-oxidative, mucous membrane protection and regeneration activities.

Western medicine usually consists of a single active ingredient and is prescribed to eradicate the causal diseases, based on the main complaint and examination data of the patients. In contrast, herbal medicines such as Japanese traditional medicine (Kampo) and Traditional Chinese Medicine (TCM) are mixtures of at least two kinds of constitutional plant extracts, are therefore applicable to various diseases [6]. "Oriental medicine" includes TCM, Korean medicine, Ayurveda (traditional Indian medicine) and Japanese Kampo medicine. TCM and medical texts were first brought to Japan from China during the 5–6th centuries. Until the 14–16th centuries, diagnosis and treatment were performed according to the theory of TCM, and thereafter developed, evolved and established independently in Japan, as a system of medicine that matches the environment and climate of Japan as well as the physical constitution and lifestyle of the Japanese population [6].

Currently, various clinical and fundamental studies have been conducted to elucidate the mechanism of the action of traditional medicines. This article presented the clinical report of Kampo medicines on the stomatitis patients in the Nihon university, and then reviewed the literature of traditional medicines for the treatment of stomatitis, based on the search by PubMed (National Center for Biotechnology Information, Bethesda, MD, USA) and Ichushi (Japan Medical Abstracts Society, Tokyo, Japan).

2. Kampo Medicines Prescribed in the Hospital of Nihon University School of Dentistry

We have surveyed approximately 400 patients with stomatitis in our hospital of the Nihon University School of Dentistry from January 2014 to October 2018. Number of patients with stomatitis progressively declined (Figure 1A), while the number of Kampo medicines prescribed to stomatitis patients was increased (Figure 1B). When the percent of Kampo medicines prescribed to stomatitis patient was calculated, it was found to be increased sharply in 2018 (Figure 1C). The most frequently prescribed Kampo medicine was Hangeshashinto (Figure 1D) (Figure 1).

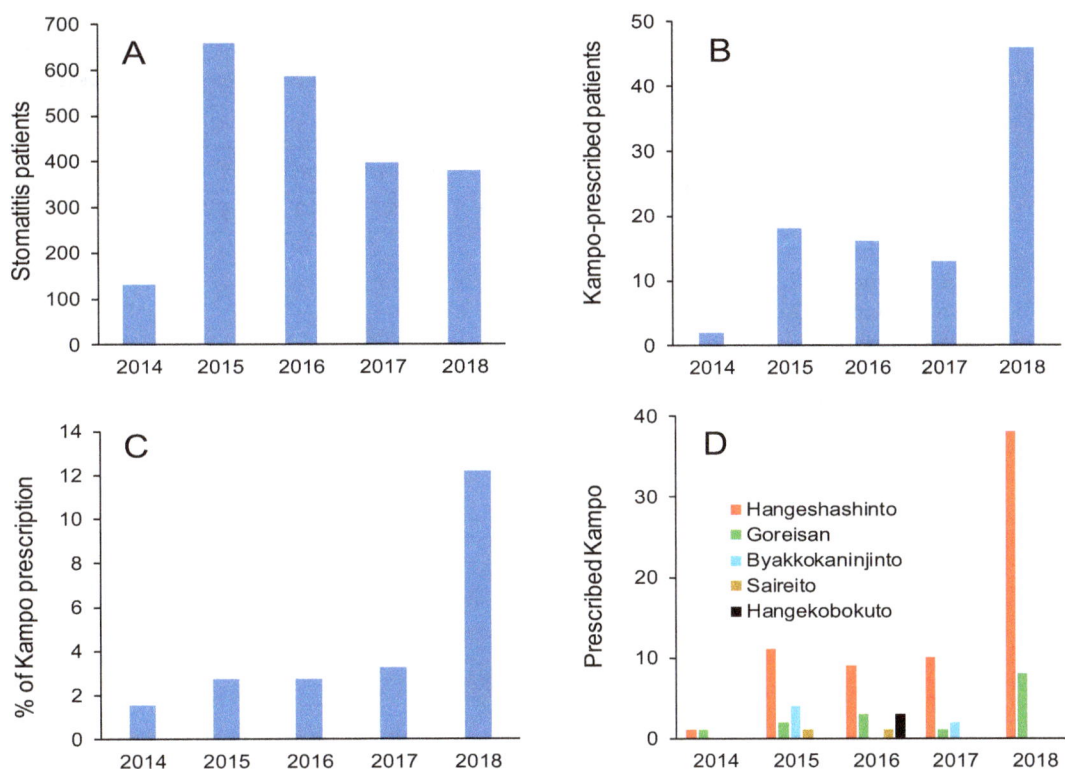

Figure 1. Changes in number of stomatitis patients (**A**), number of Kampo-prescribed stomatitis patients (**B**), percent of Kampo prescription (**C**) and number of prescribed Kampo medicines (**D**) during 2014 to 2018 (Data from hospital of Nihon University School of Dentistry).

During 12 months of years, the incidence of stomatitis was higher in winter season, peaked in March (Figure 2A), and the prescription of Kampo medicines peaked on April and May (Figure 2B), possibly to combat against the increasing numbers of stomatitis patients (Figure 2).

Byakkokaninjinto, Goreisan, Hangekobokuto, Hangeshashinto and Saireito extract granules used in our hospital contains 5, 5, 5, 7 and 11 constituent plant extracts, respectively (Table 1). It should be noted that each extract contains numerous numbers of compounds.

Clinical Oral Medicine

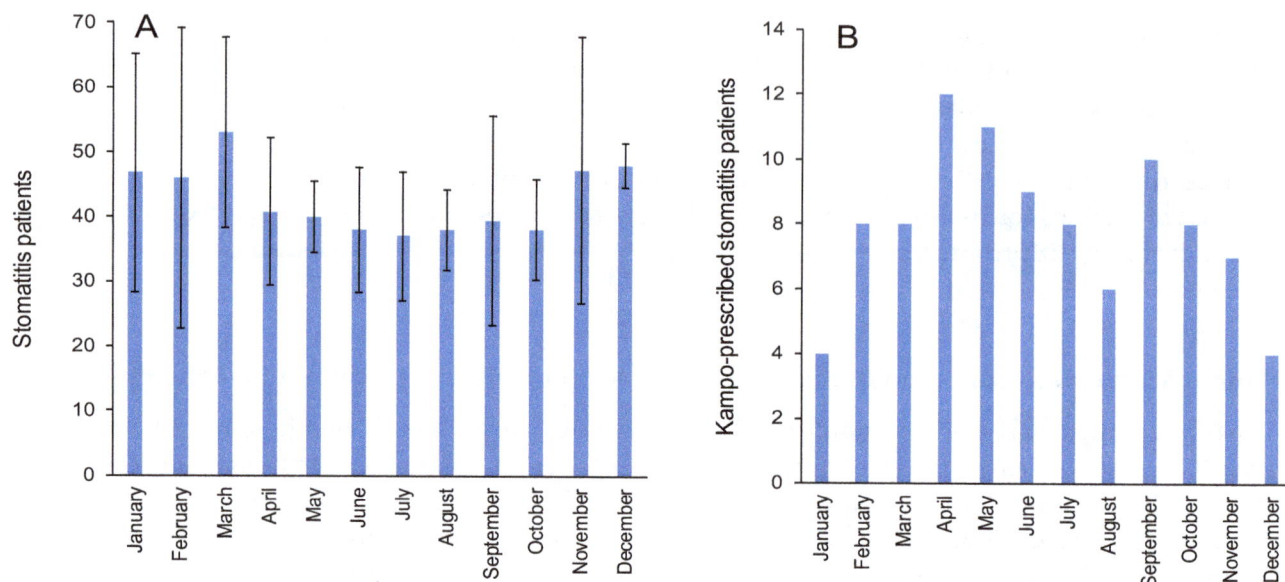

Figure 2. Number of stomatitis patients (**A**) and prescribed Kampo medicines in the hospital of Nihon University School of Dentistry (**B**).

Table 1. Kampo medicines and their constituent plant extracts used for treatment of stomatitis in the hospital of Nihon University School of Dentistry. BKTN, Byakkokaninjinto; GRS, Goreisan; HKT, Hangekobokuto; HST, Hangeshashinto; SRT, Saireito.

Constituent Plant Extracts	Kampo Medicines				
	BKNT	**GRS**	**HKT**	**HST**	**SRT**
Alisma Rhizome		○			○
Anemarrhena Rhizome	○				
Astractylodes Lancea Rhizome		○			○
Brown Rice	○				
Bupleurum Root					○
Cinnamon Bark		○			○
Coptis Rhizome				○	
Ginger			○	○	○
Ginseng	○			○	○
Glycyrrhiza	○			○	○
Gypsum	○				
Jujube				○	○
Magnolia Bark			○		
Perilla Herb			○		
Pinellia Tuber			○	○	○
Polyporus Sclerotium		○			
Poria Sclerotium	○	○			○
Scutellaria Root				○	○

During 5 years (2014–2018), 40 patients were treated with Hangeshashinto extract granules 2.5 g alone, while 27 patients were treated with hangeshashinto together with other Kampo medicines (Goreisan), gargle [sodium gualenate hydrate (azunol® gargle liquid 4%), 0.2% benzethonium chloride solution (Neostelin Green 0.2% mouthwash solution)], anti-inflammatory agent (dexamethasone, triamicinolone acetonide, loxoprofen), or antimicrobial agent (miconazole gel) (Table 2). We first dissolve Hangeshashinto in water, and patients swallow it after gargling. When bitterness is too strong for the patients, we prescribe steroid ointment or azunol gargle in addition to Hangeshashinto, since azunol gargle protects the mucous membrane [7]. If mouth rinse is difficult, we will use other medicines.

Table 2. Kampo medicines prescribed for stomatitis in the hospital of Nihon University School of Dentistry. All Kampo medicines are extract granules. BKTN, Byakkokaninjinto; BMZ, betamethasone; DX, dexamethasone, GRS, Goreisan; HKT, Hangekobokuto; HST, Hangeshashinto; SRT, Saireito; SC, Salcoat Capsule for oral spray; TAC, triamcinolone acetonide.

Kampo Medicine Prescribed	Number of Prescribed Kampo					
	2014	2015	2016	2017	2018	Total
HST 2.5 g/packet	0	8	5	9	18	40
HST 2.5 g/packet, SC 50 μg	0	1	0	0	0	1
GRS 2.5 g/packet	0	0	2	0	3	5
GRS 2.5 g + HST 2.5 g	0	0	1	0	0	1
BKTN 3 g + SC 50 μg	0	0	0	1	0	1
Azunol gargle 4% (10 mL) + HST 2.5 g	0	0	0	0	3	3
Azunol gargle 4% (10 mL) + HST 2.5 g + SC	0	0	0	0	2	2
Azunol gargle 4% (5 mL) + HST 2.5 g	0	1	2	0	0	3
TAC ointment 0.1% + Azunol + GRS 2.5 g	0	0	0	1	0	1
DX ointment 0.1% + SRT 3.0 g	0	1	0	0	0	1
DX oint 0.1% + HST 2.5 g	0	0	0	1	5	6
DX oint 0.1% + HST 2.5 g	0	0	1	0	0	1
DX oint 0.1% + GRS 2.5 g	1	0	0	0	3	4
DX oint 0.1%+ Azunol + HST 2.5 g	1	0	0	0	1	2
DX oint 0.1% + Neostelin Green gargle + HST 2.5 g	0	0	0	0	1	1
DX oint 0.1% + Neostelin + GRS 2.5 g	0	0	0	0	1	1
DX oint 0.1%+ Hachiazule gargle 0.1% + GRS 2.5 g	0	2	0	0	0	2
Neostelin green mouthwash + SRT 3 g	0	0	1	0	0	1
Neostelin green mouthwash + HST 2.5 g	0	0	0	0	3	3
Neostelin green mouthwash + GRS 2.5 g + SC 50 μg	0	0	0	0	1	1
Neostelin green mouthwash + BKTN 3 g	0	0	0	1	0	1
Miconazole gel 2% + HST 2.5 g	0	0	1	0	0	1
RACOL-NF Liquid for Enteral Use + HKT 2.5 g	0	0	1	0	0	1
BMZ/Gentamicin oint + Azonol 4% + HST 2.5 g	0	0	0	0	1	1
Loxoprofen tablet 60 mg + HST 2.5 g	0	1	0	0	0	1
Loxoprofen tablet 60 mg + HST 2.5 g + SC 50 μg	0	0	0	0	1	1
Hachiazule gargle 0.1% + BKTN 3 g	0	4	0	0	0	4
White petrolatum + Azunol 4% + HKT 2.5 g	0	0	1	0	0	1

The following is the clinical report of stomatitis patients treated with Hangeshashinto in our hospital, after obtaining the informed consent from the patient, under the condition that the patient is not identified. The patient (female, 29 years old) was subjected to first medical examination on 23 May 2018. She showed the symptoms of stomatitis every few months. Each time, she applied triamcinolone acetonide (Kenalog®, Bristol-Myers Squibb Co., Tokyo, Japan) ointment herself, but got only short-term healing. When stomatitis developed again on early May 2018, Kenalog®did not work. Herpes simplex virus was detected in the oral cavity on 21 May. Administration of acyclovir, a popular anti-HSV agent, did not improved, but rather aggravated her symptom. Upon recommendation by the doctor, she got a close examination by the first author (Y.H.) on 23 May. The pain spread to the entire oral cavity, especially inside the anterior teeth part of the lower lip, and the tongue, feeling of incongruity during meals. There was no swelling or redness in the face. An ulcer suspected of stomatitis is formed in the buccal mucosa and the inner surface of the lips in the oral cavity. There was a tender pain with palpation (Figure 3A).

She was then treated with Hangeshashinto extract granules 2.5 g × 3 packages 14 days, and neostelin green mouthwash 0.2% 40 mL. On 6 June, a new stomatitis was formed in the molar part on the right upper side, and became slightly larger, however, the application of medicines was continued. It then became smaller and disappeared on 10 June. Some redness remained on the buccal gingiva of Upper right 6, but all other parts were healed. On 17 July, there was no mouth sores on the mucosal surface (Figure 3B).

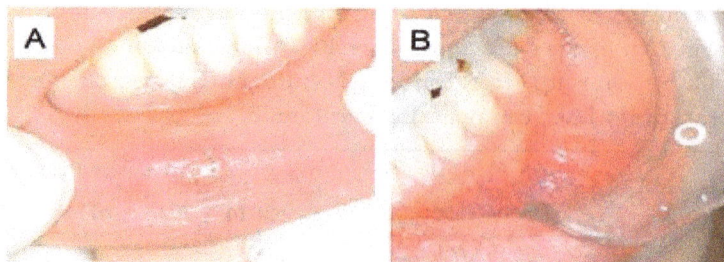

Figure 3. Therapeutic effect of Hangeshashinto on stomatitis. (**A**): Before Hangeshashinto treatment; (**B**): After Hangeshashinto treatment.

3. Data Search for Traditional Medicine for the Treatment of Stomatitis

Stomatitis is a painful oral mucosal disorder, generated from various causes. Especially stomatitis in patients undergoing chemotherapy is severe, sometimes accompanied by eating difficulties. One common stomatitis often encountered is recurrent aphtha (recurrent aphthous stomatitis: RAS). RAS developed at a rate of 5–25% in the stomatitis patients [1], and treatment of RAS with Chinese patent medicines has been reported [8]. More recently, healing effects of Kampo on chemotherapy-induced stomatitis have been published [9,10]. Changes in the number of papers that related to Chinese Traditional Medicine was searched with PubMed (Figure 4A) and Ichushi (Figure 4B) (Figure 4). The publication of TCM appeared in 1980, and increased in the number more dramatically after 2000 in both cases.

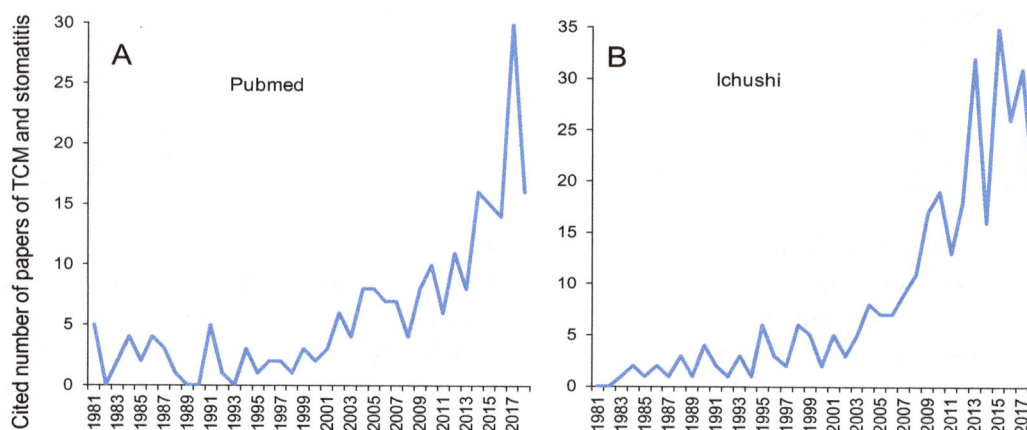

Figure 4. Increase of number of papers that cite TCM and stomatitis. (**A**): Data from Pubmed; (**B**): Data from Ichushi.

The most frequently used drugs for treatment of stomatitis, based on Pubmed search, were steroids (hydrocortisone acetate, triamcinolone acetonide, dexamethasone, beclometasone dipropionate (1 + 51 + 148 + 12 = 212 reports), followed by TCM (53 reports) > Kampo medicine (13 reports) and azunol ointment (main component: dimethyl isopropylazulene) (0 report) (Table 3). When corrected for the total numbers of references in each group, Kampo medicine was found to be the most popular for treating the stomatitis (0.92% of total application), followed by betamethasone (0.80%) > triamcinolone acetonide (0.74%) > beclometasone dipropionate (0.32%) > dexamethasone (0.22%) > hydrocortisone acetate (0.11%) > TCM (0.09%). It should be noted that Kampo medicine has been used for the purpose of treating stomatitis 10 times (= 0.92/0.09) than TCM (Table 3).

Table 3. Medicines used for treatment of stomatitis (data obtained from Pubmed on 16 January 2019).

Medicines	Number of References		% (A/B) × 100
	Alone A	+ Stomatitis B	
Azunol Ointment (Dimethyl Isopropylazulene)	18	0	0
Hydrocortisone Acetate	890	1	0.11
Triamcinolone Acetonide	6891	51	0.74
Dexamethasone	68,125	148	0.22
Betamethasone	8478	68	0.80
Beclometasone	3751	12	0.32
Kampo Medicine	1406	13	0.92
Hangeshashinto	28	10	35.71
Coptis Rhizome	150	1	0.67
Ginger	3264	1	0.03
Ginseng	8868	4	0.05
Glycyrrhiza	3244	17	0.52
Glycyrrhizin	2389	7	0.29
Jujube	802	0	0
Pinellia Tuber	94	0	0
Scutellaria Root	502	2	0.40
Traditional Chinese medicine (TCM)	61,115	53	0.09

A total of 18 Kampo medicines for the treatment of stomatitis are prescribed by hospitals and Rikkosan, Tokishakuyakusan> Kamishoyosan, Orengedokuto, Rikkunshito, Jpractitioners, according to the search with Pubmed and Ichushi. According to Pubmed, Hangeshashinto is the most frequently used [11,12], followed by Hochuekkito, uzentaihoto Unseiin > Shigyakusan, Saikokeishikankyoto, Saikokeishito, Orento, Inchinkoto, San'oshashinto, Goreisan, Keishibukuryogan and Shosaikoto (Figure 5A). The search by Ichushi reported the similar order of administration frequency: Hangeshashinto > Juzentaihoto, Hochuekkito > Rikkunshito > Orengedokuto > Orento > Rikkosan > Goreisan > Shosaikoto > Inchinkoto > Kamishoyosan > Unseiin > Tokishakuyakusan > Saikokeishito > Keishibukuryogan > San'oshashinto > Shigyakusan > Saikokeishikankyoto (Figure 5B).

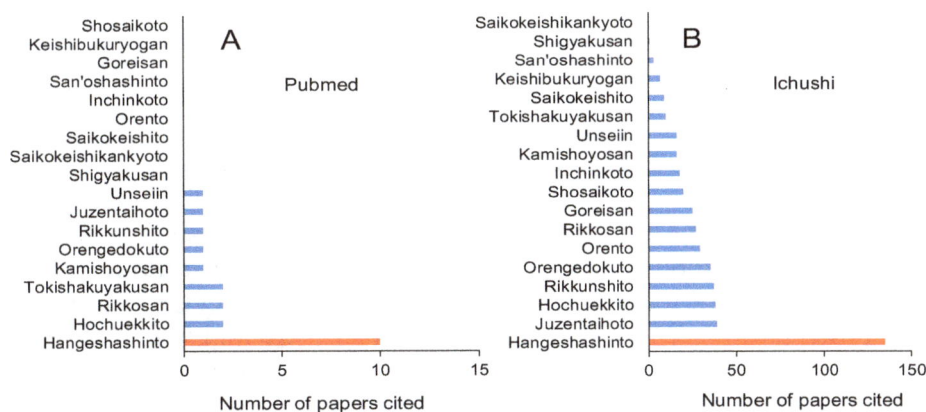

Figure 5. Hangeshashinto is the most popular kampo medicine for the treatment of stomatitis. Data obtained from Pubmed on 16 January 16 2019. (**A**): Data from pubmed; (**B**): Data from Ichushi.

Goreisan, known as "hydrostatic modulator" for edema, diarrhea, headache, nausea, and dizziness [13] is used to treat dry mouth. Rikkosan, a negative regulator of IL-1β network [14], plays a supplementary role for stomatitis by relieving the pain. Kamishoyosan (KSS), that enhances peripheral circulation and reduces stress and associated pain [15], and saikokeishikankyoto, that reduces posttraumatic stress [16], are effective to refractory and recurrent stomatitis.

While hangeshashinto is mainly administered to patients with stomatitis at the middle to late stage, orento is used for the early stage of stomatitis, such as acute aphthous stomatitis [17]. This may be due to shorter treatment time of orento required for pain relief and complete cure (2.6 and 6.3 days, respectively), as compared with those of steroid ointment (7.5 and 12.3 days, respectively) [18]. Although orento is used clinically very often, the paper of orento is limited. This may be due to the fact that early stomatitis heals much faster, as compared to intractable, recurrent stomatitis and chemotherapy-induced stomatitis. Most of fundamental and clinical research studies have been focusing on the stomatitis in the patients with head and neck cancer who received chemotherapy or radiation chemotherapy, to keep the patient's QOL and treatment continuity [19,20].

4. Application of Traditional Medicines for Pediatric Population

Kampo medicines and Hangeshashinto have been used for elderly person approximately one order higher rates, as compared with pediatric population (Table 4). Publication of TCM was approximately 44.5-fold (= 61,264/1409) as compared with Kampo medicine. Frequency of the use of TCM for elderly person was again one order higher than that for pediatrics (8494/844 = 10.1) (Table 4). This reflects that Kampo medicine and TCM are used to treat and improve the conditions of patients with many kinds of diseases.

Table 4. Medicines used for treatment of stomatitis (data obtained from Pubmed on 16 January 2019).

Cited by	Number of References	% of Control
Kampo medicine (control)	1409	100.0
Kampo medicine + elderly	242	17.2
Kampo medicine + adult	287	20.0
Kampo medicine + young	43	3.1
Kampo medicine + child	33	2.3
Kampo medicine + pediatric	26	1.8
Hangeshashinto	28	100.0
Hangeshashinto + elderly	6	21.4
Hangeshashinto + adult	6	21.4
Hangeshashinto + young	1	3.6
Hangeshashinto + child	1	3.6
Hangeshashinto + pediatric	0	0.0
TCM	61,264	100.0
TCM + elderly	8494	13.9
TCM + adult	10,349	16.9
TCM + young	2343	3.8
TCM + child	1588	2.6
TCM + pediatric	844	1.4

These traditional medicines have been used to cure the skin diseases and abdominal pain, from long ago, although there are few reports on stomatitis for pediatric population. Licorice is a crude drug prescribed in various herbal formulas in traditional Japanese and Chinese medicines, and also used worldwide as a food natural sweetener [21]. Therefore, licorice makes it easier for medication use in children.

5. Why Hangeshashinto Is So Popular for the Treatment of Stomatitis?

Among seven constitutional plant extracts, glycyrrhiza and glycyrrhizin (the major component of glycyrrhiza) have been cited most frequently as the therapeutics for stomatis (Table 3). Among 53 papers that investigated the biological activity of Hangeshashinto, 26 papers (49%) dealt with its anti-inflammatory activity, followed by mucosal protection (ten papers, 19%), based on the search by PubMed. The most well-known biological activity of glycyrrhizin was again anti-inflammatory activity (Figure 6).

Hangeshashinto

17%
4%
6%
5%
19%
49%

- Anti-inflammation
- Musosal protection
- Anti-oxidant
- Anti-stress
- Analgesic
- Others

Glycyrrhizin

28%   28%
2%
3%
4%   18%
5% 10%

- Anti-inflammation
- Organ protection
- Anti-oxidative
- Anti-hyperglycemic
- Anti-viral
- Anti-cancer
- Anti-allergic
- Anti-bacterial
- Others

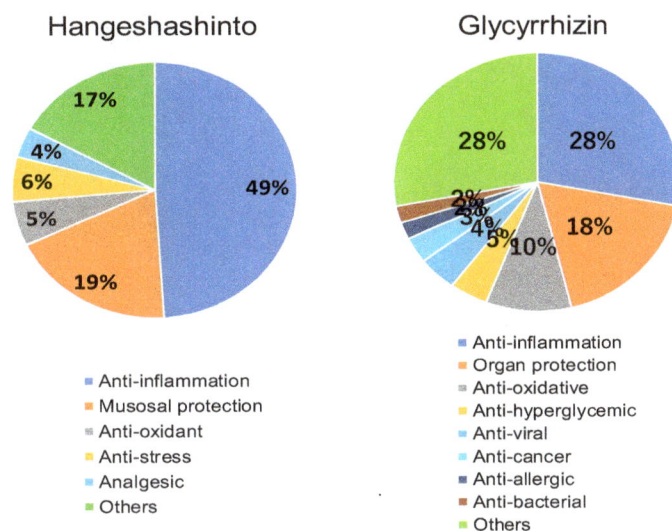

Figure 6. Prominent anti-inflammatory activity of Hangeshashinto.

We have recently reported that Hangeshashinto and Glycyrrhiza inhibited PGE_2 production in IL-1-β-stimulated human periodontal ligament fibroblast (selectivity index [SI (CC_{50}/EC_{50}) = 285 and 59, respectively) [22,23]. This suggests that anti-stomatitis activity of Hangeshashinto may be at least in part by Glycyrrhiza.

It has become increasingly apparent that oral health is co-related well with general health. Generally, the anti-HIV activity of Kampo medicine, prepared by hot water extraction, is generally weak [24]. However, alkaline extract of licorice extract [25], green tea, oolong tea and orange flower [26], that contain significant amount of lignin-carbohydrate complex, shows higher anti-viral activity than hot water extract. Supplementation of alkaline extract may further expand the therapeutic ranges of Kampo medicine (Figure 7).

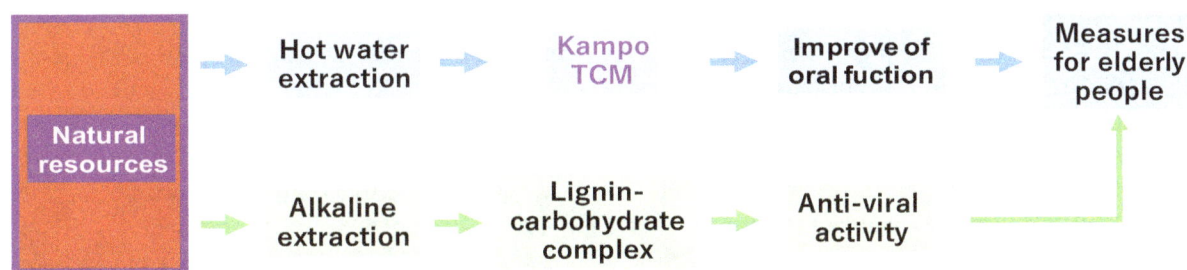

Natural resources
→ Hot water extraction → Kampo TCM → Improve of oral fuction → Measures for elderly people
→ Alkaline extraction → Lignin-carbohydrate complex → Anti-viral activity

Figure 7. Supplementation of alkaline extract to Kampo prescription extends its therapeutic potential.

6. Conclusions

Literature searches demonstrated that among 18 Kampo medicines, Hangeshashinto is most frequently used in Japan, possibly due to the presence of glycyrrhiza that contains anti-inflammatory glycyrrhizin. It was surprising that Hangeshashinto has not been used in China. Since Kampo medicines are prepared by hot water extraction, they have low levels of lignin–carbohydrate complexes (LCC) that are extracted by alkaline extracts and shows the prominent antiviral activity among three major polyphenols. By adding an alkaline extract rich in LCC to Kampo medicine, its therapeutic potential will become much broader. Up to now, traditional medicines have few cases of adaptation to children, but inclusion of sweet licorice ingredient will make it easier for children to take without resistance. Hangeshashinto is applicable for the treatment of stress gastritis, and seems to be the best Kampo medicine for the treatment of stomatitis, judging from the huge number of publications.

Author Contributions: Y.H., writing the paper; H.S. and T.K. data collection; H.S., writing the paper.

Acknowledgments: The authors acknowledge Tsumura Co. Ltd for the supply of Kampo.

Abbreviations

BKTN   Byakkokaninjinto
BMZ   betamethasone
DX   dexamethasone
GRS   Goreisan
HIV   Human immunodeficiency virus
HKT   Hangekobokuto
HST   Hangeshashinto
LCC   Lignin-carbohydrate complex
SRT   Saireito
SC   Salcoat Capsule for oral spray
TAC   Triamcinolone Acetonide
TCM   Traditional Chinese Medicine

References

1.   Edgar, N.R.; Saleh, D.; Miller, R.A. Recurrent aphthous stomatitis: A Review. *J. Clin. Aesthet. Dermatol.* **2017**, *10*, 26–36.

2.   Kunikullaya, U.K.; Kumar, M.A.; Ananthakrishnan, V.; Jaisri, G. Stress as a cause of recurrent aphthous stomatitis and its correlation with salivary stress markers. *Chin. J. Physiol.* **2017**, *60*, 226–230. [CrossRef] [PubMed]

3.   Tugrul, S.; Koçyiğit, A.; Doğan, R.; Eren, S.B.; Senturk, E.; Ozturan, O.; Ozar, O.F. Total antioxidant status and oxidative stress in recurrent aphthous stomatitis. *Int. J. Dermatol.* **2016**, *55*, e130–e135. [CrossRef]

4.   Yoshino, F.; Yoshida, A.; Nakajima, A.; Wada-Takahashi, S.; Takahashi, S.S.; Lee, M.C. Alteration of the redox state with reactive oxygen species for 5-fluorouracil-induced oral mucositis in hamsters. *PLoS ONE* **2013**, *20*, e82834. [CrossRef] [PubMed]

5.   Sonis, S.T. Mucositis: The impact, biology and therapeutic opportunities of oral mucositis. *Oral Oncol.* **2009**, *45*, 1015–1020. [CrossRef] [PubMed]

6.   Wanga, P.-L.; Kaneko, A. Introduction to Kampo medicine for dental treatment—Oral pharmacotherapy that utilizes the advantages of Western and Kampo medicines. *Jpn. Dent. Sci. Rev.* **2018**, *54*, 197–204. [CrossRef]

7.   Kato, S.; Saito, A.; Matsuda, N.; Suzuki, H.; Ujiie, M.; Sato, S.; Miyazaki, K.; Kodama, T.; Satoh, H. Management of afatinib-induced stomatitis. *Mol. Clin. Oncol.* **2017**, *6*, 603–605. [CrossRef]

8.   Zhou, P.; Mao, Q.; Hua, H.; Liu, X.; Yan, Z. Efficacy and safety of Chinese patent medicines in the treatment of recurrent aphthous stomatitis: A systematic review. *J. Am. Dent. Assoc.* **2017**, *148*, 17–25. [CrossRef]

9.   Takeda, H.; Sadakane, C.; Hattori, T.; Katsurada, T.; Ohkawara, T.; Nagai, K.; Asaka, M. Rikkunshito, an herbal medicine, suppresses cisplatin-induced anorexia in rats via 5-HT2 receptor antagonism. *Gastroenterology* **2008**, *134*, 2004–2013. [CrossRef]

10. Kono, T.; Suzuki, Y.; Mizuno, K.; Miyagi, C.; Omiya, Y.; Sekine, H.; Mizuhara, Y.; Miyano, K.; Kase, Y.; Uezono, Y. Preventive effect of oral goshajinkigan on choronic oxaliplatin-induced hypoesthesia in rats. *Sci. Rep.* **2015**, *5*, 16078. [CrossRef]

11. Kono, T.; Kaneko, A.; Matsumoto, C.; Miyagi, C.; Ohbuchi, K.; Mizuhara, Y.; Miyano, K.; Uezono, Y. Multitargeted effects of hangeshashinto for treatment of chemotherapy-induced oral mucositis on inducible prostaglandin E_2 production in human oral keratinocytes. *Integr. Cancer Ther.* **2014**, *13*, 435–445. [CrossRef]

12. Matsumoto, C.; Sekine-Suzuki, E.; Nyui, M.; Ueno, M.; Nakanishi, I.; Omiya, Y.; Fukutake, M.; Kase, Y.; Matsumoto, K. Analysis of the antioxidative function of the radioprotective Japanese traditional (Kampo) medicine, hangeshashinto, in an aqueous phase. *J. Radiat. Res.* **2015**, *56*, 669–677. [CrossRef] [PubMed]

13. Terasawa, K. Evidence-based reconstruction of Kampo medicine: Part II—theconcept of Sho. *Evid. Based Complement. Altern. Med.* **2004**, *1*, 119–123. [CrossRef]

14. Horie, N.; Hashimoto, K.; Hino, S.; Kato, T.; Shimoyama, T.; Kaneko, T.; Kusama, K.; Sakagami, H. Anti-inflammatory potential of Rikkosan based on IL-1β network through macrophages to oral tissue cells. *In Vivo* **2014**, *28*, 563–569. [PubMed]

15. Yamaguchi, K. Traditional Japanese herbal medicines for treatment of odontopathy. *Front. Pharmacol.* **2015**, *6*, 176. [CrossRef]

16. Numata, T.; Gunfan, S.; Takayama, S.; Takahashi, S.; Monma, Y.; Kaneko, S.; Kuroda, H.; Tanaka, J.; Kanemura, S.; Nara, M.; et al. Treatment of posttraumatic stress disorder using the traditional Japanese herbal medicine saikokeishikankyoto: A randomized, observer-blinded, controlled trial in survivors of the great East Japan earthquake and tsunami. *Evid. Based Complement. Altern. Med.* **2014**, *2014*, 683293. [CrossRef]

17. Oka, S. The effects of Oren-to on Stomatitis. *Pharm. Med.* **2007**, *25*, 35–38. (In Japanese)

18. Sunagawa, M.; Yamaguchi, K.; Tsukada, M.; Ebihara, N.; Ikemoto, H.; Hisamitsu, T. Kampo (traditional Japanese herbal) formulae for treatment of stomatitis and oral mucositis. *Medicines (Basel)* **2018**, *5*, 130. [CrossRef] [PubMed]

19. Yamashita, T.; Araki, K.; Tomifuji, M.; Kamide, D.; Tanaka, Y.; Shiotani, A. A traditional Japanese medicine–Hangeshashinto (TJ-14)–alleviates chemoradiation-induced mucositis and improves rates of treatment completion. *Support Care Cancer* **2015**, *23*, 29–35. [CrossRef]

20. Ohnishi, S.; Takeda, H. Herbal medicines for the treatment of cancer chemotherapy-induced side effects. *Front. Pharmacol.* **2015**, *6*, 14. [CrossRef]

21. Sakagami, H. Chapter 1. Introductory chaper: Fugure prespect of licorice, popular crude drug and food sweetener. In *Biological Activities and Action Mechanisms of Licorice Ingredients*; Intech: Houston, TX, USA, 2017; pp. 3–12. ISBN 978-953-51-5195-1.

22. Kato, T.; Segami, N.; Sakagami, H. Anti-inflammatory activity of hangeshashinto in IL-1β-stimulated gingival and periodontal ligament fibroblasts. *In Vivo* **2016**, *30*, 257–264. [PubMed]

23. Ara, T.; Sogawa, N. Effects of shinbuto and ninjinto on prostaglandin E2 production in lipopolysaccharide-treated human gingival fibroblasts. *PeerJ* **2017**, *5*, e4120. [CrossRef]

24. Kato, T.; Horie, N.; Matsuta, T.; Umemura, N.; Shimoyama, T.; Kaneko, T.; Kanamoto, T.; Terakubo, S.; Nakashima, H.; Kusama, K.; et al. Anti-UV/HIV activity of Kampo medicines and constituent plant extracts. *In Vivo* **2012**, *26*, 1007–1013. [PubMed]

25. Ohno, H.; Miyoshi, S.; Araho, D.; Kanamoto, T.; Terakubo, S.; Nakashima, H.; Tsuda, T.; Sunaga, K.; Amano, S.; Ohkoshi, E.; et al. Efficient utilization of licorice root by alkaline extraction. *In Vivo* **2014**, *28*, 785–794. [PubMed]

26. Sakagami, H.; Sheng, H.; Yasui, T.; Fukuchi, K.; Oizumi, T.; Ohno, H.; Yamamoto, M.; Fukuda, T.; Kotohda, K.; Yoshida, H.; et al. Chapter 18. Therapeutic potential of solubilized nanolignin against oral diseases. In *Nanostructures for Oral Medicicne*; Elsevier: New York, NY, USA, 2017; pp. 545–576. ISBN 978-0-323-47720-8.

11

The Association of Periodontitis and Peripheral Arterial Occlusive Disease

Mark Kaschwich [1,2,*], Christian-Alexander Behrendt [1], Guido Heydecke [3], Andreas Bayer [2], Eike Sebastian Debus [1], Udo Seedorf [3] and Ghazal Aarabi [3]

[1] Department of Vascular Medicine, University Heart Center Hamburg, University Medical Center Hamburg-Eppendorf, 20251 Hamburg, Germany; ch.behrendt@uke.de (C.-A.B.); s.debus@uke.de (E.S.D.)

[2] Department of Surgery, University Medical Centre Schleswig-Holstein, Campus Luebeck, Ratzeburger Allee 160, 23538 Luebeck, Germany; andreas.bayer@uksh.de

[3] Department of Prosthetic Dentistry, Center for Dental and Oral Medicine, University Medical Center Hamburg-Eppendorf, 20246 Hamburg, Germany; g.heydecke@uke.de (G.H.); u.seedorf@uke.de (U.S.); g.aarabi@uke.de (G.A.)

* Correspondence: mark.kaschwich@uksh.de

Abstract: Background: Observational studies support an association between periodontitis (PD) and atherosclerotic vascular disease, but little is known specifically about peripheral arterial occlusive disease (PAOD). Objectives: To systematically review the evidence for an association between PD and PAOD. Data Sources: Medline via PubMed. Review Methods: We searched the Pubmed database for original studies, case reports, case series, meta-analyses and systematic reviews that assessed whether there is an association between PD (all degrees of severity) and PAOD (all degrees of severity). The reporting of this systematic review was in accordance with the Preferred Reporting Items for Systematic Reviews and Meta-Analyses (PRISMA) statement following the Population, Intervention, Control, and Outcome (PICO) format. Results: 17 out of 755 detected studies were included in the qualitative synthesis. Nine studies demonstrated associations between PD and PAOD, and two studies reported associations between tooth loss and PAOD. Six studies addressed the pathomechanism regarding PD as a possible trigger for PAOD. No study that dismissed an association could be detected. Odds ratios or hazard ratios ranged from 1.3 to 3.9 in four large cohort studies after adjusting for established cardiovascular risk factors. Conclusions: The presented evidence supports a link between PD and PAOD. Further studies which address the temporality of PD and PAOD and randomized controlled intervention trials examining the causal impact of PD on PAOD are needed. Although our results cannot confirm a causal role of PD in the development of PAOD, it is likely that PD is associated with PAOD and plays a contributing role.

Keywords: oral disease; periodontitis; PD; peripheral arterial occlusive disease; PAOD; systematic review

1. Introduction

As a consequence of demographic changes and the proliferation of the western lifestyle, peripheral arterial occlusive disease (PAOD) has developed into a widespread disease with globally over 200 million persons affected [1–3]. PAOD preferably effects the peripheral limb vessels of the lower extremity. It limits a person's ability to walk, may require revascularization, or worse yet, can result in the loss of a limb. But it is not simply a disease of the legs. PAOD is one of multiple clinical manifestations of atherosclerotic vascular disease. It is a clinical manifestation of a systemic disease, that is frequently associated with ischemic heart disease, stroke, abdominal aortic aneurysms, and other serious health issues [4]. In addition to its clinical aspects that limit the patient's quality of life, it has a profound cost impact on the healthcare system [5].

Despite the benefit of modern medicine, to date, there is no curative treatment available, and all non-invasive or invasive approaches aim to address the symptoms or disease progression. Hence, screening and prevention programs have gained more attention to identify new PAOD risk factors. It is well known that PAOD is associated with tobacco use, diabetes, high cholesterol, and higher age [3]. With respect to prevention of PAOD, the identification of additional risk factors is of high clinical importance.

Nowadays, there is scientific consensus that the development of PAOD is also associated with chronic subclinical inflammation [6–8]. The inflammatory genesis has been demonstrated to be multifactorial, and there is evidence that local inflammatory processes can spread systemically and trigger inflammation of the vessel wall [9]. One inflammatory focus in humans is the oral cavity, and it was proposed that chronic oral inflammations, e.g., periodontitis (PD) and caries, lead to degradation of the tooth-supporting structures [8] and may, in concert with other established risk factors, be able to trigger PAOD. PD is caused by the outgrowth of oral microorganisms, which induce a destructive host inflammatory response that contributes to progressive periodontal tissue destruction and loss of the alveolar bone around the teeth, resulting in gingival pocket formation and clinical attachment loss and, if untreated, tooth loss [10]. Tailored options are available for periodontitis treatment at various stages [11]. Approximately 47% of adults aged ≥30 years in the United States have chronic periodontitis (CP), with 30% having moderate and 8.5% severe PD [12]. PD is a complex inflammatory disease, with genetic and epigenetic factors having a role along with lifestyle and environmental factors, such as smoking, oral hygiene, nutrition, and stress, as well as other widespread systemic diseases, such as diabetes. Hereditary factors, age-dependent mutagenesis, and epigenetic changes have also been involved in the development of certain head and neck cancers, such as squamous cell carcinomas [13]. Chronic PD and obesity have been shown to be associated with pro-atherogenic lipid profiles, which are also risk factors for PAOD [14].

PD has been shown to be associated with atherosclerotic vascular disease. At least four basic pathogenic mechanisms are currently hypothesized that may explain how PD may promote atherosclerosis [15]: (1) Oral bacteria enter the blood stream and invade the arterial wall by chronic low level bacteremia; (2) inflammatory mediators released from the sites of the oral inflammation into the blood stream cause an acute phase reaction, which is pro-atherogenic; (3) specific components of oral pathogens trigger a host immune response, thereby promoting autoimmunity; (4) specific bacterial toxins that are produced by oral pathogenic bacteria have pro-atherogenic effects. A connection between PD as a trigger for the development of PAOD has been controversially discussed for years.

Therefore, the goals of this systematic review were: (1) to collect evidence for an association between PD or tooth loss and PAOD from the published literature and (2) to look for clinical studies that investigated the pathomechanism that might be involved in a potential cause-effect relationship between PD and PAOD.

2. Results

Seven hundred and fifty-one studies were detected by the search formula (shown in the method section), and four additional studies were identified through other sources and added in December 2018. Seven hundred and two studies were excluded following the screening algorithm (see Methods section). Full-text articles were assessed for eligibility. Thirty-six studies were excluded because no full-text article was available, the paper did not match the eligibility criteria, or it had limitations regarding the definition of PAOD or PD. Following application of the eligibility criteria, 17 studies out of the detected 755 studies were included in the qualitative synthesis. Nine studies demonstrated associations between PD and PAOD and two studies associations between tooth loss and PAOD. Six studies addressed the pathomechanism regarding PD as a trigger for PAOD and were included in the discussion. No study that dismissed an association was detected. Figure 1 summarizes the search-results using the Preferred Reporting Items for Systematic Reviews and Meta-Analyses (PRISMA) flow diagram.

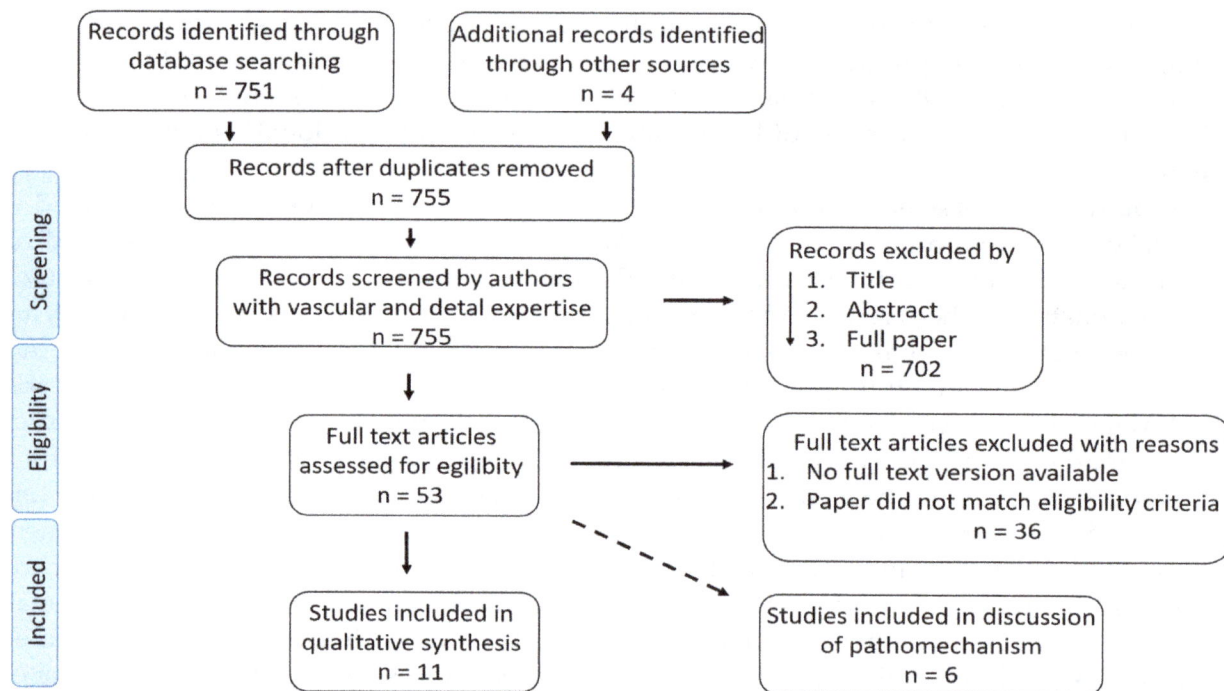

Figure 1. Preferred Reporting Items for Systematic Reviews and Meta-Analyses (PRISMA) flow diagram, the detected studies regarding the pathomechanism were also inserted into the PRISMA diagram (represented by a dashed line).

2.1. Association between PD or Tooth Loss and PAOD

The first study to demonstrate an association between PD and PAOD was a longitudinal study published by Mendez et al. in 1998 [16]. One thousand, one hundred and ten men were followed for up to 30 years, and a 2.27-fold increased incidence rate (95% CI: 1.32–3.9, $p = 0.003$) of developing PAOD was observed in men with clinically significant PD at baseline compared to men with no or only mild PD at baseline. Subsequently, an evaluation of the prospective Health Professionals Follow-up Study [17], which was based on 45,136 male health professionals free of cardiovascular diseases at baseline and 342 incidences of PAOD that had occurred during 12 years of follow-up, showed that incident tooth loss caused by PD was significantly associated with elevated risk of PAOD (relative risk (RR) for history of PD: 1.41, RR for any tooth loss during follow-up: 1.39, after controlling for traditional risk factors of cardiovascular disease) [17].

In a cross-sectional evaluation of data from the National Health and Nutrition Examination Survey (NHANES), 172 of 3585 participants were diagnosed to have PAOD. PD was significantly associated with PAOD with an odds ratio (OR) of over two in men and women [18]. Moreover, systemic markers of inflammation, such as C-reactive protein (CRP), white blood cell count, and fibrinogen, were also associated with PAOD and PD.

Munoz-Torres et al. [19] assessed the association between baseline number of teeth and recent tooth loss and the risk of PAOD in over 70,000 women participating in the Nurses' Health Study. During 16 years of follow-up, a significant association between incident tooth loss and the hazard of PAOD (hazard ratio (HR) = 1.31 95% CI: 1.00–1.71) could be demonstrated.

A recently reported meta-analysis that included a total of 4,307 participants from seven independent studies, confirmed these findings. The study showed a significantly increased risk of PD in PAOD patients compared with non-PAOD patients (RR = 1.70, 95% CI = 1.25–2.29, $p = 0.01$). PAOD patients also had more missing teeth than non-PAOD participants (weighted mean difference, WMD = 3.75,

95% CI = 1.31–6.19, p = 0.003), while no significant difference was found with respect to the clinical attachment loss between PAOD patients and non-PAOD participants (WMD = −0.05, 95% CI = −0.03–0.19, p = 0.686) [20].

Association between PD and PAOD was not only detected in cross-sectional and longitudinal studies, but also in several case-control studies. A strong association was observed by Soto-Barreras et al. [21] based on a small case-control study that included 30 patients with PAOD and 30 healthy controls. Patients with ≥30% of the teeth with an attachment loss ≥4 mm had a six-fold increased risk of PAOD compared to controls (OR = 8.18, 95% CI = 1.21 to 35.23, p = 0.031). The results also indicated that PAOD patients had higher CRP levels (p = 0.0413) and a higher mean decayed missing filled teeth (DMFT) index value (p = 0.0002) along with an elevated number of missing teeth (p = 0.0459) compared to the control group. The study also addressed the potential mechanism of the association. The CRP level was significantly higher (p = 0.0413), and there was also a difference in the decayed-missing-filled-teeth (DMFT) index (p = 0.0002), with a higher number of missing teeth (p = 0.0459) in the PAOD group compared to the control group. However, there were no significant differences regarding the frequency of bacteria in serum and subgingival plaque samples.

A strong association between PAOD and PD was also reported by Calapkorur et al. [22] who found an OR of 5.8 after adjusting for confounders (age, gender, diabetes, hypertension, and body mass index (BMI)) based on a case-control study including 40 patients with PAOD and 20 healthy controls. In a multicenter, population-based, case-control study that included 212 young women with PAOD and 475 healthy women from the Netherlands, PD was associated with PAOD with an OR of 3.0 (95% CI: 1.4–6.3) [23].

In a case-control, retrospective study based on chart reviews, Molloy et al. [24] evaluated self-reported systemic conditions and smoking history of 2006 selected patients attending the University of Minnesota dental clinics. In addition, the number of missing teeth and the degree of alveolar bone loss were recorded. After adjustments for age, sex, diabetes, and smoking, vascular disease and vascular surgery were significantly associated with alveolar bone loss and the number of missing teeth. The association could be demonstrated not only in people of mostly European descent but also in Asians. Ahn et al. observed an OR of 2.03 (95% CI: 1.05–3.93) for the association between severe PD and PAOD in a Korean community cohort of adults aged over 40 years (N = 1343) [25].

Chen et al. [26], observed that PD was significantly associated with PAOD (OR: 5.45, 95% CI: 1.57–18.89 after adjusting for age, gender, diabetes, and smoking) in a Japanese case-control sample of 25 patients with aorto-iliac and/or femoro-popliteal occlusive disease and 32 generally healthy patients who were employed as controls. Table 1 summarizes the results presented above.

Table 1. Summary of the strength of the association between PD or tooth loss and PAOD. RR = risk ratio; OR = odds ratio; HR = hazard ratio; WMD = weighted mean difference. * PAOD patients had more missing teeth than non-PAOD participants. ** conditions that were significantly related to bone loss or number of missing teeth.

Ref	Study Design	Strength of the Association between PD or Tooth Lost and PAOD	Participants	Limitations
[20]	systematic review and meta-analysis	RR = 1.70 (95% CI: 1.3–2.3; p = 0.01) * WMD = 3.75 (95% CI: 1.3–6.2; p = 0.003)	4.307	
[22]	cross-sectional study	OR = 5.8 (95% CI: 1.5–21.9; p = 0.009)	60	
[19]	cohort study	HR = 1.3 (95% CI: 1.0–1.7)	79.663	no adjustment for smoking only women
[25]	cross-sectional study	OR = 2.0 (95% CI: 1.0–3.9; p = 0.036)	1.343	
[21]	case-control study	OR = 8.2 (95% CI: 1.2–35.2; p = 0.031)	60	
[26]	case-control study	OR = 5.5 (95% CI: 1.6–18.9; p = 0.007)	57	
[18]	cross-sectional study	OR = 2.3 (95% CI: 1.2–4.2; p = 0.004)	3.585	
[24]	case-control study	**vascular disease p-value 0.014; **vascular surgery p-value 0.001	2.006	
[17]	cohort study	RR = 1.41 (95% CI: 1.1–1.8)	45.136	only men
[23]	case-control study	OR = 3.0 (95% CI: 1.4–6.3)	687	only women
[16]	cohort study	OR = 2.27 (95% CI: 1.3–3.9; p = 0.003)	1.110	only men

2.2. Pathomechanism

For this systematic review, six studies were found that addressed the potential pathomechanism that may be involved in the association and may explain how PD could induce or aggravate PAOD (see supplementary Table S1 for details). These studies suggest at least three basic mechanisms (Figure 2): (1) Periodontal pathogenic bacteria were demonstrated to enter the bloodstream and to invade atherosclerotic lesions at damaged sites of the arterial wall [27,28]; (2) experimental data showed that inflammatory mediators, such as serum amyloid A and anti-inflammatory mediators, are released from the oral sites affected by PD into the bloodstream, thereby modulating systemic inflammation [29,30]; (3) it was demonstrated in patients with PD that autoimmunity to the host protein heat shock protein 60 (HSP60) resulted from the host immune response to the bacterial HSP60 homolog GroEL produced by *Phorphyromonas gingivalis* (the main oral pathogens involved in PD) [31].

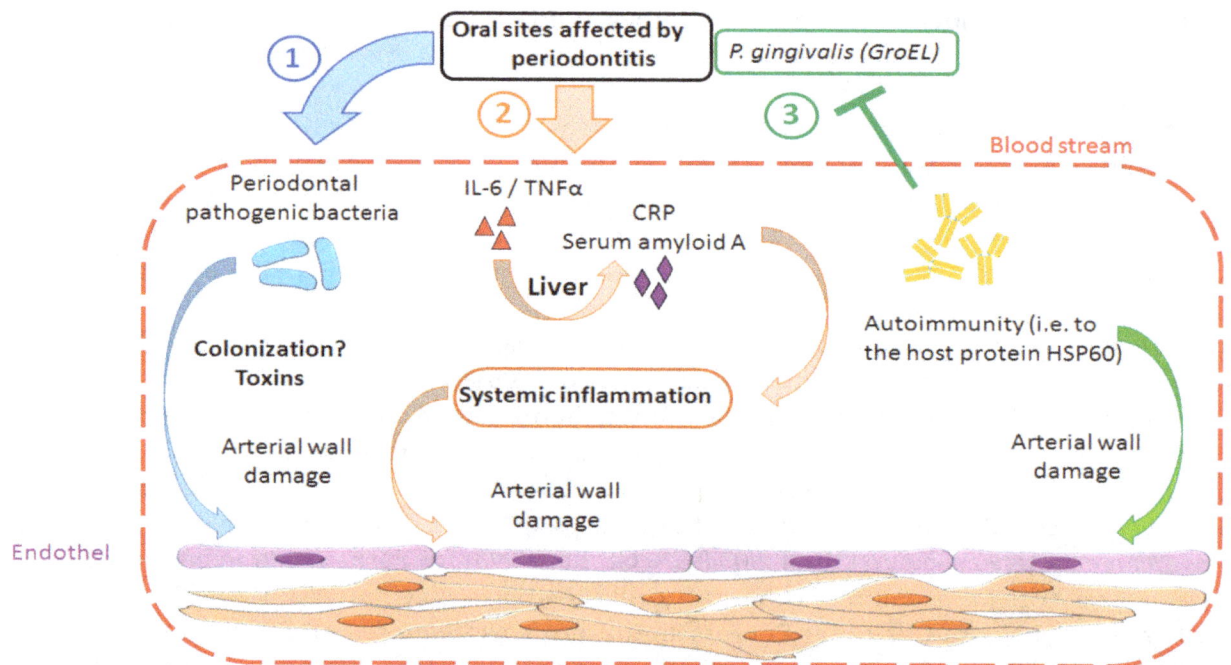

Figure 2. Potential pathomechanism that may be involved in the association of PD and PAOD; (1) periodontal pathogenic bacteria enter the bloodstream, invade and damage the arterial wall; (2) release of inflammatory mediators into the bloodstream, such as serum amyloid A, interleukin-6 (IL-6), tumor necrosis factor α (TNFα), and C-reactive protein (CRP) causing a systemic inflammation that also damages the arterial wall; (3) autoimmunity to host proteins (i.e., heat shock protein 60, HSP60) resulting from the host immuno response to the bacterial proteins, such as the HSP60 homolog GroEL.

In a blinded randomized controlled trial, Li et al. [32] could show that treatment of PD lowered the number of circulating CD34+ cells relative to untreated controls. The reduction of circulating CD34+ cells correlated with the treatment-induced decrease in sites showing bleeding on probing and the number of periodontal pockets with a depth of ≥4 mm, suggesting that treatment of PD reduced the level of systemic inflammation. On the other hand, treatment of PD did not improve endothelial function in this study.

3. Discussion

This systematic review supports that PD is associated with PAOD, which may lead to the hypothesis that PD may be a risk factor for PAOD. To date, many studies describe associations between periodontitis or oral disease and atherosclerosis in general. Therefore, we wanted to specifically focus on studies that concern peripheral vascular disease (PAOD) as a potential consequence of periodontitis in this systematic review. However, it has to be stated that the published literature is not absolutely certain about the term PAOD for "peripheral artery occlusive disease". In publications, it is frequently used for lower extremity artery disease (LEAD). Indeed, other peripheral localizations, including the carotid and vertebral, upper extremities, mesenteric and renal arteries, are also frequently affected, mainly by atherosclerosis, and complete the family of peripheral arterial diseases [6]. In addition, there is sometimes no differentiation between extracranial and cerebral atherosclerotic pathologies. Hence, for this systematic review, we excluded studies that were linked to carotid/cerebral sclerosis, coronary sclerosis as well as vascular sclerosis in general. We also excluded animal studies as we wanted to focus on clinical evidence for an association between the two pathologies.

All studies that were included in this systematic review could detect an association between PD or tooth loss and PAOD irrespective of study design, outcome measure, and study population.

This supports that the consistency of the association is high. It must be noted, however, that there is inherent bias, since risk factors for PAOD also can cause PD. Standardized effect sizes, which provide a measure of the strength of the association, have mostly been determined by logistic regression analyses and reported as ORs together with 95% CIs. After making adjustments for age, gender, and other cardio vascular disease (CVD) risk factors, the reported ORs ranged from somewhat over two in NHANES [18] to over eight in the small case-control study published by Soto-Barreras et al. [21]. In general, the smaller case-control studies yielded higher ORs than the larger cohort studies. Measures of hazard ratios or relative risk estimates are available from only a few studies. Data from the Nurses' Health Study demonstrated a significant association between incident tooth loss and PAOD and reported a hazard ratio of 1.3 for PAOD in women with PD vs. women without PD. The meta-analysis published by Yang et al. 2018 [20] reported a statistically significant relative risk of 1.7 for PAOD in people with PD vs. those without PD.

Taken together, these results suggest that severe PD increases the risk for PAOD to a similar extent as PD increases the risk for cardiovascular events, which with respect to the latter was shown to be $\approx$1.20-fold in adjusted models from meta-analyses of prospective cohort studies [33,34]. Smoking, a profound risk factor for PAOD, is associated with PAOD with odds ratios ranging between 1.7 and 7.4 [3]. With respect to diabetes, a twofold increased rate of macroalbuminuria and a threefold increased rate of end-stage renal disease were found in diabetics who also had severe periodontitis compared to diabetics without severe periodontitis [35]. Moreover, cardiorenal mortality resulting from ischaemic heart disease and diabetic nephropathy was three times higher in diabetics with severe PD compared to periodontally healthy diabetics [36]. The risk of PD for preterm delivery ranged between 4.45 and 7.07, depending on the gestational age [37]. Severe maternal PD was also shown to be associated with preterm low birth weight with an odds ratio of 7.5 [38]. All referenced studies considered a wide range of suspected confounders and included corresponding adjustments. Thus, PD may be a risk factor for multiple, widespread diseases. On the other hand, the possibility that some of the weak associations may be due to residual confounding by unrecognized confounders should not be neglected.

If PD is a causal or, at the least, an important contributor involved in the pathogenesis of PAOD, one would expect that PD precedes the onset of PAOD. However, only very limited information exists with respect to the temporality of both diseases. According to results from the prospective Health Professionals Follow-up Study, tooth loss seemed to precede PAOD, since the incidence of PAOD was most strongly associated with tooth loss in a period of 2 to 6 years prior to the occurrence of PAOD [17]. The fact that tooth loss in the previous 2 to 6 years was more strongly associated with PAOD than tooth loss in the previous 2 years or 6 to 8 years suggests that 6 years may be too distant and 2 years may be too recent for tooth loss to have an impact on PAOD. However, these reported time-dependent differences in the strength of the association were based on only the disparity of only a few PAOD incidences and may, thus, have been chance findings.

The plausibility of a causal or, at least, an important involvement of PD in the development of PAOD mostly relates to experimental data showing that inflammation is involved in the pathophysiology of atherosclerosis, which in turn is involved in the development of PAOD. This inflammation could be caused by a direct involvement of periodontal pathogenic bacteria, which enter the vascular wall via the bloodstream. The study by Figuero et al. used nested polymerase chain reaction (PCR) to detect three periodontal pathogens in subgingival, vascular, and blood samples. Although positive test results were obtained in high fractions of the subgingival samples (>70%) and the vascular and blood samples (7 to 11.4%), patients with and without PD did not differ with respect to the levels of the targeted bacteria. Therefore, a direct involvement of the bacteria seems inconclusive at this stage.

The studies by Nishida et al. 2016 [30] and Armingohar et al. 2015 [29] support that inflammatory mediators, such as serum amyloid A and anti-inflammatory mediators, such as interleukin-10, which are released from the oral sites affected by PD into the bloodstream, thereby modulating systemic inflammation may be involved in the pathomechanism of PD-induced PAOD. In addition, autoimmunity induced by PD via the immune response of the host to the bacterial HSP60 homolog GroEL produced by *P. gingivalis* (the main oral pathogen involved in PD) could play a role [31]. Support for this mechanism comes from the study by Choi et al., who successfully established *P. gingivalis*–specific T-cell lines from atheroma lesions isolated from PD patients. However, the study included only two patients, and the origin of the lesions remained unclear.

It is evident from the results section that our search-strategy yielded only a few publications that dealt with the pathomechanism of the association between PD and PAOD. A large fraction of the published mechanistic studies concerned animal, in vitro and ex vivo studies describing the link between PD and vascular sclerosis in general rather than that between PD and PAOD specifically. These studies were, however, not eligible for this review based on the pre-defined exclusion criteria shown in Figure 3. Roles of oral infections in the pathomechanism of atherosclerosis, in general, were discussed in great detail in a recent review published by Aarabi et al. [15]. Briefly, there is a wealth of support for at least four plausible pathogenic mechanisms: (1) low-level bacteremia by which oral bacteria enter the bloodstream and invade and damage the arterial wall; (2) systemic inflammation induced by inflammatory mediators, which are released from the sites of the oral inflammation into the bloodstream; (3) autoimmunity to host proteins which results from the host immune response to specific components of oral pathogens; (4) pro-atherogenic effects resulting from specific bacterial toxins that are produced by oral pathogenic bacteria. In addition, recent genome-wide association studies supported that PD and PAOD share at least one important predisposing genetic risk haplotype that is located at chromosome 9p21.3 in a locus known as *ANRIL/CDKN2B-AS1* [39,40]. The risk haplotype affects the structure and expression of ANRIL, which is a long non-coding RNA (lncRNA) that, such as other lncRNAs, regulates genome methylation, thereby affecting the expression of multiple genes by *cis* and *trans* mechanisms. How precisely ANRIL contributes to the risk of PD and PAOD on the molecular level is currently unclear.

So far, many, but not all, studies demonstrated the presence of bacterial DNA in a large number of atheromas, but only very few could demonstrate the successful isolation of viable bacteria from an atherosclerotic plaque. In fact, to the best of our knowledge, there is not a single study available that could demonstrate isolation and cultivation of viable *P. gingivalis* from atherosclerotic tissue. In addition, it should be noted that long-term treatment with antibiotics, such as roxithromycin and rifalazil, showed no benefit in patients with an established diagnosis of PAOD [41,42]. Nevertheless, it seems prudent at this stage to recommend that patients with PAOD should be routinely referred to a dentist, and periodontitis should be appropriately treated if present.

4. Methods

4.1. Literature Search

This systematic review considered all studies listed in PubMed until 30 September 2018. For additional studies, we double-checked in EMBASE and supplemented with additional hits obtained from Google Scholar. Grey literature was not part of the review process. It was reported in accordance with the Preferred Reporting Items for Systematic Reviews and Meta-Analyses statement

(PRISMA) [43]. For the PRISMA checklist, see http://www.prisma-statement.org. We employed the Population, Intervention, Control, and Outcome (PICO) format to answer the following PICO questions:

Is PD associated with the occurrence of PAOD?

Population = All patients with PD (all degrees of severity) who were detected in the selected literature

Intervention = None

Comparison = Patients with and without PD

Outcome = PAOD of the lower extremity

We first determined a list of synonyms and MeSH-terms (Medical Subject Headings) for PAOD and PD. Using these lists, we defined the following search-formula.

(peripheral arterial disease OR peripheral artery disease OR PAD OR occlusive vascular disease OR IC OR intermittent claudication OR CLI OR peripheral arterial occlusive disease OR peripheral artery occlusive disease OR PAOD OR lower limb ischemia OR DFS OR vascular surgery)

AND (periodontitis OR gum disease OR pyorrhea OR periodontal disease OR periodontal infection OR periodontal conditions OR chronic periodontitis OR periodontal health OR tooth loss OR attachment loss OR probing pocket depth)

4.2. Study Selection and Data Extraction

All studies were reviewed by two independent authors, one with vascular expertise (MK) and one with oral health expertise (US). Reviewers were blinded to each other results. Both reviewers screened all papers selected by the search formula to identify inclusion criteria. Any disagreements between reviewers at each stage of selection were resolved by consensus. Cohen's kappa coefficient (κ) demonstrated good agreement between the two reviewers ($\kappa = 0.9$) (Appendix A Figure A1). The studies were processed according to the PRISMA flow diagram shown in Figure 1. To sort the studies, we developed a screening-algorithm (Figure 3).

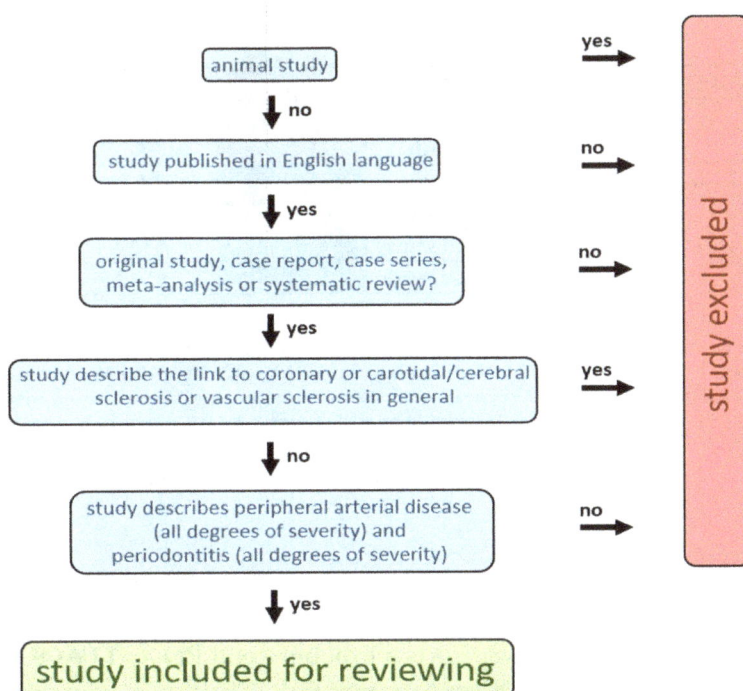

Figure 3. Screening algorithm.

Following this algorithm, we decided whether the eligibility criteria were met; first by title, and if the title led to an uncertainty regarding the eligibility criteria, additionally by the abstract. If there was still uncertainty, the whole paper was read. Animal studies, studies that were published in non-English, studies that did not correspond to original papers, case reports, case series, meta-analyses, or systemic reviews were excluded. In addition, studies on coronary or carotidal/cerebral sclerosis or vascular sclerosis were excluded in general because the aim of this systematic review was to focus on PAOD. Studies describing an association between PD (all degrees of severity) and PAOD (all degrees of severity) were included and further processed according to the PRISMA flow diagram (Figure 1). Studies that were identified by additional manual searches were also added. No duplicates were identified. Citations were managed throughout the different stages of preparing the review with the Mendeley reference management software.

4.3. Quality Assessment

The risk of bias was assessed by using the Newcastle–Ottawa Scale [44] for case-control studies and cohort studies. For the quality assessment of cross-sectional studies, we used a modified version of the Newcastle–Ottawa Scale [45]. The results of the quality assessment are shown in Figure 4.

author	study design	Quality score	Selection	Comparability	Outcome/[1]Exposure/[2]Outcome
Munoz-Torres FJ et al. 2017	cohort study	4	*	*	**
Hsin-Chia Hung et al. 2003	cohort study	5	*	*	***
Mendez M et al. 1998	cohort study	7	**	**	***
Soto-Barreras U et al. 2013	case-control study	4	*	**	*
Chen Y.-W. et al. 2008	case-control study	7	***	**	**
Molloy J et al. 2004	case-control study	3	*	*	*
Bloemenkamp D et al. 2002	case-control study	7	***	**	**
Lu B et al. 2008	cross-sectional study	9	****	**	***
M. Unlu Calapkorur et al. 2017	cross-sectional study	9	****	**	***
Ahn Y-B et al. 2016	cross-sectional study	9	****	**	***

Thresholds for converting the Newcastle-Ottawa scales to AHRQ standards (good, fair, and poor):
Good quality: 3 or 4 stars in selection domain AND 1 or 2 stars in comparability domain AND 2 or 3 stars in outcome/exposure domain
Fair quality: 2 stars in selection domain AND 1 or 2 stars in comparability domain AND 2 or 3 stars in outcome/exposure domain
Poor quality: 0 or 1 star in selection domain OR 0 stars in comparability domain OR 0 or 1 stars in outcome/exposure domain

Figure 4. Results of the quality assessment.

5. Conclusions

In conclusion, the present evidence supports a link between PD and PAOD. Further studies which address the temporality of PD and PAOD are warranted. Thus, a causal, or at least, an important contributing role of PD in the development of PAOD can currently not be confirmed but may be suspected. Clearly, the ultimate proof of causality would depend on data from randomized controlled invention trials to show that treatment of PD can diminish or even prevent PAOD. Such data does, to the best of our knowledge, currently not exist.

Appendix A

Cohens Kappa coefficient

$$\kappa = 0{,}90$$

$$p_0 = 0{,}99$$
$$p_e = 0{,}88$$

		Reviewer II (US)		sum
		included	excluded	
Reviewer I	included	45	1	46
(MK)	excluded	8	701	709
sum		53	702	755

Figure A1. Cohens Kappa coefficient calculation.

References

1. Vos, T.; Flaxman, A.D.; Naghavi, M.; Lozano, R.; Michaud, C.; Ezzati, M.; Shibuya, K.; Salomon, J.A.; Abdalla, S.; Aboyans, V.; et al. Years lived with disability (YLDs) for 1160 sequelae of 289 diseases and injuries 1990–2010: A systematic analysis for the Global Burden of Disease Study 2010. *Lancet* **2012**, *380*, 2163–2196. [CrossRef]
2. Sampson, U.K.A.; Fowkes, F.G.R.; McDermott, M.M.; Criqui, M.H.; Aboyans, V.; Norman, P.E.; Forouzanfar, M.H.; Naghavi, M.; Song, Y.; Harrell, F.E., Jr.; et al. Global and Regional Burden of Death and Disability from Peripheral Artery Disease: 21 World Regions, 1990 to 2010. *Glob. Heart* **2014**, *9*, 145–158. [CrossRef]
3. Fowkes, F.G.R.; Rudan, D.; Rudan, I.; Aboyans, V.; Denenberg, J.O.; McDermott, M.M.; Norman, P.E.; Sampson, U.K.; Williams, L.J.; Mensah, G.A.; et al. Comparison of global estimates of prevalence and risk factors for peripheral artery disease in 2000 and 2010: A systematic review and analysis. *Lancet* **2013**, *382*, 1329–1340. [CrossRef]
4. Creager, M.A. The Crisis of Vascular Disease and the Journey to Vascular Health. *Circulation* **2016**, *133*, 2593–2598. [CrossRef] [PubMed]
5. Malyar, N.; Fürstenberg, T.; Wellmann, J.; Meyborg, M.; Lüders, F.; Gebauer, K.; Bunzemeier, H.; Roeder, N.; Reinecke, H. Recent trends in morbidity and in-hospital outcomes of in-patients with peripheral arterial disease: A nationwide population-based analysis. *Eur. Heart J.* **2013**, *34*, 2706–2714. [CrossRef] [PubMed]
6. Aboyans, V.; Ricco, J.B.; Bartelink, M.E.L.; Björck, M.; Brodmann, M.; Cohnert, T.; Collet, J.P.; Czerny, M.; De Carlo, M.; Debus, S.; et al. 2017 ESC Guidelines on the Diagnosis and Treatment of Peripheral Arterial Diseases, in collaboration with the European Society for Vascular Surgery (ESVS). *Eur. Heart J.* **2018**, *39*, 763–816. [CrossRef] [PubMed]
7. Hamburg, N.M.; Creager, M.A. Pathophysiology of Intermittent Claudication in Peripheral Artery Disease. *Circ. J.* **2017**, *81*, 281–289. [CrossRef]
8. Taleb, S. Inflammation in atherosclerosis. *Arch. Cardiovasc. Dis.* **2016**, *109*, 708–715. [CrossRef]
9. Miao, C.-Y.; Li, Z.-Y. The role of perivascular adipose tissue in vascular smooth muscle cell growth. *Br. J. Pharmacol.* **2012**, *165*, 643–658. [CrossRef]
10. Armitage, G.C. Periodontal diagnoses and classification of periodontal diseases. *Periodontol. 2000* **2004**, *34*, 9–21. [CrossRef]

11. Matarese, G.; Ramaglia, L.; Fiorillo, L.; Cervino, G.; Lauritano, F.; Isola, G. Implantology and Periodontal Disease: The Panacea to Problem Solving? *Open Dent. J.* **2017**, *11*, 460–465. [CrossRef] [PubMed]

12. Thornton-Evans, G.; Eke, P.; Wei, L.; Palmer, A.; Moeti, R.; Hutchins, S.; Borrell, L.N. Periodontitis among adults aged ≥30 years—United States, 2009–2010. *MMWR Suppl.* **2013**, *62*, 129–135. [PubMed]

13. Ferlazzo, N.; Currò, M.; Zinellu, A.; Caccamo, D.; Isola, G.; Ventura, V.; Carru, C.; Matarese, G.; Ientile, R. Influence of MTHFR Genetic Background on p16 and MGMT Methylation in Oral Squamous Cell Cancer. *Int. J. Mol. Sci.* **2017**, *18*, 724. [CrossRef] [PubMed]

14. Cury, E.Z.; Santos, V.R.; da Silva Maciel, S.; Gonçalves, T.E.D.; Zimmermann, G.S.; Mota, R.M.S.; Figueiredo, L.C.; Duarte, P.M. Lipid parameters in obese and normal weight patients with or without chronic periodontitis. *Clin. Oral Investig.* **2018**, *22*, 161–167. [CrossRef] [PubMed]

15. Aarabi, G.; Heydecke, G.; Seedorf, U. Roles of Oral Infections in the Pathomechanism of Atherosclerosis. *Int. J. Mol. Sci.* **2018**, *19*, 1978. [CrossRef] [PubMed]

16. Mendez, M.V.; Scott, T.; LaMorte, W.; Vokonas, P.; Menzoian, J.O.; Garcia, R. An Association between Periodontal Disease and Peripheral Vascular Disease. *Am. J. Surg.* **1998**, *176*, 153–157. [CrossRef]

17. Hung, H.-C.; Willett, W.; Merchant, A.; Rosner, B.A.; Ascherio, A.; Joshipura, K.J. Oral Health and Peripheral Arterial Disease. *Circulation* **2003**, *107*, 1152–1157. [CrossRef]

18. Lu, B.; Parker, D.; Eaton, C.B. Relationship of periodontal attachment loss to peripheral vascular disease: An analysis of NHANES 1999–2002 data. *Atherosclerosis* **2008**, *200*, 199–205. [CrossRef]

19. Muñoz-Torres, F.J.; Mukamal, K.J.; Pai, J.K.; Willett, W.; Joshipura, K.J. Relationship between Tooth Loss and Peripheral Arterial Disease among Women. *J. Clin. Periodontol.* **2017**, *44*, 989–995. [CrossRef]

20. Yang, S.; Zhao, L.S.; Cai, C.; Shi, Q.; Wen, N.; Xu, J. Association between periodontitis and peripheral artery disease: A systematic review and meta-analysis. *BMC Cardiovasc. Disord.* **2018**, *18*, 141. [CrossRef]

21. Soto-Barreras, U.; Olvera-Rubio, J.O.; Loyola-Rodríguez, J.P.; Reyes-Macías, J.F.; Martinez-Martinez, R.E.; Patiño-Marin, N.; Martinez-Castanon, G.-A.; Aradillas-García, C.; Little, J.W. Peripheral Arterial Disease Associated with Caries and Periodontal Disease. *J. Periodontol.* **2013**, *84*, 486–494. [CrossRef] [PubMed]

22. Çalapkorur, M.U.; Alkan, B.A.; Tasdemir, Z.; Akcali, Y.; Saatci, E. Association of peripheral arterial disease with periodontal disease: Analysis of inflammatory cytokines and an acute phase protein in gingival crevicular fluid and serum. *J. Periodontal Res.* **2017**, *52*, 532–539. [CrossRef] [PubMed]

23. Bloemenkamp, D.G.; van den Bosch, M.A.; Mali, W.P.; Tanis, B.C.; Rosendaal, F.R.; Kemmeren, J.M.; Algra, A.; Visseren, F.L.; Van Der Graaf, Y. Novel risk factors for peripheral arterial disease in young women. *Am. J. Med.* **2002**, *113*, 462–467. [CrossRef]

24. Molloy, J.; Wolff, L.F.; Lopez-Guzman, A.; Hodges, J.S. The association of periodontal disease parameters with systemic medical conditions and tobacco use. *J. Clin. Periodontol.* **2004**, *31*, 625–632. [CrossRef] [PubMed]

25. Ahn, Y.-B.; Shin, M.-S.; Han, D.-H.; Sukhbaatar, M.; Kim, M.-S.; Shin, H.-S.; Kim, H.-D. Periodontitis is associated with the risk of subclinical atherosclerosis and peripheral arterial disease in Korean adults. *Atherosclerosis* **2016**, *251*, 311–318. [CrossRef] [PubMed]

26. Chen, Y.-W.; Umeda, M.; Nagasawa, T.; Takeuchi, Y.; Huang, Y.; Inoue, Y.; Iwai, T.; Izumi, Y.; Ishikawa, I. Periodontitis May Increase the Risk of Peripheral Arterial Disease. *Eur. J. Vasc. Endovasc. Surg.* **2008**, *35*, 153–158. [CrossRef]

27. Armingohar, Z.; Jørgensen, J.J.; Kristoffersen, A.K.; Abesha-Belay, E.; Olsen, I. Bacteria and bacterial DNA in atherosclerotic plaque and aneurysmal wall biopsies from patients with and without periodontitis. *J. Oral Microbiol.* **2014**, *6*, 23408. [CrossRef]

28. Figuero, E.; Lindahl, C.; Marín, M.J.; Renvert, S.; Herrera, D.; Ohlsson, O.; Wetterling, T.; Sanz, M. Quantification of Periodontal Pathogens in Vascular, Blood, and Subgingival Samples from Patients with Peripheral Arterial Disease or Abdominal Aortic Aneurysms. *J. Periodontol.* **2014**, *85*, 1182–1193. [CrossRef]

29. Armingohar, Z.; Jørgensen, J.J.; Kristoffersen, A.K.; Schenck, K.; Dembic, Z. Polymorphisms in the interleukin-10 gene and chronic periodontitis in patients with atherosclerotic and aortic aneurysmal vascular diseases. *J. Oral Microbiol.* **2015**, *7*, 26051. [CrossRef]

30. Nishida, E.; Aino, M.; Kobayashi, S.-I.; Okada, K.; Ohno, T.; Kikuchi, T.; Hayashi, J.-I.; Yamamoto, G.; Hasegawa, Y.; Mitani, A. Serum Amyloid A Promotes E-Selectin Expression via Toll-Like Receptor 2 in Human Aortic Endothelial Cells. *Mediat. Inflamm.* **2016**, *2016*, 7150509. [CrossRef]

31. Choi, J.-I.; Chung, S.-W.; Kang, H.-S.; Rhim, B.Y.; Kim, S.-J.; Kim, S.-J. Establishment of *Porphyromonas gingivalis* Heat-shock-protein-specific T-cell Lines from Atherosclerosis Patients. *J. Dent. Res.* **2002**, *81*, 344–348. [CrossRef] [PubMed]
32. Li, X.; Tse, H.F.; Yiu, K.H.; Li, L.S.W.; Jin, L. Effect of periodontal treatment on circulating CD34+ cells and peripheral vascular endothelial function: A randomized controlled trial. *J. Clin. Periodontol.* **2011**, *38*, 148–156. [CrossRef] [PubMed]
33. Leng, W.-D.; Zeng, X.-T.; Kwong, J.S.; Hua, X.-P. Periodontal disease and risk of coronary heart disease: An updated meta-analysis of prospective cohort studies. *Int. J. Cardiol.* **2015**, *201*, 469–472. [CrossRef] [PubMed]
34. Humphrey, L.L.; Fu, R.; Buckley, D.I.; Freeman, M.; Helfand, M. Periodontal Disease and Coronary Heart Disease Incidence: A Systematic Review and Meta-analysis. *J. Gen. Intern. Med.* **2008**, *23*, 2079–2086. [CrossRef] [PubMed]
35. Shultis, W.A.; Weil, E.J.; Looker, H.C.; Curtis, J.M.; Shlossman, M.; Genco, R.J.; Knowler, W.C.; Nelson, R.G. Effect of Periodontitis on Overt Nephropathy and End-Stage Renal Disease in Type 2 Diabetes. *Diabetes Care* **2007**, *30*, 306–311. [CrossRef] [PubMed]
36. Saremi, A.; Nelson, R.G.; Tulloch-Reid, M.; Hanson, R.L.; Sievers, M.L.; Taylor, G.W.; Shlossman, M.; Bennett, P.H.; Genco, R.; Knowler, W.C. Periodontal disease and mortality in type 2 diabetes. *Diabetes Care* **2005**, *28*, 27–32. [CrossRef]
37. Jeffcoat, M.K.; Geurs, N.C.; Reddy, M.S.; Cliver, S.P.; Goldenberg, R.L.; Hauth, J.C. Periodontal infection and preterm birth: Results of a prospective study. *J. Am. Dent. Assoc.* **2001**, *132*, 875–880. [CrossRef]
38. Offenbacher, S.; Katz, V.; Fertik, G.; Collins, J.; Boyd, D.; Maynor, G.; McKaig, R.; Beck, J. Periodontal Infection as a Possible Risk Factor for Preterm Low Birth Weight. *J. Periodontol.* **1996**, *67*, 1103–1113. [CrossRef]
39. Belkin, N.; Damrauer, S.M. Peripheral Arterial Disease Genetics: Progress to Date and Challenges Ahead. *Curr. Cardiol. Rep.* **2017**, *19*, 131. [CrossRef]
40. Aarabi, G.; Zeller, T.; Heydecke, G.; Munz, M.; Schäfer, A.; Seedorf, U. Roles of the Chr.9p21.3 ANRIL Locus in Regulating Inflammation and Implications for Anti-Inflammatory Drug Target Identification. *Front. Cardiovasc. Med.* **2018**, *5*, 47. [CrossRef]
41. Jaff, M.R.; Dale, R.A.; Creager, M.A.; Lipicky, R.J.; Constant, J.; Campbell, L.A.; Hiatt, W.R. Anti-Chlamydial Antibiotic Therapy for Symptom Improvement in Peripheral Artery Disease. Prospective Evaluation of Rifalazil Effect on Vascular Symptoms of Intermittent Claudication and Other Endpoints in *Chlamydia pneumoniae* Seropositive Patients (PROVIDENCE-1). *Circulation* **2009**, *119*, 452–458. [CrossRef] [PubMed]
42. Joensen, J.B.; Juul, S.; Henneberg, E.; Thomsen, G.; Ostergaard, L.; Lindholt, J.S. Can long-term antibiotic treatment prevent progression of peripheral arterial occlusive disease? A large, randomized, double-blinded, placebo-controlled trial. *Atherosclerosis* **2008**, *196*, 937–942. [CrossRef] [PubMed]
43. Moher, D.; Shamseer, L.; Clarke, M.; Ghersi, D.; Liberati, A.; Petticrew, M.; Shekelle, P.; Stewart, L.A. Preferred reporting items for systematic review and meta-analysis protocols (PRISMA-P) 2015 statement. *Syst. Rev.* **2015**, *4*, 1. [CrossRef] [PubMed]
44. Wells, G.A.; Shea, B.; O'Connell, D.; Peterson, J.; Welch, V.; Losos, M.; Tugwell, P. The Newcastle-Ottawa Scale (NOS) for Assessing the Quality of Nonrandomised Studies in Meta-Analyses. Ottawa Hospital Research Institute. Available online: http://www.ohri.ca/programs/clinical_epidemiology/oxford.asp (accessed on 23 July 2015).
45. Herzog, R.; Álvarez-Pasquin, M.J.; Díaz, C.; Del Barrio, J.L.; Estrada, J.M.; Gil, A. Are healthcare workers' intentions to vaccinate related to their knowledge, beliefs and attitudes? A systematic review. *BMC Public Health* **2013**, *13*, 154. [CrossRef] [PubMed]

12

Kampo Therapies and the Use of Herbal Medicines in the Dentistry in Japan

Shuji Watanabe [1,2], Toshizo Toyama [1], Takenori Sato [1], Mitsuo Suzuki [1,3], Akira Morozumi [4], Hiroshi Sakagami [5] and Nobushiro Hamada [1,*]

[1]   Division of Microbiology, Department of Oral Science, Kanagawa Dental University, 82 Inaoka-cho, Yokosuka 238-8580, Japan; swatanabe2010@nifty.com (S.W.); toyama@kdu.ac.jp (T.T.); t.sato@kdu.ac.jp (T.S.); suzuki@d2clinic.jp (M.S.)
[2]   Odoriba Medical Center, Totsuka Green Dental Clinic, 1-10-46 Gumizawa, Totsuka-ku, Yokohama 245-0061, Japan
[3]   Dental Design Clinic, 3-7-10 Kita-aoyama, Minato-ku, Tokyo 107-0061, Japan
[4]   Morozumi Dental Clinic, 1-3-1 Miyamaedaira, Miyamae-ku, Kawasaki 216-0006, Japan; morozumident@gmail.com
[5]   Meikai University Research Institute of Odontology (M-RIO), 1-1 Keyakidai, Sakado, Saitama 350-0283, Japan; sakagami@dent.meikai.ac.jp
*   Correspondence: hamada@kdu.ac.jp

Abstract: Dental caries and periodontal disease are two major diseases in the dentistry. As the society is aging, their pathological meaning has been changing. An increasing number of patients are displaying symptoms of systemic disease and so we need to pay more attention to immunologic aggression in our medical treatment. For this reason, we focused on natural products. Kampo consists of natural herbs—roots and barks—and has more than 3000 years of history. It was originated in China as traditional medicine and introduced to Japan. Over the years, Kampo medicine in Japan has been formulated in a way to suit Japan's natural features and ethnic characteristics. Based on this traditional Japanese Kampo medicine, we have manufactured a Kampo gargle and Mastic Gel dentifrice. In order to practically utilize the effectiveness of mastic, we have developed a dentifrice (product name: IMPLA CARE) and treated implant periodontitis and severe periodontitis.

Keywords: periodontitis; Kampo; traditional medicine; *Jixueteng*; *Juzentaihoto*; technical terms; gargle; tongue diagnosis; mastic; pathogenic factors

1. Introduction

Kampo medicine in Japan is the Oriental medicine which was originally brought from China through east Asia and the Korean peninsula as the ancient Chinese medicine. During the Nara period of Japan (AD 710-784), Japanese envoys were sent to Tang Dynasty (AD616-907) under the name of Kentoshi and it became a channel that Chinese medicine was directly brought to Japan. In the Kamakura period (AD1185-1333), it made a progress to become more practical medicine by being adopted more to Japan's natural environment, rather than a simple copy of Chinese medicine. In the Muromachi period (AD 1336-1573), a Japanese whose name was Sanki Tashiro studied in China during its Ming dynasty (AD1368-1644) and created the academic foundation of the Japanese Kampo medicine. Kampo was first used in higher social classes but since the 15th century it has provided general people natural material-based medicine. In the Edo period (AD 1603-1867), Western medicine was introduced to Japan from Netherland and was called Rangaku, innovating special characteristics such as abdominal diagnosis and contributed to the developments of medical diagnosis and treatment [1–3]. On the other hand, the traditional medicine which was primarily using herbal medicines was called Kampo medicine. In 1883, the Japanese government promulgated the regulation of the medical license that only those doctors who have mastered the Western medicine could prescribe the Kampo medicines and the Kampo medicine declined since then except for the practice by some facilities or individuals. In 1927, the book of Kokan Igaku (traditional Japanese and Chinese medicine) by Kyushin Yumoto was published and it triggered the subsequent revival of Kampo medicine. Following that in 1950, the academic society of "Japan Society of Oriental Medicine" of Kokan Igaku was established, which became the association of Oriental medicine including acupuncture and moxibustion treatments. Under the guidance of the Japan Medical Association, Kitasato University Oriental Medicine Research Centre was founded in 1972 and it has played a central role in the education of Oriental Medicine. Further in 2001, the model curriculum of medical education newly incorporated a course of study for "being capable of explaining Japanese and Chinese medicines." At present, all medical schools in Japan have the courses of study for Kampo medicine or Oriental medicine as part of their education program.

Kampo medicine has a unique character, which is different from Western medicine. Kampo uses as a combination drug of various herbal plants that have complementary physiological activities. In fact, 148 Kampo formulations are used for medicinal treatments and are covered by the Japanese National Health Insurance Program [4]. Since 2012, seven kinds of Kampo formulations were approved by Japan Dental Association within the National Health Insurance Drug Price Standard related with dental treatment [5]. In 2015, Kampo Education Plan of Dentistry was sent from the Japan Dental Association to all dental universities [6]. At the same time, the first author of this article (S.W.) established the Yokohama Kampo Dentistry Study Group for the continuing education of Kampo. This group has held 18 research sessions and symposiums by calling a special lecturer of Kampo and is planning to publish a side reader of 11 Kampo preparations for dental students from the Nanzando publishing company. There are two academic societies on Kampo in Japan: The Japan Society for Oriental Medicine and Japan Dental Society of Oriental Medicine. The latter showed previously different direction about *qigong* and massage but now changing to the same direction with the former.

Kampo prescriptions in dentistry has special characteristics due to the diverse symptoms such as the pain caused by the bad bite alignment or malocclusion (exogenous cause) and unidentified complaints. For Kampo prescriptions, it is important to understand the symptoms, by considering these special characteristics. It has also become known that the negative feedback functionality would not work when malocclusion and occlusal destruction become chronic with the sympathetic-nerve predominant state. We expect that Western medicine and the Oriental medicine will be used selectively and in parallel in many of the clinical cases in dentistry to ensure the best results for primary cares and that it would contribute to the dentistry medicine going forward.

In this review article, we firstly focus on the basic theory of Kampo medicine and then its biological activities and clinical effects in the dental treatments.

2. Basic Theory of Kampo Medicine

2.1. Concept of Oriental Medicine

Western medicine is a proof medicine that is based on the medical evidence, while Oriental medicine is a traditional medicine that has accumulated the evidence based on the experiences [7]. The modern medicine has made great advances by accumulating scientific evidences but it was at the same time a challenge to the limit of the medicine and it has added a new dimension of problems such as the side effects of medicines to cope up with the aggravation of diseases. In recent years, medical evidences of Kampo prescription (traditional medicine in Japan based on the traditional Chinese medicine), which is one of the pharmacotherapies of Oriental medicine, has become widely known. It is making it possible to include Kampo in the pharmacotherapy of the modern medicine, in consideration of its role as biological response modifiers (BRMs) of the vital balance. Oriental medicine was generated from the concept that the natural world consists of the opposing axis of *Yin* (Table A1) or "non-resistant" and *Yang* or "resistant," where the relativity of these axes maintains the qualitative balance of the workings of mother nature [3]. This principle is therefore called the *"Yin-Yang theory."* In the Kampo therapy, the body state and each internal organ are divided into *Yin* or *Yang* and it treats the patient so the *yin-yang* is balanced and can maintain the homeostasis (Figure 1).

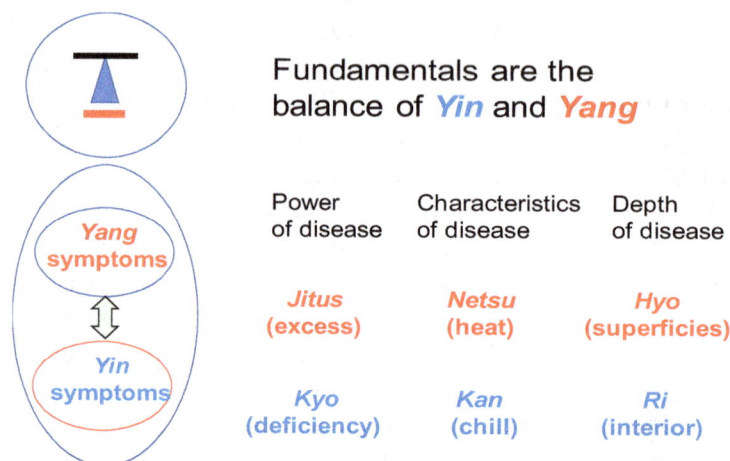

Figure 1. Concepts of Kampo therapy. Kampo therapy begins with the knowledge of constitutional characteristics of patient's body. *In-Yo* or *Yin-Yang*: When the switch-over between two representative autonomic nerves, the sympathetic nerves *(yang)* and the parasympathetic nerves *(yin)*, is good, the *yin-yang* balance is kept well. *Kyo-Jits* or asthenia and sthenia show physical strength, constitutional characteristics of body and the strength of resistance against disease. The reaction differs, depending on their *Kyo-Sho* or *Jitsu-Sho*. It is categorized into *Jitsu-Sho* (excess symptom), *Kyo-Sho* (deficiency symptom) and *Chukan-Sho* (symptom in-between the two). *Kan-Netsu* or chills and fever: *Kan* is *Yin* while *Netsu* is *Yang*. They are always in a relative relation. When *Yin* deteriorates, *Yang* predominates, called *Netsu-sho* (heat syndrome).

2.2. Differences from the Western Medicine

Oriental medicine and Western medicine are both medical sciences, fundamentally and equally. Oriental medicine identifies the disease mainly based on the pathological condition at the time of diagnosis. It understands that a part of the body appeals the problem and it spreads to the entire body and shows the symptom in that part. Therefore, the treatment aims at alleviating the symptom while improving the pathological condition itself. This pathological condition is called *Sho* or Kampo Diagnosis.

The Western medicine diagnoses based on the demonstrated symptom and it emphasizes the importance of the examinations in order to find out the condition of the appearing symptoms, then gives it a name and treats it accordingly. On the other hand, Kampo medicine improves the symptom by improving the pathological condition presented in the form of *Sho* [2,8]. *Sho* is the measure to know the characteristics, size and depth of the disease, which would indicate the cause of the disease and the treatment, is given by finding out the cause of the pathological condition by *Sho*. From this, Oriental medicine makes it possible to treat the patient as expressed in the phrase "Different treatments for one disease; identical treatment for different diseases." It means that different treatments will be given for the same disease name of patients if the *Sho* (Kampo diagnosis) is different. Likewise, the same treatment will be given to the different disease names of patients, if the *Sho* is the same. Here in this article, the disease name means the name of the disease under the modern medical science (Figure 2).

2.3. The Categories of Sho

Shoko (Kampo medical conditions, symptoms in Western medical terms) consists of *Yin-Yang* with *Kyo-Jitsu*, *Kan-Netsu* and *Hyo-Ri*. They reflect the current pathogenic condition. Table 1 shows the definitions and classifications of *Yin-Yang*, *Kyo-Jitsu* (asthenia and sthenia) and *Kan Netsu* (chills and fever). Table 2 shows the definitions of *Yin-Kyo*, *Yo-Kyo*, *Yin-Jitsu* and *Yo-Jitsu*. Figure 3 shows the condition categories of *Yin-Yang*, *Kyo-sho* and *Netsu-Kan* in the body.

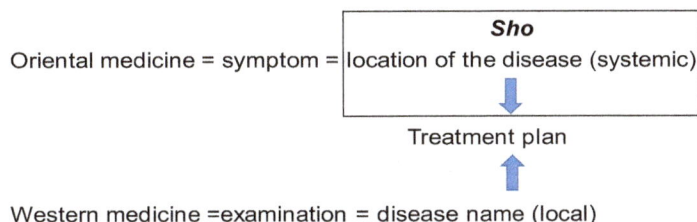

```
                                    ┌──────────────────────────────────────┐
                                    │                  Sho                   │
  Oriental medicine = symptom =     │ location of the disease (systemic)     │
                                    │                  ⬇                     │
                                    └──────────────────────────────────────┘
                                              Treatment plan
                                                  ⬆
  Western medicine = examination = disease name (local)
```

Figure 2. Characteristics of Oriental medicine and Western medicine therapy. *Sho* (Kampo Diagnosis): Capturing the *Shoko* (yin-yang, *Kyo-Jitsu* or deficiency and excess, *Kan-Netsu* or chills and fever, *Hyo-Ri* or superficies and interior) as the holistic symptom caused by the pathological condition and it shows the condition of the patient at the time of diagnosis. *Sho* changes depending on the bodily sensation.

Table 1. Definitions and classifications of *Yin-Yong*, *Kyo-Jitsu* and *Kan-Netsu*.

Categories	Yin-Yang	Kyo-Jitsu (Asthenia and Sthenia)	Kan-Netsu (Chills and Fever)
Definitions	Ability to resist the disease. The treatment differs, depending on whether the *sho* is *yang* and *yin*. *Yin* disease: The resistant power against the disease is weak. Treatment is given to recover the exhaustion of the body. It is called *honchi* or the systemic meridian treatment	The state of deficiency is *kyo-sho* or asthenia and excess is *jitsu-sho* or sthenia. *Kyo* (Asthenia): Deficiency of what is required for the body and shows the *sho* of *Yin-kyo* syndrome or *yang-kyo* syndrome	Actual feeling of chill and heat *Kyo-netsu* (asthenic heat): Heat coming from poor metabolism and retained inside the body, slight fever, internal fever, showing *yin*-syndrome.
Classification (According to the Orthodox Theory)	*Yang* disease: The resistant power against the disease is strong. Treatment which positivity attacks the disease is effective. It is called *hyochi* or local and symptomatic treatment.	*Jitsu* (Sthenia): Low metabolic rate due to the accumulation of toxic substance in the body and shows the *sho* of *yin-jitsu* or *yang-jitsu*.	*Jitsu-netsu* (sthenic heat): Chills that occurs by increasing the heat in the body. Observes pyrexia and showing *Yang*-syndrome.

Table 2. Definitions of *Yin-Kyo*, *Yo-Kyo*, *Yin-Jitsu* and *Yo-Jitsu*.

Categories	Yin-Kyo (yin deficiency)	Yo-Kyo (yang deficiency)	Yin-Jitsu (Yin excess)	Yo-Jitsu (Yang excess)
Definitions	*Yin* is insufficient and *yan* becomes relatively overactive; shows fever called asthenic fever; feverish symptom.	*Yang* is insufficient and *yin* relatively becomes overactive; asthenia cold; feeling chills.	Coldness comes from outside to constantly maintain the homeostasis of *yin* and *yang* and shows the state of chills, called *Jitsu-Kan* or sthenic cold; body is chilled and feeling cold.	Heat comes from outside to constantly maintain the homeostasis of *yin* and *yang*; and shows the state of heat, called *Jitsu-Netsu* or sthenic heat; feeling hot and excessive sw eating.

On the other hand, *Hyo-Ri* (superficies and interior) indicates where the disease exists in the body and shows the depth of *Sho*, depending on the part of the body. *Hyo-ri* is a unique concept of Kampo medicine, which indicates the seriousness of the disease, based on the location and depth of the disease. According to the classic literature "Shokan-ron," *Yin* and *Yang* are further divided into 3 layers by the degree of development and it calls them the "Three *Yin*" and the "Three *Yang*" of diseases [8]. The Three *Yang* stage indicates *Hyo* or the surface of the body such as skin but also includes the parts of the body that show the *Hyo* symptoms such as chill, fever, headache, joint pain and sweat. The three *Yin* stage indicates *Ri*. Mostly *Sho*'s of the internal organs, including heart, lungs and digestive apparatus, are shown, where the symptoms are, for example, abdominal pain, constipation, diarrhoea, fullness of the abdomen, stomach tension. The middle part between the *Hyo-Ri* is called *Han-Hyo-Ri* or mesodermal.

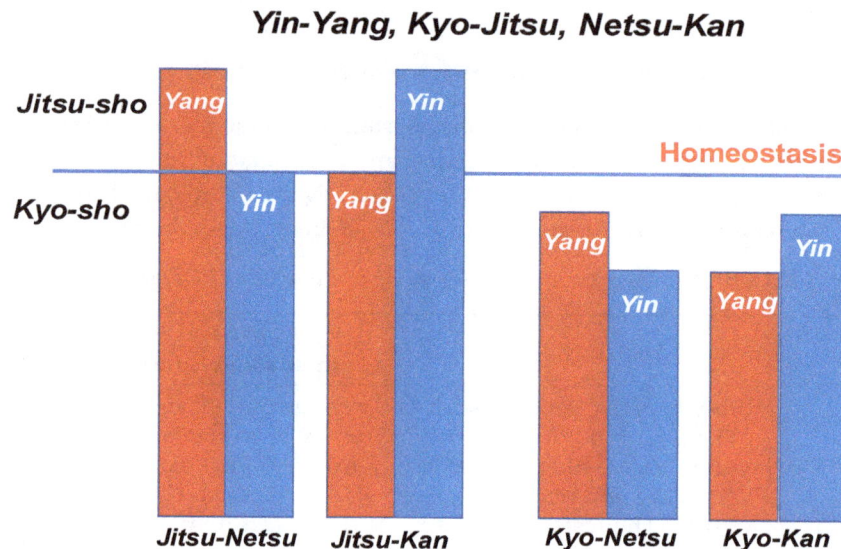

Yin-Yang, Kyo-Jitsu, Netsu-Kan

Figure 3. Condition categories of *Yin-Yang*, *Kyo-sho* and *Netsu-Kan* in the body.

2.4. Cause of Illness

Disease in Kampo medicine is the disorder of harmony of spirit and body. The living body has physiological functions to maintain the homeostasis of the organism against the changes of internal and external environment. This function is called *Shoki* or healthy *Ki*. *Shoki* is a function which would defend the body against disease and would induce natural healing ability, where the natural healing ability would seek for the harmony of *Ki, Ketsu and Sui* (vital energy, blood circulation and aqua). In contrast, the factor that attempts to destroy the homeostasis is called *Ja* or *Byoja* or stress or pathogen. It induces the climate, emotion or virus to cause various physical abnormalities which would lead to diseases. Causes of disease are categorized into endogenous, exogenous and other factors.

Endogenous factor means that the cause of disease comes from the inside of body. It may be common emotions of human beings. It is a physiological phenomenon and may be quintessential in life. However, it can cause abnormality in the functions of internal organs, when mental stress persists or when a sudden strong shock hits us, because it would collapse the balance of *Yin, Yang, Ki* and *Ketsu* on such occasions. It is called the *Seven Emotions* –joy, anger, anxiety, worry, grief, apprehension and fear.

Exogenous factor means that *ja* invades the body from outside. Diseases occur influenced by the mental or physical changes when the body cannot accept the natural environment such as pathogens, severe natural environment and sudden climate changes. It is called the *Six Pathogenic Agents* - wind, cold, heat, humidity, dryness and fire (fever).

These are other factors, which would cause diseases due to other causes such as inadequate eating-drinking, fatigue, overwork, injury, poisoning, parasite and heredity.

2.5. Explanation of Ki, Ketsu, Oketsu and Sui

The concept of *Ki* (vital energy), *Ketsu* (blood/blood circulatory function) and *Sui* (aqua) is the fundamental concept to understand the Kampo medicine [2,8] (Figure 4).

Ki indicates *yang* and *Ketsu* and *Sui* indicate *yin*. Patients reversibly show *Jitsu-Sho* (excessive) and *Kyo-Sho* (deficiency) (Table 3).

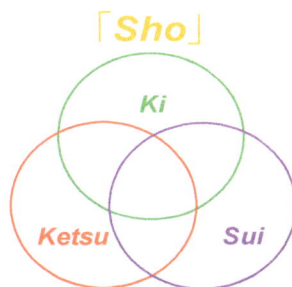

Figure 4. Diagrams of biological factors in *Sho*.

Table 3. Classifications of *Ki*, *Ketsu* and *Sui*.

Yin	Yang
Ketsu Sui	Ki

2.5.1. *Ki*, Vital Energy

Ki is the source of energy of the entire biological activities and it circulates blood and bodily fluid in the whole body [8]. Therefore, the inhibition of the workings of *Ki* would inhibit the workings of *Ketsu* (blood circulation) and *Sui* (bodily liquid) and thus a disease would occur. *Ki* belongs to *yang*. When these elements are excessively active, it is called *Jitsu* or excess and is called *Kyo* or deficiency when these are deficient. Excessive *Ki* is called *Ki-Gyaku* (*ki-Jitsu*) or hyperactive *ki*. It is called *Ki-Tai* when stagnated due to over excess, while *Ki-Kyo* when under hypersecretion.

2.5.2. *Ketsu*, Blood Circulation

Blood circulates through the body and supplies nutrition to the five parenchymatous viscera (heart, liver, spleen, lung and kidney) and the six hollow viscera [gallbladder, stomach, small intestine, large intestine, urinary bladder and triple heater (*sansho*, a passage that controls the flow of air, blood and water)]. *Ki* and *ketsu* are interdependent each other –*Ki* warms up the body in *Yang and ketsu* nourishes the body in *Yin*. There are three states of *Ketsu*, namely, *Ketsu-Netsu* (*Ketsu-Jitsu*) (blood-heat), *Oketsu* (*Ketsu-Tai*) (blood stagnation) and *Ketsu-Kyo* (blood deficiency). Symptoms of blood-heat shows hematemesis, bloody stools, nose bleeds, for example and shows bleeding from tissue, constipation and yellowish urine [8]. When heated blood (*ketsu-netsu*) goes up to the upper body, it causes not only *oketsu* (blood stagnation) but also affects emotions such as irritation. Blood deficiency is the decay of the recuperation ability of blood. It causes so-called anaemia but also shows other dysfunction such as anorexia and weakening of digestion and absorption and these are governed by *Ki*. Blood will not circulate the body if *Ki* is insufficient to operate the blood vessels. This *Ki* in each part of the body is called *Ei-ki* or *Yin*-energy. *Ki* initiates functions of each organ of the body. *Ketsu* belongs to *Yin*. The concept of *Oketsu* or blood stagnation is the most important concept. *Oketsu* is a pathological change that would cause diseases when the blood is stagnated in the entire body or in a local tissue (Figure 5).

Sansho (triple heater), one of the 12 main acupuncture channels in the body, responsible for moving energy between the upper body and the lower body.

2.5.3. Oketsu

Pathological condition of *Oketsu* (blood stagnation) is expressed in a unique way to Kampo medicine and it is the most important concept [8]. In the modern medicine, it is perhaps more commonly understood as one of the syndromes of disability of microcirculation mechanism (Figure 6). However, Kampo medicine does not simply diagnose the symptoms but it considers important to identify the pathological condition which caused the symptom and the following are considered the pathogenic *Sho* of *Oketsu* such as the changes in the blood vessels due to inflammation, accentuation of blood coagulation factors, blood congestion, polycythaemia, menstruation, pregnancy or child-delivery.

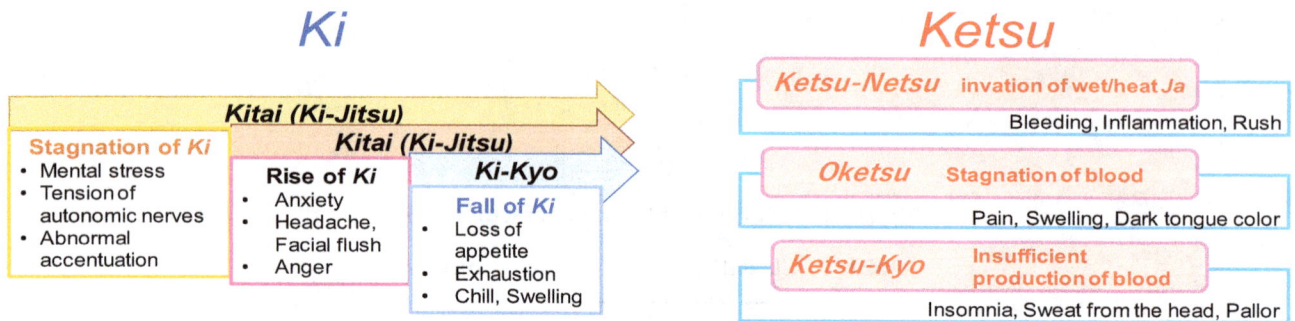

Figure 5. The concepts of *Ki* and *Ketsu*.

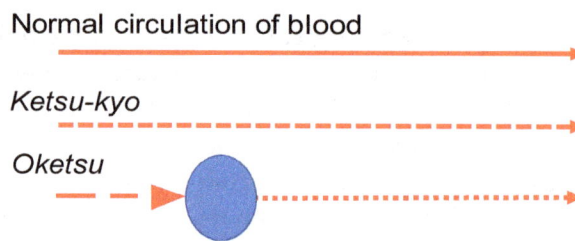

Figure 6. The Symptoms of *Oketsu*, in blood stagnation.

When the following symptoms are observed, we diagnose them *Oketsu*; the patient feels mouth dryness and would moisten the mouth with water but does not want to drink water; the patient feels stomach fullness though the abdominal distension is not observed; burning fever is felt locally or universally; purple spots appear on the skin or membrane; purple spots are appearing on the skin or membrane; dark purple spots appear on the edge of the tongue and lips are pale; stool is black; easy bleeding. The endogenous factor is in imbalance of autonomic nerve and the exogenous factor is coldness and bruise.

2.5.4. *Sui, Aua*

Sui is also called *Shin-Eki*. *Shin* is the relatively thin and pure fluids such as fluid component of blood, tissue fluids, sweat and urine, while *Eki* is relatively thick and sticky fluids among the intracellular and secretory fluids [8]. Each shows *Sho* of *Sui-Tai* (*Sui-Jitsu*) and *Sui-Kyo*. *Sui-tai* means stagnation of the body fluid (Figure 7).

Unevenly distributed *Sui* or aqua causes a local oedema. When it is linked with blood-heat, it becomes *Tan-In*-diseases and the fluid becomes sticky phlegm. As the blood-heat is understood as the inflammatory blood, it can appear when physical infection control is conducted. *Ko-Katsu* or mouth dryness is a symptom appearing when water is temporarily exhausted due to insufficient intake of water. Fever, thirst and tongue dryness are also systemically observed. It is called *Sui-Kyo* or aqua deficiency, which occurs from the temporal water exhaustion and shows dehydration. Xerostomia is a symptom of chronical insufficiency of water. Patients would feel mouth dryness and appeal lip dryness and cracks but would not want to drink water. It is mainly caused by the endogenous factors and systemically showing *Yin-Kyo* or *Yin*-deficiency and is diagnosed as *Oketsu-Sho*. It also shows the deterioration of kidney functions that is the symptom of deterioration of *Ki*.

Sui (*Shin-Eki*)

Dry Mouth
(hyperhidrosis
polyuria,
diarrhea)

Xerostomia
(internal heat-
***Yin* deficiency,**
renal failure-
***Jin-Kyo*)**

Suo-Kyo
(temporary
insufficiency)

Insufficientcy
(Chronical
insufficiency)

Stagnation
(*Sui-Tai*)

Wet
(*Sui-Tai*)

Retention
(*mucus, phlegm*)
oliguria,
constipation

Localization
(swelling,
edema)

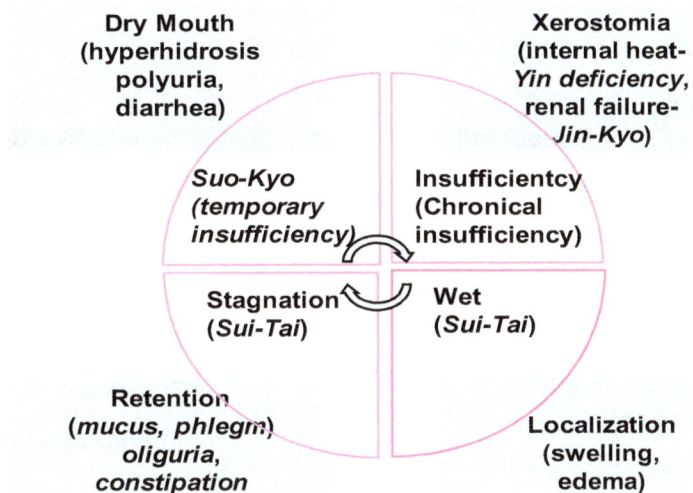

Figure 7. The concepts of *Sui* (*Shin-Eki*).

2.5.5. Views on Periodontal Disease and Toothache

In the progress of periodontitis, the gingival blood circulation induces the loss of capillary vessels and become anaemia. This status is so-called *Ketsu-Kyo* (blood deficiency) in Kampo. *Ketsu-Kyo* affects the nutritional disorder of gingiva and reduces oral immune system. Consequently, microcirculatory dysfunction induces the loss of oral biological activity, increasing the numbers of compromised hosts. This status is called *Oketsu* (blood stasis) in Kampo. *Oketsu* was observed in 70% to 80% of the randomly chosen periodontal patients above age 40 (Figure 8).

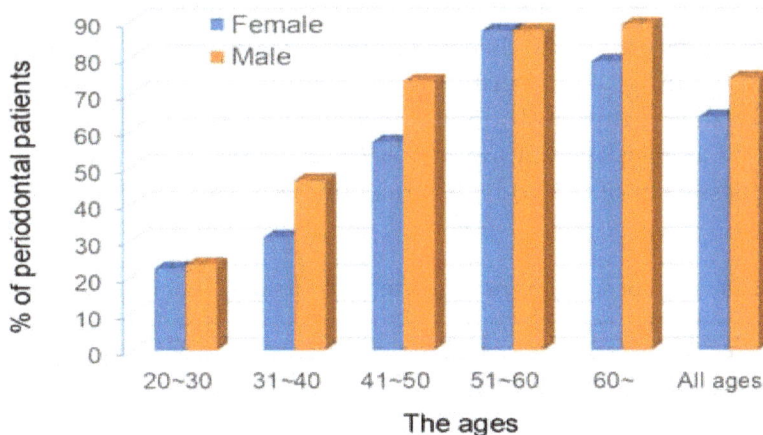

Figure 8. The proportions of poor blood circulation (*Oketu*) in the ages of the periodontal patients. Cited from [9] with permission.

Although there are Kampo medicines which contain analgesic effect but they are not comparable to the western medicines. In oriental medicine, pain is understood as the change of symptom to maintain the homeostasis of organism. The flows of *ki, ketsu, sui* (vital energy, blood circulation function and aqua) deteriorate and it causes the unwell condition from stagnation. Therefore, Kampo medicine emphasizes to recuperate the body condition to normal. The background of pain would include not only infections and injuries but also the environmental and mental stress, where psychological factor would cause anxiety and anger and can go back to the emotions in the past. Chinese proverb says that good circulation brings no pain (= stagnation), meaning that if it flows, no pain.

Occlusal trauma, occlusal destruction and traumatic occlusion are intraoral fragility and could cause systemic symptoms (Figure 9).

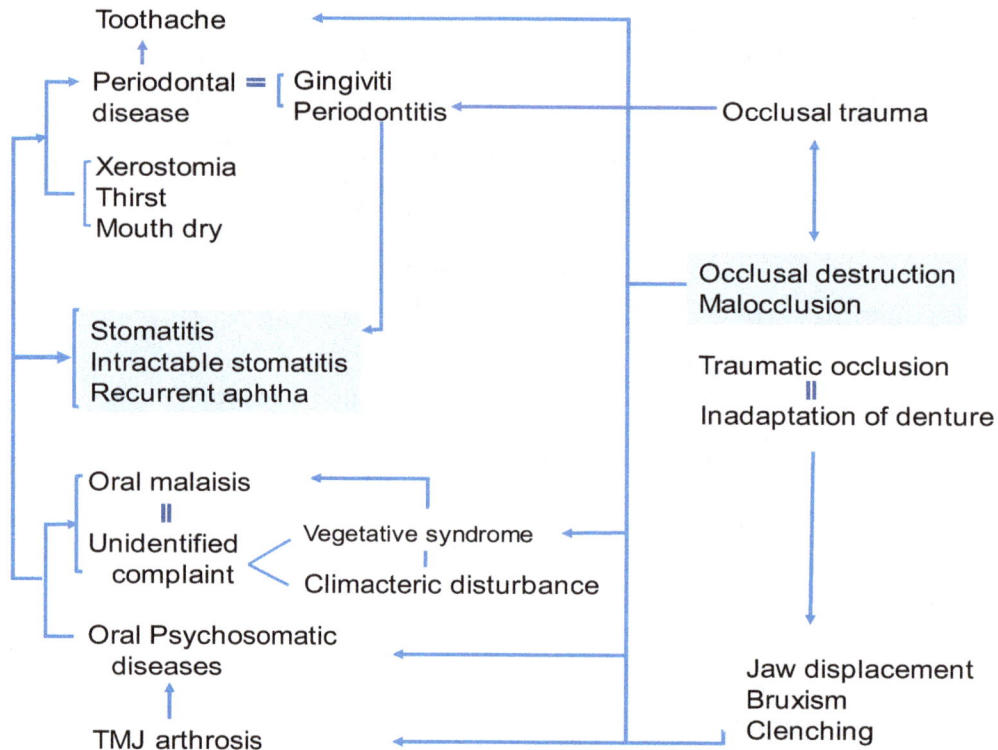

Figure 9. The correlations between occlusal-related troubles and oral diseases. (Watanabe S, unpublished data)

3. Tongue Diagnosis

Clinical tongue conditions reflect the diseases of internal organs. The important points of clinical observations are colours, coatings and volume of the tongue [8]. The tension of the tongue (shape and lustre) change to the depending on the fall and rise of *Ki-Ketsu and* the location and the depth of the pathogen in body. Coating of the tongue mostly indicates the stomach condition, especially, dampness-dryness, coldness-heat of the body. Normal and abnormal conditions are shown in Tables 4 and 5.

Table 4. The correlations between the colours and shapes in tongue.

Colour Tone	
	• **Pale tongue:** Paler colour than normal tongue; showing deficiency of *Ki* and *Ketsu.*
	• **Reddish tongue:** *Netsu-Sho* (heat) symptom; redder than normal tongue colour and often shows dryness of mouth and lips.
	• **Purplish tongue:** Systemic *Oketsu* due to stagnation of *Ki and Ketsu;* especially it is very likely when the dorsal lingual veins are over swelling.
	• If the tongue is wet, it is *Kan-Sho* (cold) symptom and the body is chilled. If dry, it shows *Netsu-Sho.*
Shape	
	• **Swelled tongue:** Tongue is swollen and shows tooth marks on peripheral; showing *Ki-Kyo* and *Sui-Tai* (deficiency of *Ki* and fluid stagnation).
	• **Thin tongue:** Tongue is dry and in deep purple colour; shows *Sui-Kyo, Yin-Yo-Kyo* (deficiency of *Sui, Kyo* of both *Yin* and *Yang.*
	• **Trembling tongue:** When moving the tongue, it trembles; it vibrates; showing *Netsu-Sho* and *Ki-Kyo (Ki* deficiency).

Table 5. The correlations between the colours and volumes in tongue.

Colour Tone	
	• *White tongue coating*: Pale white colour is considered normal but shows the changes in body condition, depending on the wetness
	• *Yellow tongue coating:* Shows stomach/intestine function deficiency; fever; lack of water due to fever
	• *Greyish black tongue coating*: Yellow tongue coating symptom progressed and disease worsened; related to infectious disease, high fever, dehydration
Volume	
	• *Thin tongue coating*: Normal
	• *No tongue coating*: Abnormal; chronical disease; protracted illness
	• *Thick tongue coating*: Abnormal; exacerbation of disease, growth of bacteria due to defective metabolism of tongue coating

Kampo promotes the metabolism involved in the physical growth, development and physiological activity. Kampo moderate *Ketsu* and *Sui*, so that the blood runs in blood vessels and prevents blood from leaking outside. Kampo produces *Ki* that works to produce *Ketsu* and *Sui*, thus converting fluids into sweat and urine.

Changes in the internal organs (liver, heart, lienogastric, lung and kidney) are reflected on the tongue (Figure 10). It tells the *Sho* of disease, namely, *Kyo, Jitsu, Hyo* and *Ri*. Tongue diagnosis is very important among the empirical diagnostic techniques. Systematic diagnosis theory has been formed based on the empirical evidences over several thousands of years. The rise and fall of *Ki, Ketsu* and *Sui* reflect the advance or retreat of illness. Severity of the disease can be seen on the tongue. Therefore, pathological changes of a disease are shown in the change of the tongue at its early stage. It is called *Mibyo* or pre-symptomatic in Kampo medicine. It is important diagnostic criteria and is recognized as a clue to find the cause of the illness at an early stage in the primary care.

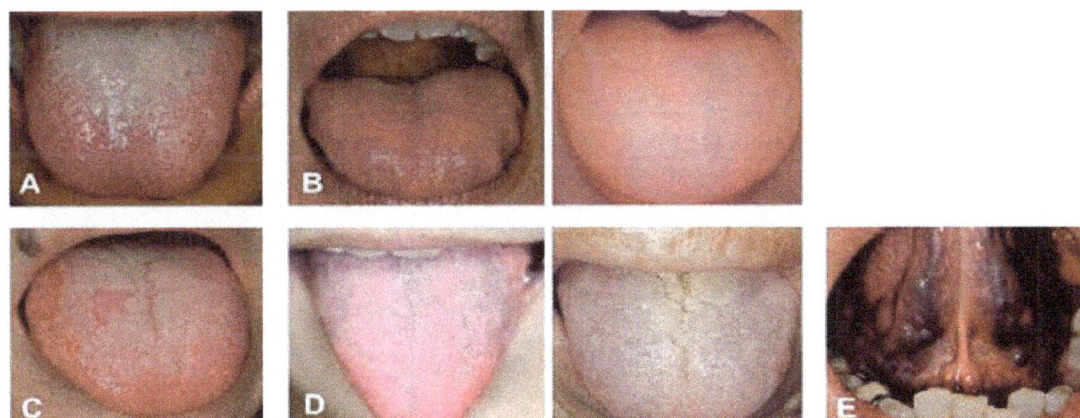

Figure 10. Tongue diagnosis of patients. (**A**) *Clinical observation of Healthy tongue*. Properly moistened: tongue coating white colour, thinly spread across the tongue. Light pink colour, Shape: fitting within the mouth. Back of tongue: sublingual vein is not over swelling. (**B**) *Abnormal tongue (Sui)*. Tongue peripheral impression, swelling tongue (oedema). Left: *Sui-Tai* or water stagnationis oedema, tongue peripheral impression. Pressure impression by the teeth on the edge of the tongue where water is sustained. Right: *Sui-Kyo* (insufficient water): oedema, water is not flowing well; big and swollen. (**C**) *Abnormal Ki (vital energy)*. Map-like tongue, insufficient Ki, slow circulation of *Ki*. Warming: Workings of warm-up and circulation; central of *Ki*. Defence: Workings to promote natural healing; protects skin and membrane and defends the body from the cause of disease. (**D**) *Abnormal tongue (Ketsu-Kyo and Kyo-Netsu)*. *Ketsu* (blood circulation) indicate the body of the tongue and sublingual vein that are in reddish purple, colour change of the tongue coating (*Ketsu-Kyo, Kyo-Netsu*). Left: *Ketsu-Kyo*: Tongue is thin and lean; Nutrition, water and blood circulation were insufficient. Right: *Kyo-Netsu*: Sticky blood; stagnated; Nutrition. water and blood body fluids were insufficient. Body is dry, since

the heat remains to circulate internally. (E) *Abnormal tongue (Okesu)*. Blood heat condition in tongue. Ischemia (tongue: cyanosis) and over-swelling of sublingual veins. Systemically impaired flow of blood. These photos were taken, after obtaining the informed consent from the patients, under the condition that the patients are not identified. (Watanabe S, unpublished data)

4. Therapeutic Effect of *Juzentaihoto*

Periodontitis is the most common chronic inflammatory disease in humans and is characterized by alveolar bone loss and connective tissue destruction. Periodontitis is exacerbated by risk factors including age, gender, smoking, systematic diseases and psychological stress [10]. The stress response mediates the interaction between unfavourable psychological conditions and inflammatory periodontal disease. There is a higher prevalence of chronic destructive periodontal disease in individuals with psychological stress, which may be associated with acute necrotizing periodontal disease [11]. Psychological stress downregulates the cellular immune response, which may link the stress to periodontal disease [12]. Herbal medicines, such as *Juzentaihoto* (JTT), have good therapeutic effects for stress-related systematic diseases and minimal side effects. JTT consists of 10 herbs: *Ginseng radix*, *Astragali radix*, *Angelicae radix*, *Rehmanniae radix*, *Atractylodis lanceae rhizoma*, *Cinnamomi cortex*, *Poria*, *Paeoniae radix*, *Ligustici rhizome* and *Glycyrrhizae radix*. JTT is traditionally used for anaemia, rheumatoid arthritis, chronic fatigue syndrome and inflammatory bowel disease. It is widely used to prevent cancer metastasis and infection in immunocompromised patients [13]. We had examined the efficacy of JTT to prevent periodontitis.

4.1. Biological Activity (in Vitro)

4.1.1. Bactericidal Effect of JTT on *P. gingivalis*

We evaluated the bactericidal effect of JTT on *P. gingivalis*. Treatment of *P. gingivalis* with 0.1 to 10 mg/mL JTT reduced the number of viable cells in a dose-dependent manner. In particular, bacterial reduction by 10 mg/mL JTT was greater than that of 0 (control), 0.1 and 1 mg/mL JTX treatment at 60 minutes [14] (Figure 11), suggesting that JTT may suppress virulence factors from periodontal bacteria and prevent the progression of periodontitis. Some herbs from JTT and their ingredients have antimicrobial effects [15]. Compounds from *Glycyrrhizae radix* inhibit the growth of *P. gingivalis* [16]. *Glycyrrhizae radix* may have an important role in the bactericidal effect of JTT on *P. gingivalis*.

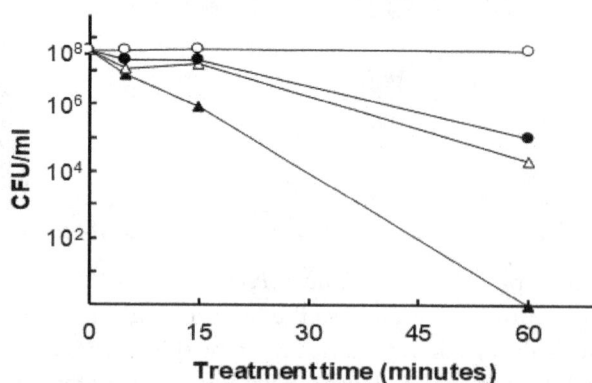

Figure 11. Antibacterial effect of JTT on *P. gingivalis*. Bacterial cells were treated with 10 mg/mL (▲), 1 mg/mL (△) or 0.1 mg/mL of JTT (●) or 0 mg/mL of JTT (○) for the indicated period. At the end of the incubation period, a 10-fold serial dilution was performed in phosphate-buffered saline (PBS; pH 7.4) and spread onto a BHI blood agar plate broth supplemented with hemin (5 µg/mL), vitamin K_1 (0.2 µg/mL) and yeast extract (5 mg/mL). The number of CFU (colony forming unit) was determined after 7 days of incubation under anaerobic conditions (CO_2: 10%, H_2: 10%, N_2: 80%) at 37°C. Cited from [14] with permission.

4.1.2. Anti-osteoclastogenesis Effect of JTT

We investigated whether JTT inhibits the osteoclast differentiation using a mouse co-culture system, according to the guideline of the intramural Committee of Ethics on Animal Experiments. Bone marrow cells (1.5×10^5 cells/well) obtained from the tibiae of 5–8-week-old BALB/c mice and pre-adipose cell line MC3T3-G2/PA6 cells (1.5×10^4 cells/well) were co-cultured for 7 days in the presence of 10 nM 1a,25-$(OH)_2D_3$ (calcitriol) and 10 nM dexamethasone in α modification of Minimum Essential Medium (α-MEM) supplemented with 20% FBS (foetal bovine serum) in 48-well plates under a 5% CO_2 atmosphere. Osteoclast was defined as tartrate-resistant acid phosphatase (TRAP)-positive multinucleated cells containing three or more nuclei. Treatment with JTT at concentrations of 10, 1 and 0.1 µg/mL significantly inhibited osteoclast formation (Figure 12A) [14]. A low concentration (0.1 µg/mL) of JTX significantly inhibited the osteoclast formation compared to control (Figure 12B). *Angelicae gigantis radix*, one of the components in JTT, significantly decreased osteoclast formation [17]. Therefore, JTT can be a therapeutic drug that prevents periodontitis.

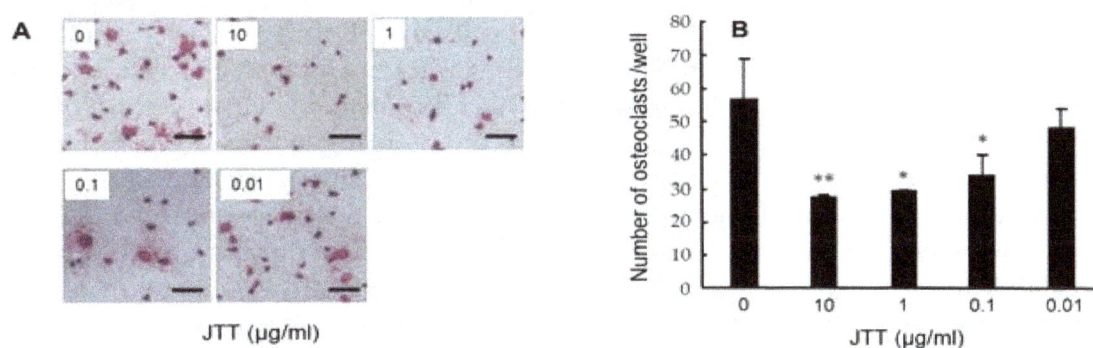

Figure 12. JTT inhibits osteoclast differentiation of BALB/c mouse bone marrow cells co-cultured with MC3T3-G2/PA6 cells. After incubation for 7 days, co-cultured cells were stained for TRAP (**A**) and determination of TRAP-positive multinucleated cells containing three or more nuclei (**B**). Results are expressed as the mean ±SD of triplicate cultures. $**p < 0.01$, $*p < 0.05$. Cited from [14] with permission.

4.2. Clinical of JTT

Kampo medicine and adjustment of denture were effective for a patient (80 years old, female, cervical cancer operated 25 years ago with good prognosis), with symptom of spinal canal stenosis, cervical vertebra stenosis, dizziness, unsteadiness and oppression on the chest. She was diagnosed as inadaptation of the denture, oral malaise (tongue), dysfunction of masticatory and xerostomia. Her *oketsu* (blood stagnation) was improved by taking JTT mornings and evenings – 2 doses before meals. Swelling and oedema of the tongue was improved by taking *Goreisan* (GRS) before going to bed. Medical consultation resulted in the improvement of mental condition. Two Kampo medicines, GRS (that improves *Sui-Tai* or fluid retention symptom caused by poor metabolism of water) and JTT [that enhances *ki* (vital energy) and *ketsu* (blood circulation function) and improve fatigue, anaemia, low appetite, night sweat, cold hands and feet which accompany the decondition] were administered in this case. In the initial diagnosis, prescription of GRS showed no progress in 2 weeks, then additionally JTT *was* administered. After 1 month later (Figure 13A), the filling pain when chewing with denture stopped jaws gliding and oppression on throat while sleeping. Two months later, she could bite off and eat food. She had no sensation of tongue torsion, stopped waking up at night due to the neck pain. Administration of GRS stopped due to frequent urination. Four months later (Figure 13B), upon the mounting of dentures, she felt neck strain and torsion of denture and tongue. The administration of GRS was restarted. Eight months later (Figure 13C), she became able to chew any food, with no sensation of tongue swells. She did not wake up at night. Twelve months later (Figure 13D), the administration of GRS was stopped but that of JTT was continued (Figure 13).

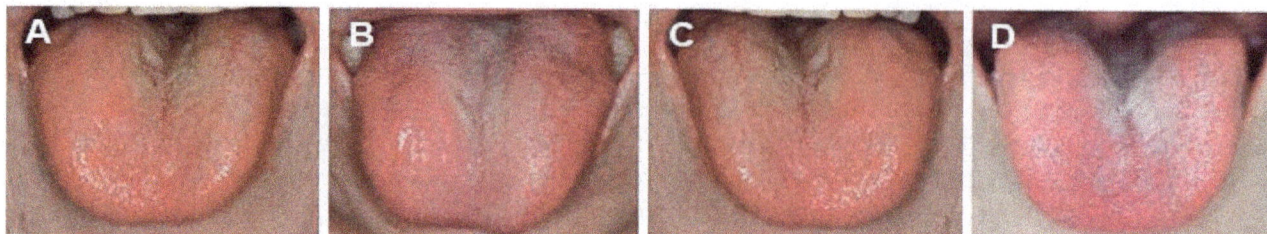

Figure 13. Changes of the tongue surfaces at 1 (**A**), 4 (**B**), 8 (**C**) or 12 (**D**) months after GRS + JTT treatment. (Presented in Kanagawa Dental College Society 53rd General Assembly: A case in which Kampo and denture adjustment was successful for patients complaining of denture). Photos were taken, after obtaining the informed consent from the patient. (Watanabe S, unpublished data)

When making dental prosthesis, it is necessary to pay attention to the intraoral environment. In the case above, we observed the lower jaw denture floated due to tongue oedema and swelling and that the denture instability caused the occlusal pain and dysfunction of masticatory. We therefore prescribed Kampo medicines that would improve these symptoms. In this clinical case, we considered that the improvement of *sui-tai* (fluid stagnation) should be the target of *Hyo-Chi*, a local and symptomatic treatment, to improve the tongue oedema, so GRS was administered. However, we could not get the expected results, so JTT was also administered in the morning and before going to bed and it presented the trend of improvements from the next day. JTT is a Kampo medicine for *hon-chi*, that is, the systemic treatment of the fundamental cause of the disease. It is often observed in the dentistry and intraoral medicine that patient's conditions change until the symptom finally surfaces due to the chronical deficiencies. Especially, the entire body is psychologically and mentally affected when malocclusion exists. Under the situation that malocclusion lasts long, it is known that glucocorticoid appears in blood chronically due to the chronical stress from the malocclusion which would induce the malfunction of negative feedback. The Oriental medicine explains that the symptoms of *Ki* and *Ketsu* occur and they worsen as the time elapses. In our case above, GRS manifested its effect at early timing by the simultaneous administration of JTT. It not only cured the oedema of the tongue but also mentally stabilized the patient.

JTT is known to improve the pathological condition of the blood circulation and mental stability. When the condition of the disease is found difficult to improve, Kampo medicine of *hon-chi* (treatment of fundamental cause), in combination would relieve the symptoms.

5. Therapeutic Effects of *Jixueteng*

5.1. Bactericidal Effect of *Jixueteng*

Jixueteng is prepared from the dried stems of *Spatholobus suberectus* (*S. suberectus*) Dunn of the family Leguminosae. *Jixueteng* has beneficial pharmacological properties such as increasing circulation, analgesia and the number of red and white blood cells [18]. *Jixueteng* contains various types of flavonoids such as flavone, isoflavones, flavanones, flavanonols and chalcone [19]. Flavonoids are natural products that show antibacterial [20] and antioxidant activities [21]. Production of reactive oxygen species (ROS) is decreased by *Jixueteng* in a dose-dependent manner [22]. Therefore, we focused on the bactericidal effect of *Jixueteng* on oral bacteria. The gram-positive species, *Streptococcus mutans* Ingbritt (*S. mutans*) and the gram-negative species, *Aggregatibacter actinomycetemcomitans* ATCC 29523 (*A. actinomycetemcomitans*), *Fusobacterium nucleatum* ATCC 25586 (*F. nucleatum*), *Porphyromonas gingivalis* ATCC 33277 (*P. gingivalis*) and *Veillonella parvula* GAI-0580 (*V. parvula*), were grown in BHI broth and suspended in PBS to an optical density of 1.0 at 600 nm. Fifty μL of bacterial suspension was exposed for 1, 15 and 60 min in the presence of 0, 0.2, 2.0 or 8% *Jixueteng* extract. The same volume of PBS was used as a control. At the end of the incubation period, a 10-fold serial dilution was inoculated onto BHI sheep blood agar plates and incubated anaerobically at 37°C for 7 days. The bactericidal effect of *Jixueteng* was determined by counting the number of bacterial cells. *Jixueteng* extract reduced the number of viable bacterial cells, such as *S. mutans* (Figure 14A), *P. gingivalis* (Figure 14B), *V. parvula* (Figure 14C) and *F. nucleatum* (Figure 14D) (Figure 14). In particular, the bactericidal effects of *Jixueteng* against *F. nucleatum* (Figure 14D) was higher than those of other oral bacteria. After treatment with 8% *Jixueteng* extract for 60 min, the number of *P. gingivalis* was decreased from 4.61×10^9 to 2.90×10^6 per millilitre (Figure 14B) [23]. Gram-negative periodontal pathogens are late colonizers of dental plaque and promote inflammatory tissue destruction in the oral cavity [24]. Thus, *Jixueteng* extract may act selectively on periodontal bacteria and break down dental plaque accumulation.

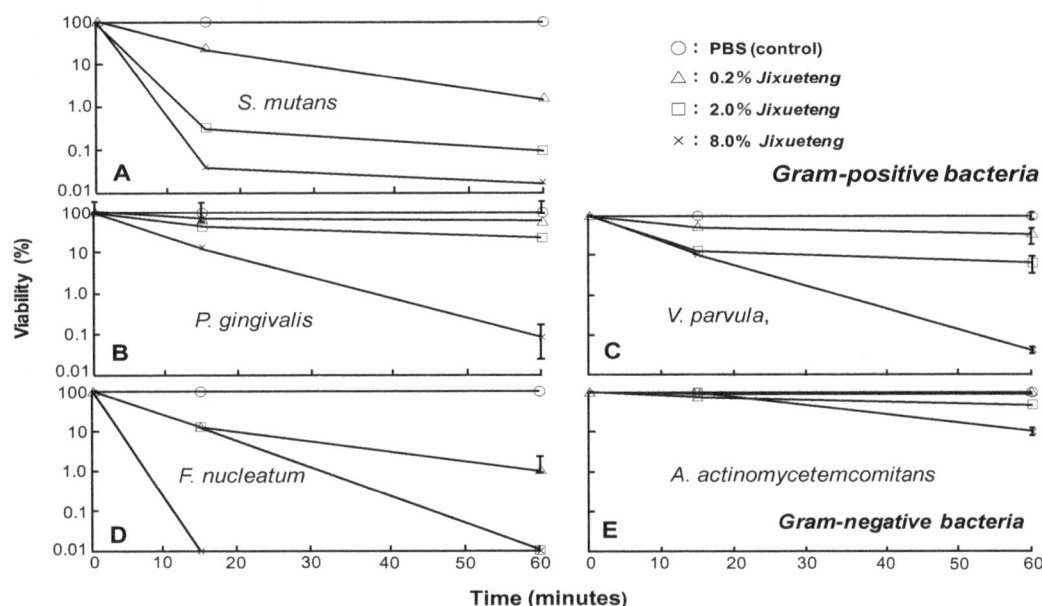

Figure 14. Bactericidal effect of *Jixueteng* against Gram-positive and -negative bacteria. Gram-positive bacteria (*S. mutans*) (**A**) and gram-negative bacteria (**B**: *P. gingivalis*, **C**: *V. parvula*, **D**: *F. nucleatum*, **E**: *A. actinomycetemcomitans*.) were treated by 0.2, 2 and 8% of the *Jixueteng* extract for 1, 15 or 60 min. The suspensions were treated by PBS as a control. Cell viability was expressed as a percentage relative to control. Cited from [23] with permission.

5.2. Inhibitory Effect of Jixueteng on Osteoblast Differentiation

In periodontitis, several cytokines, such as interleukin (IL)-1, prostaglandin (PG) E_2 and RANKL (receptor activator of NF-κB ligand), promote osteoclast differentiation. RANKL, a tumour necrosis factor (TNF)-family member, binds to its receptor RANK, which is on the surface of osteoclasts and preosteoclasts. The interaction between RANK and RANKL signalling is important for osteoclastogenesis [25]. To examine the influence of *Jixueteng* on osteoclastogenesis, we used mouse co-cultured cells in the presence of 1α,25-$(OH)_2D_3$ and dexamethasone. *Jixueteng* extracts were added to co-cultured cells at a final concentration of 0.1%, 0.01%, 0.001% and 0.0001% and cultivated for 7 days under 5% CO_2 atmosphere. After 7 days, cells were fixed and stained for TRAP. TRAP-positive multinucleated cells containing three of more nuclei were counted as osteoclasts. The treatment of *Jixueteng* extract (at concentrations of 0.1% and 0.01%) significantly inhibited osteoclast formation ($P < 0.01$). Addition of 0.1% extract completely inhibited TRAP-positive cells and multinucleated osteoclasts. In addition, the inhibitory effect of *Jixueteng* on osteoclast survival was determined by mouse co-cultured cells in the presence of RANKL and PGE_2. The number of osteoclasts was decreased with 0.001 to 0.1 mg/mL *Jixueteng* in a dose-dependent manner [26]. These results suggest that *Jixueteng* inhibits osteoclastogenesis and reduces osteoclast activity in periodontitis.

5.3. Inhibitiory Effect of Alveolar Bone Resorption by Jixueteng on Mice Experimental Periodontitis

Flavonoids are effective ingredients for the inhibition of inflammatory bone resorption [27]. We evaluated the inhibitory effect of alveolar bone resorption by *Jixueteng* using an experimental periodontitis model, under the guideline of the intramural Committee of Ethics on Animal Experiments. Fifty-four male C57BL/6N 4-week-old mice were used. Mice were given sulfamethoxazole (1 mg/mL) and trimethoprim (200 mg/mL) in their drinking water for 4 days to reduce original oral flora followed by 3 days of an antibiotic-free period before bacterial infection. The bacteria used was *P. gingivalis* A, which was inoculated in BHI broth under anaerobic conditions. Animals were randomly divided into the following three groups: Group A received only 5% carboxymethylcellulose (CMC) (sham-infected group), group B was infected orally with *P. gingivalis* and group C was administered *Jixueteng* extract in drinking water and was infected orally with *P. gingivalis*. Each mouse in group B and group C was infected orally with *P. gingivalis*, which was suspended in 5% CMC and received 0.1 ml $(1.0 \times 10^{10}$ cells/mL) of bacterial suspension. The bacterial infection was given by oral gavage (three times) at 48 h intervals. The mice were sacrificed 2, 4 and 6 weeks after the final bacterial infection to examine the change in alveolar bone resorption every 2 weeks. The left sides of the horizontal alveolar bone resorption around the maxillary molars were evaluated morphometrically as dry specimens to measure horizontal alveolar bone loss. The distance between the cemento-enamel junction (CEJ) and the alveolar bone crest (ABC) was measured at seven palatal sites per mouse. Measurements were made under a dissecting microscope (40× magnification) fitted with a digital high-definition system, standardized to provide measurements in millimetres. The right sides of the upper jaws were analysed for histology. The samples were fixed, decalcified and embedded in paraffin. The paraffin section was cut serially into 5-mm sections in a mesial–distal direction. The sections were stained for haematoxylin–eosin (H–E) and TRAP. In particular, TRAP-positive multinucleated cells were defined as osteoclasts and examined under an optical microscope (40× magnification). The number of osteoclasts was counted in the area of the periodontal tissue between the mesial root of the first molar and the distal root of the third molars. We found apparent horizontal bone loss in C57BL/6N mice challenged with *P. gingivalis* (group B) but not in the control (group A) or the *Jixueteng*-administered group (group C) (Figure 15A). Figure 15B shows the mean values ± standard error (SEM) of the CEJ to ABC derived from seven measurement sites in weeks 2, 4 and 6 after infection. Induction of alveolar bone loss was more reproducible with an infection by *P. gingivalis* by oral gavage (group B) ($p < 0.01$) than in the sham-infected control (group A) 4 weeks after infection, whereas no difference was observed 2 weeks after infection. In all experimental groups, the maximum resorption of alveolar bone was observed at the end of the experiment and the mean bone levels of the sham-infected control (group A) and *P. gingivalis* infection group (group B) were 0.194 ± 0.001 mm and 0.228 ± 0.010 mm, respectively. Alveolar bone loss was significantly lower in the *Jixueteng* group (group C) ($p < 0.01$) than that of group B in weeks 4 and 6. The mean bone level of group C in week 6 was 0.188 ± 0.003 mm, which was comparable to that of the control group A (Figure 15) [28].

By histopathological examination, osteoclasts were observed along the alveolar septum in mice periodontal tissues (Figure 16). Table 6 shows the number of osteoclasts in the alveolar bone crest. No significant difference in the number of osteoclasts was observed among the experimental groups 2 weeks after infection.

Table 6. Effects of *Jixueteng* on osteoclast formation in periodontal tissues.

Groups	Number of Osteoclasts		
	2W	4W	6W
Control	14.25 ± 1.71	16.00 ± 1.00	10.33 ± 0.58
P. gingivalis	18.50 ± 5.45	29.00 ± 8.25 **	23.33 ±1.53 **
Jixueteng + *P. gingivalis*	15.75 ± 7.41	17.00 ± 2.94	12.33 ± 3.21

** Significantly different ($p < 0.01$) from Group A and C. The number of osteoclasts was examined in the section from right maxillary specimen stained of tartrate-resistant acid phosphatase. The results were expressed as mean ± standard deviation. Group A, control (non- infected with *P. gingivalis*); group B, orally infected with *P. gingivalis*; group C, administered *Jixueteng* and orally infected *with P. gingivalis*. Cited from [28] with permission.

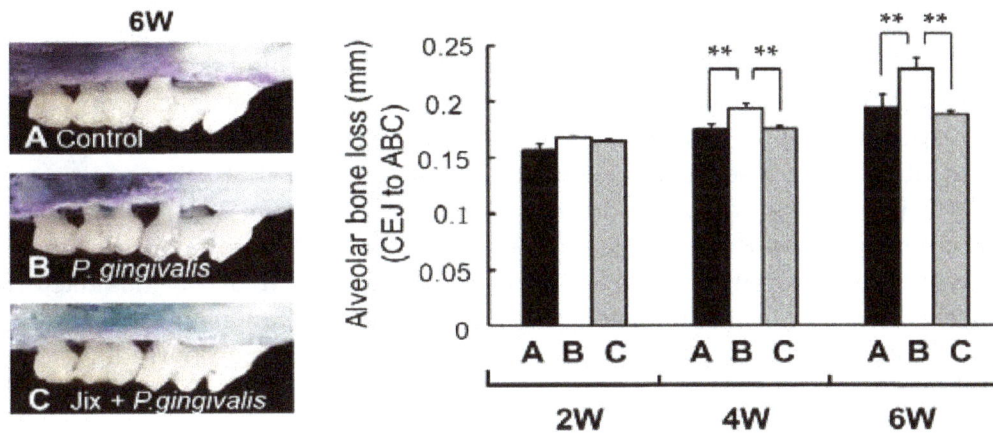

Figure 15. Morphometric bone levels of 6 week after *P. gingivalis* infection (left) and alveolar bone levels at 2, 4 and 6 weeks after *P. gingivalis* infection (right). **A**, non-infected control; **B**, infected with *P. gingivalis*; **C**, Jixueteng administered group along with *P. gingivalis* infection. Bone levels were evaluated by measuring the distance from the cemento-enamel junction (CEJ) to the alveolar bone crest (ABC) at seven palatal sites per mouse. Values indicate the mean bone loss levels ± standard error of the mean (n = 6/group). **: significantly different (*p* < 0.01). Cited from [28] with permission.

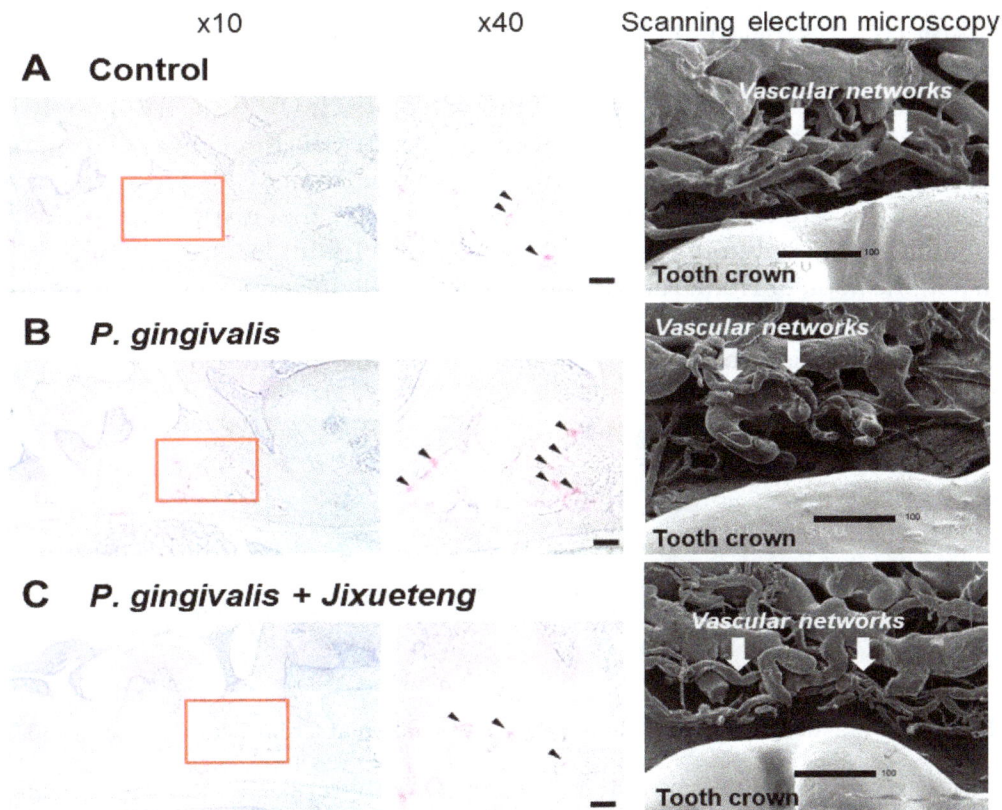

Figure 16. Histopathological examination of mice periodontal tissues. Specimens obtained from the maxillary bone of mice were evaluated with TRAP staining. Osteoclasts (arrows) were observed along the alveolar septum of the maxillary molars. **A**, con-infected control; **B**, infected with *P. gingivalis*; **C**, administered *Jixueteng* and infected with *P. gingivalis*. Original magnification: × 10 and × 40. Bars: 100 μm. Scanning electron microscopy shows that compared to the normal group (**A**), morphological degeneration of vessels in vascular networks and abnormality of the vascular lumen caused by *P. gingivalis* infection were observed (**B**). However, improvement in degeneration of these vascular networks and prolongation of the vascular plexus were observed by administration of *Jixueteng* (**C**). Cited from [28] with permission.

After 4 weeks, the number of osteoclasts in the *P. gingivalis*-infected group B was significantly higher than that of sham-infected group (group A) and the *Jixueteng*-administered group (group C) ($p < 0.01$) [28]. *P. gingivalis* has virulent factors that induce inflammatory responses and alveolar bone resorption [29]. This bacterium also invades and survives in host cells, inducing a network of inflammatory responses [30]. *P. gingivalis* also increases the likelihood of systemic diseases such as diabetes and cardiovascular disease [31]. We previously reported that *Jixueteng* improves gingival vascular networks in a *P. gingivalis*-induced periodontitis [28] (Figure 15). *Jixueteng* may inhibit the adherence and colonization of *P. gingivalis* in mice oral cavities. Therefore, our findings suggest that *Jixueteng* reduces the inflammatory destruction in periodontitis. *Jixueteng* has bactericidal effects against oral bacteria, inhibits the osteoclastogenesis and reduces the alveolar bone resorption induced by *P. gingivalis*. *Jixueteng* reduces the inflammatory tissue destruction in periodontitis and *Jixueteng* may be a useful ingredient to prevent periodontitis.

6. Therapeutic Effects of *Mastic*

6.1. History of Mastic (Kampo Name: Yo-Nyuko olibanum)

Mastic is the resin collected from the naturally growing trees in only Chios Island in southeast Aegean Sea of Greece. It was initially called frankincense. Mastic has a long history, it is written in the Old Testament (Genesis 37:25) and many ancient Greek literatures mentioned the medical effect of mastic. Christopher Columbus, before he stayed in Portugal, visited Chios Island during his voyage to the Orient as recorded in his diary in 1474–1475 and he described about mastic; it is sticky sap extracted from tree and becomes resin when solidified. There has been a habit of chewing this in Greece since more than 5000 years ago and it was known that those people who had this habit rarely had digestive diseases. In China's classical Kampo medicine masterpiece of "Zu-Kei Honzo" (masterpiece of plant diagrams) also described it as *Kun-roku-ko*, kuduruka. The substance called frankincense today is the resin from the trees of *Boswellia* genus of the *Burseraceae* family that grow in north-eastern Africa or Arabian coast and it is different from the mastic from Greece. Traditional frankincense to present is the same kuduruka in the book of Honzo and they grow in the Mediterranean coast areas. Resin from the tree that belongs to the *Anacardiaceae* family is considered *MASTICHE RESINA*. This is called "mastic" or *Yo-Nyuko* in Kampo and is known as *Pistacia lentiscus* locally (Figure 17).

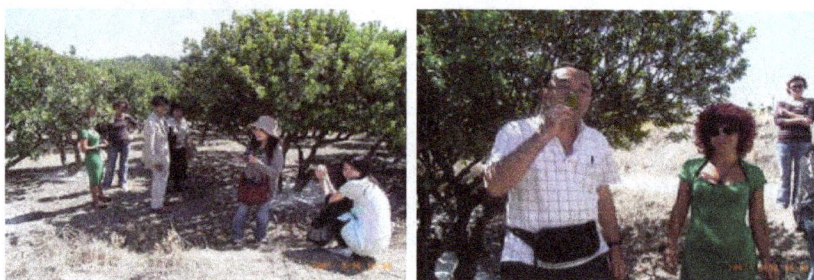

Figure 17. Mastic tree (*Pistacia lentiscus*). (photos taken at Chios island, Greece, 2007)

It is empirically proven that herbs that are used in folk therapies, including the herbal medicines constituting Kampo, have multifunctional medicinal effects. Mastic resin has a unique shape and various efficacy and has been used to promote health from old time. In addition, mastic resin has been used in chewing gums as a material for oral health and hygiene and indicated antiplaque activities. Recently in Japan, mastic has been receiving attention as material for oral cares and many companies are developing and selling mastic-formulated oral gels for toothbrushing paste.

Mastic has been forming a market of high-end products of oral cares. Also, dentists have been paying attentions to its effect and mastic is securing its position in the clinical medicine as the primary care product for oral cavity cares. To cope with the improvements of adult diseases and systemic diseases associated with the oral hygiene in the aging society of Japan and further to improve the oral health in Asia, a group of dentists launched an NPO called "Mastic Clinical Study Group." It has been running the public awareness building programs of the oral hygiene including preventive dentistry. Presently, many dentists are making use of mastic in the clinical studies and are promoting its use in the treatment of patients and to spread the awareness of the primary cares.

6.2. Component of Mastic

Essential oils, obtained by hydrodistillation of aerial parts of *Pistacia lentiscus* var *chia*, were determined for their oil composition using gas chromatography-mass spectrometry (GC/MS). Most abundant component was α-pinene (72.93% of the total oil composition), followed by β-myrcene (13.57%) > β-pinene (2.58%) > limonene (0.89%) > linalool (0.73%) > camphene (0.58%), methylanisol (0.58%) > α-pinene oxide (0.56%) > sabinene (0.30%), β-caryophyllene (0.30%) > verbenone (0.26%) > pinocarveol (0.21%) > myrtenol (0.18%) > pinocarvone (0.10%) [32].

6.3. Biological Activity of Mastic Gum (Resin)

6.3.1. Antimicrobial Activity

Compared with the group, which used the PBS mouthwash, the group that used the mastic-formulated gums showed the significant inhibition of the increase of oral bacteria (Figure 18). Compared with the group that used the gums without mastic formulation, it inhibited the increase of the pathogenic bacteria and the effect was equivalent of benzalkonium chloride.

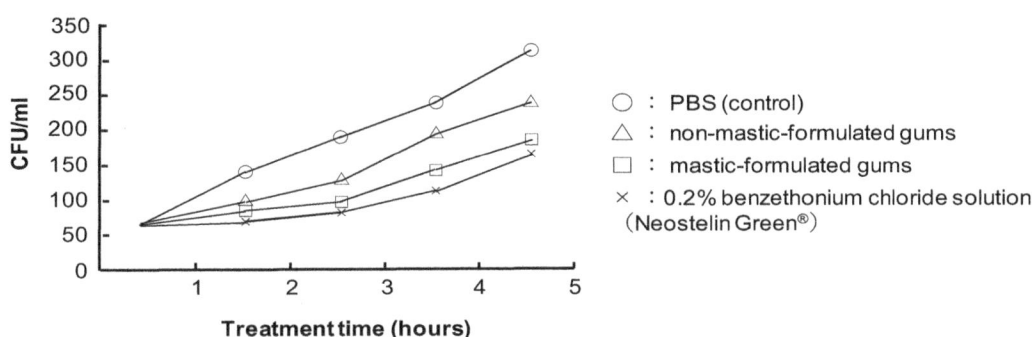

Figure 18. Bactericidal effect of mastic gum against oral bacteria. (Hamada N, unpublished data)

Stick examined the antibacterial effect against gram-negative bacteria. The result of the examination of the minimum inhibitory concentration (MIC) of mastic resin oil against the oral bacterial groups showed it had antibacterial effect (< 0.05%) for adult periodontal bacteria, *P. gingivalis*. Mastic rein oil also showed great selective effect at < 0.05% against *Fusobacterium nucleatum* (Tables 7 and 8). *F. nucleatum* is an important periodontal bacterium that derives the bacterial agglutination on the dental plaque formation. Mastic rein oil can reduce the dental plaque and promote the prevention of periodontitis.

Mastic showed selective antimicrobial activity against *Porphyromonas gingivalis* and *Prevotella melaninogenica*, as compared with that against the growth of *Actinomyces viscosus*, *Streptococcus gordonii*, *Streptococcus mutans*, *Capnocytophaga ochracea*, *Fusobacterium nucleatum*, *Prevotella intermedia*, *Staphylococcus aureus*, *Escherichia coli* and *Candida albicans* [33]. When mastic gum was fractionated with successive extractions with organic solvents with increasing water-solubility into hexane, ethyl acetate, n-butanol extracts and remaining water layer, the ethyl acetate extractable fraction showed eight or nine times higher anti-bacterial activity against *Streptococcus mutans* (IC_{50} = 104 μg/mL), as compared with other fractions (831–936 μg/mL). The most sensitive bacterium was *P. gingivalis* (IC_{50} = 32.7 μg/mL), followed by *S. mutans* (IC_{50} = 104 μg/mL), *S. aureus* (IC_{50} = 609.4 μg/mL), *F. nucleatum* (IC_{50} = 759.6 μg/mL) and *E. coli* (IC_{50} = 907.4 μg/mL) [34]. Ethyl acetate extract of mastic, which has higher antibacterial activity than unfractionated mastic, may be appropriate for the treatment of periodontal diseases.

Table 7. Minimum inhibitory concentration (MIC) of mastic resin oil. (Hamada N, unpublished data).

Oral Bacteria	MIC (%)
Streptococcus mutans	0.4
Streptococcus sanguinis	0.4
Streptococcus mitis	0.4
Lactobacillus species	0.2
Staphylococcus aureus	0.8
Bacillus species	0.2
Actinomyces species	0.2
Porphyromonas gingivalis	< 0.05
Porphyromonas endodontalis	1.6
Prevotella intermedia	1.6
Fusobacterium nucleatum	< 0.05
Aggregatibacter actinomycetemcomitans	0.2

Table 8. Plaque formation on the tooth surface and effect of inhibition of gingivitis of mastic gums. (Hamada N, unpublished data).

Group	Plaque Index		Gingivitis Index	
	Baseline	1 week	Baseline	1 week
Mastic gum (n = 10)	1.06 ± 0.29	2.69 ± 0.29 **	0	0.44 ± 0.15*
Placebo gum (n = 10)	1.19 ± 0.19	3.15 ± 0.24 **	0	0.66 ± 0.23*

These data are represented as mean ± standard deviation. No statistical difference was observed between the groups at baseline. $p < 0.05$* $p < 0.001$** comparison with the baseline using Student' test. The data are determined as the lowest concentrations of mastic resin oil.

The MIC of polymers from mastic gum of *Pistacia lentiscose* (MW: 50-130 kD), isolated by gel permeation chromatography against gram-negative bacteria (*Escherichia coli* type 1, *Salmonella typhimurium*, *Serratia marscens*. *Pseudomonas aeruginosa*, *Alcaligenes faecalis*, *Enterobacter aerogenes*, *Pseudomonas fluorescens*, *Proteus vulgaris*, *Porphyromonas*. *gingivalis*) and gram-positive bacteria (*Bacillus cereus*, *Staphylococcus aureus*, *Streptococcus faecalis*, *Staphylococcus epidermidis*, *Bacillus subtilis*, *Corynebacterium sp*) was 200–250 and 1000 µg/mL, respectively. The MIC of polymer of β-myrcene (MW 50–500 kD), synthesized by incubation with cyclohexane and *sec*-butyl lithium, against gram-negative and -positive bacteria was 100 and 1000 µg/mL, respectively [35]. Chewing mastic gum decreased the total viable bacteria, *S. mutans* and *lactobacilli* in saliva in orthodontically treated patients with fixed appliances, suggesting the usefulness of chewing mastic gum in preventing caries lesions [36].

6.3.2. Antiviral Activity

Anti-HIV activity was determined by the selectivity index (SI), based on the ratio of 50% cytotoxic concentration (CC_{50}) against mock-infected CD4-positive human T-cell line MT-4 cells to 50% protective concentration (EC_{50}) against HIV-infected MT-4 cells. All mastic extracts did not prevent HIV-induced cytopathic effects on MT-4 cells (SI <1), whereas three anti-HIV agents (azidothymidine, dideoxycytidine, curdlan sulphate) showed excellent anti-HIV activity (SI = 5624, 3868, 7142). All mastic extracts partially but significantly reduced the HSV-induced cytopathic effects on Vero cells, recovering the cell viability up to 43.2 ± 5.3% of mock-infected cells [34].

6.3.3. Anti-tumour Activity

Mastic showed very low antitumor activity against four human oral squamous cell carcinoma cell lines (Ca9-22, HSC-2, HSC-3, HSC-4) (CC_{50} = 13.5–24.4 µg/mL) as compared with three human normal oral cells (gingival fibroblast HGF, periodontal ligament fibroblast HPLF, pulp cells HPC) (CC_{50} = 28.1–84.8 µg/mL), with the tumour-specificity value (TS, determined by the ratio of CC_{50} against normal cells to CC_{50} against tumour cells) of only 1.4 to 2.4. Among 5 extracts, ethyl acetate extract showed the highest TS values (TS = 2.6), although its values were two-order lower than that of doxorubicin (TS = 244.7) [34]. However, mastic showed approximately 5-fold higher cytotoxicity against human leukemic cell lines: promyelocytic HL-60 (19 µg/mL), myeloblastic ML-1 (25 µg/mL), myeloblastic KG-1 (27 µg/mL), erythroleukemia K-562 (30 µg/mL), as compared with normal cells (HGF, HPLF, HPC) (93–155 µg/mL). Mastic induced apoptotic cell death (internucleosomal DNA fragmentation, caspase-3 activation, decline in the intracellular concentration of putrescine) in HL-60 promyelocytic leukaemia, while it inhibited the spontaneous apoptosis of oral polymorphonuclear leukocytes. Mastic showed hydroxyl radical scavenging activity, suggesting the beneficial effects of mastic on oral health [33]. Mastic gum (200 mg/kg) inhibited the growth of colorectal tumour xenografts by approximately 35%, when the optimal experimental conditions were chosen [37].

Recently, apoptosis induction by mastic in COLO205 human colonic adenocarcinoma [38], MCF-7 human breast cancer cells [39], LT97 human colon adenoma cells [40], FTC-133 (human follicular thyroid carcinoma) [41], H-SY5Y, SK-N-BE(2)C human neuroblastoma [42] and YD-10B human oral squamous carcinoma [43] has been reported, however, most of these studies have not mentioned the tumour-specificity of mastic.

6.3.4. Anti-inflammatory Activity

Essential oil of mastic showed a strong iron chelating activity (IC_{50} = 20 µg/mL) and actively scavenged hydroxyl radical (IC_{50} = 3 µg/mL) and protected *tert*-butyl hydroperoxide-treated lymphocyte [44]. Mastic inhibited the production of nitric oxide (NO) and prostaglandin (PG)E_2, as well as expression of inducible NO synthase (iNOS) and cyclooxygenase (COX)-2 protein and mRNA, induced by lipopolysaccharide (LPS)-activated mouse macrophage-like RAW264.7 cells. Mastic scavenged hydroxyl radical more potently than NO and superoxide radicals. The narrow range of effective concentration of mastic due to its cytotoxicity may limit its potential application as an anti-inflammatory agent [45].

6.3.5. Inhibition of CYPs

Five days oral treatment with *Pistacia lentiscus* oil 100 µL per mice did not show any undesirable effect on the function of kidney and liver but significantly inhibited the enzyme activity and expression of CYP1A1, CYP1A2, CYP2E1 and CYP3A4, especially in the liver tissue [46]. The result suggests the possibility that when mastic is used in combination with other pharmacological agents, the biological action of the latter may be more enhanced.

Among five masic fractions, *n*-hexane extract exhibited the highest CYP3A4-inhibitory activity (IC_{50} = 3.1 µg/mL), followed by methanol extract (macerated) (IC_{50} = 4.1 µg/mL), *n*-butanol extract (IC_{50} = 12.1 µg/mL), unfractionated sample (IC_{50} = 14.3 µg/mL), ethyl acetate extract (IC_{50}=14.8 µg/ml) (C) and, finally, methanol extract (refluxed) (IC_{50} = 24.4 µg/ml). Washing out these CYP3A4 inhibitory substance with *n*-hexane may reduce these pharmacological action or side-effects of combined drugs [34].

6.3.6. Oral Application of Mastic Gel

Salivary bacteria create healthy microbiomes when the intraoral condition becomes good. In order to maintain the good intraoral environment, we developed a gel toothpaste with mastic (*Boswellia carterii*, Kampo name: Yo-Nyuko), a mouthwash with Kampo herbs formulated (Figure 19).

Since the patient had lost the freedom of his hands thus the prevention infection control after treatment would be difficult, it was decided to try treatments using dental laser and Kampo mouth wash and mastic gel to improve the gingival tissue [47–49]. Then, we show a clinical case using the mastic gel in oral cavity. The following is the clinical report of patients treated with mastic in our dental clinic, after obtaining the informed consent from the patient, under the condition that the patient is not identified (Figure 20).

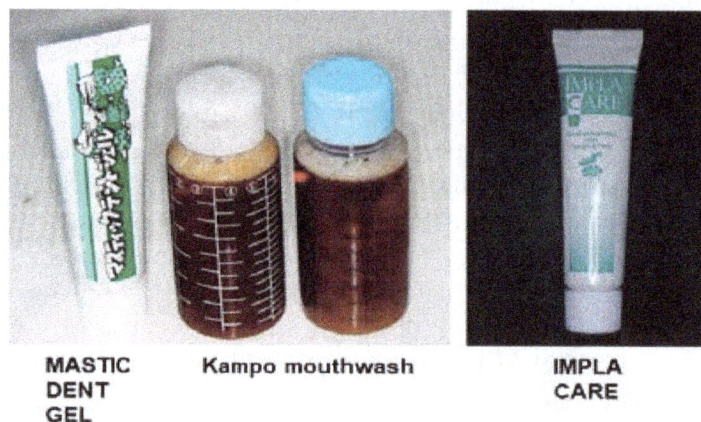

Figure 19. Toothpaste and mouth-rinse including mastic and IMPLA CARE. (unpublished data)

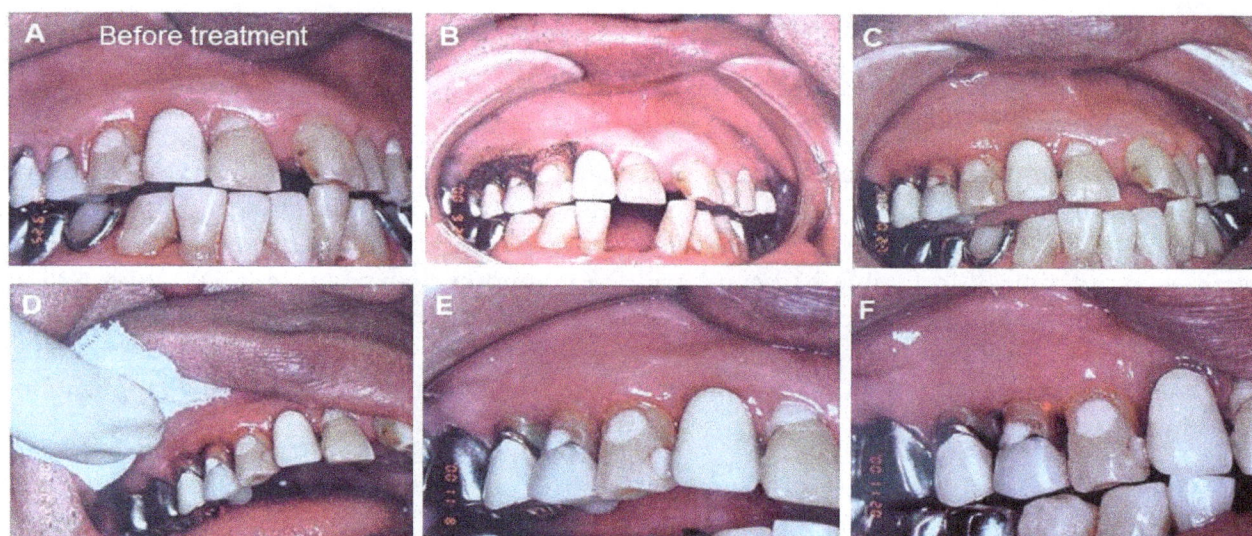

Figure 20. The clinical observation of periodontal tissue around the upper 4th and 5th teeth before and after treatment with laser and mastic gel. (**A**) Before treatment (at the first visited time); (**B**) First time after the laser treatment. Mastic gel was applied after carbonized laser treatment. (**C**) Second times after the laser treatment. After the laser treatment, chlorhexidine was used to prevent bacterial infection and mastic gel was applied at the gingiva. (**D**) Third times after the laser treatment. Mastic gel was applied after light coagulation layer was added by laser. (**E**) Fourth times after the laser treatment. Mastic gel was applied around the inflammatory gingival area. (**F**) Inflammatory gingival area between upper 4th and 5th are improved by using the mastic gel. Photos were taken, after obtaining the informed consent from the patient. (Watanabe S, unpublished data)

The patient was a 66 years old male. Showing bleeding due to the mobility of upper right 4th and 5th teeth. He visited us due to his chief complaint of mastication disorder. He had a stroke 3 years ago and is currently seeing the physician once a month. The condition is stable. As his hands tremble, the mouth cleaning was poor and the breath was bad. Poor oral hygiene, bleeding from the gums (+++), red swelling on the gums and inflammation were observed. As it was necessary to create the environment that treatment can be done, Kampo mouthwash and application of mastic gel toothpaste was conducted for three times a day before and after the treatment. Next, we showed the improvement of the chief complaint by the initial treatment. When the patient came to the clinic, his 4th and 5th teeth in upper right were showing medium level of mobility but it was judged from the observation using X-ray that the bone absorption was not bad.

We used the dentifrice that mastic was formulated and expected the effect of preventing the fixation of pathogen bacteria before and after the treatment. Considering that the oral hygiene significantly influences the management of the entire body, the biological study of the natural products is critically important from now on [50–52].

7. Development of A Dentifrice Gel Containing A Mastic Resin and *Jixueteng*

Periodontitis is the second most common dental disease worldwide after dental decay. Periodontitis is caused by microorganisms that adhere and grow on tooth surfaces and by an aggressive immune response against these microorganisms. The mouth contains a wide variety of oral bacteria, which is an ideal environment for their growth. Nutrition is supplied from food residues and saliva, nitrogen and amino acids mix in gingival crevicular fluids. Periodontitis is triggered by a complex microbial biofilm in the subgingival area that houses over 700 bacterial species and phylotypes [47]. Bacteria from the red complex group, such as *P. gingivalis*, predominate in gingivitis and periodontal disease patients by PCR analysis. Three microorganisms are mainly associated with periodontal disease, *Treponema denticola*, *Tannerella forsythia* and *P. gingivalis* and they usually form a complex called red complex bacteria (RCB). These bacteria are Gram negative, non-spore-forming anaerobic organisms and they may be found as pure or mixed infections [48]. RCB possess several virulence factors including fimbriae, proteinases, exopolysaccharides and hemin-binding proteins [49]. RCB have been detected in both subgingival plaque and in the apical root canal and cause periodontal and endodontic diseases [48,53,54]. *P. gingivalis* is a pathogen that causes periodontal disease, which is a common chronic inflammatory disease [55–57].

Jixueteng is a herbal medicine with pharmacological properties, such as increasing circulation, analgesia and the number of red and white blood cells and is composed of the dried stems of *Spatholobus suberectus* Dunn and *Millettia dielsiana* Harms, both family Leguminosae [58,59]. *Jixueteng* has potent local anti-infection effects on oral indigenous bacteria and inhibits alveolar bone loss [23,39]. These findings suggest that *Jixueteng* is a safe and effective therapeutic agent for periodontal disease because of its antibacterial and immune activities and its ability to improve circulation. However, *Jixueteng* has not been clinically used in the oral field and its effects on reactive oxygen species (ROS) in inflamed regions and the detailed mechanisms underlying these pharmacological actions remain unclear. ROS is involved in various physiological and pathological events. Overproduction of ROS causes oxidative damage to biomolecules, such as lipids, proteins and DNA, which ultimately results in many chronic diseases in humans such as atherosclerosis, cancer, diabetes, rheumatoid arthritis, post-ischemic perfusion injury, myocardial infarction, cardiovascular diseases, chronic inflammation, stroke, septic shock, aging and other degenerative diseases [60,61].

Because, *Jixueteng* extract inhibits osteoclast differentiation and survival in a dose-dependent manner, neutralizes oxygen species and improves blood flow, we developed a dentifrice containing *Jixueteng* in this study. However, *Jixueteng* alone did not have a satisfactory bactericidal effect on periodontopathic bacteria and fungi. Therefore, the antimicrobial effect was supplemented with a mastic, which effectively suppresses pathogenic bacteria. Furthermore, as a result of searching for plant-derived components that suppress periodontopathic bacteria, we found that antibacterial lotuses had comprehensive and effective antibacterial effects on pathogenic bacteria and fungi. We are commercializing a dentifrice containing these ingredients and named it "IMPLA CARE" (Figure 19).

At our hospital, dental hygienists do not invasively remove dental calculus in primary care. Patients were supplied with an IMPLA CARE at night-time and the dental calculus was removed after the gums were healthy and tight. Improving gingiva before treatment with IMPLA CARE reduced the risk of bacteraemia. IMPLA CARE was important for subsequent treatment, postoperative management and may help prevent systemic diseases such as diabetes, cerebral infarction and myocardial infarction. We investigated natural products with antimicrobial activity. First, the minimum inhibitory concentrations (MIC) of *Jixueteng*, *Sasa veitchii* and lotus on oral bacteria were measured. The natural products were dissolved in sterilized phosphate-buffered saline (PBS; pH 7.4) and two-fold serial dilutions were aliquoted in small volumes in microwell plates. Bacterial cells were grown in brain heart infusion (BHI) broth supplemented with hemin (5 μg/mL), vitamin K_1 (0.2 μg/mL) and yeast extract (5 mg/mL) under anaerobic conditions (CO_2: 10%, H_2: 10%, N_2: 80%) at 37°C for 18 h. Bacterial cells were washed and suspended in PBS to an optical density of 1.0 at 600 nm. The bacterial suspension was exposed for 40 h to two-fold serial dilutions of the natural products. The same volume of PBS was used as a control. *Jixueteng* had bactericidal effects on *S. mutans*, *L. casei*, *S. gordonii*, *F. nucleatum* and *S. aureus*. *Sasa veitchii* had a strong bactericidal effect on the fungus *C. albicans* (Table 9). Therefore, the IMPLA CARE contained a mixture of *Jixueteng*, *Sasa veitchii*, grapefruit and lotus in the mastic resin.

Table 9. Minimum inhibitory concentration (MIC) of five natural products. (Hamada N, unpublished data).

Tested bacteria	Jixueteng	Sasa Veitchii	Grapefruit	Propolis	Lotus
Streptococcus mutans	4	> 8192	512	256	8192
Streptococcus gordonii	8	4	2048	8192	> 8192
Lactobacillus casei	4	> 8192	512	256	8192
Staphylococcus aureus	32	> 8192	4096	> 8192	> 8192
Actinomyces viscosus	32	4	4096	256	8192
Porphyromonas gingivalis	> 8192	512	4096	> 8192	> 8192
Prevotella nigresecens	> 8192	128	> 8192	> 8192	> 8192
Fusobacterium nucleatum	16	8	4096	2048	> 8192
Escherichia coli	> 8192	> 8192	1024	16	8192
Candida albicans	64	8	8192	2048	> 8192

Six patients with periodontal disease, peri-implant inflammation or both were examined. Results were measured after using IMPLA CARE and 1–3 times daily tooth brushing and 1–3 months of light massage of the affected part with fingers (Tables 9 and 10). Periodontal disease improved in all patients (Table 11, Figure 21).

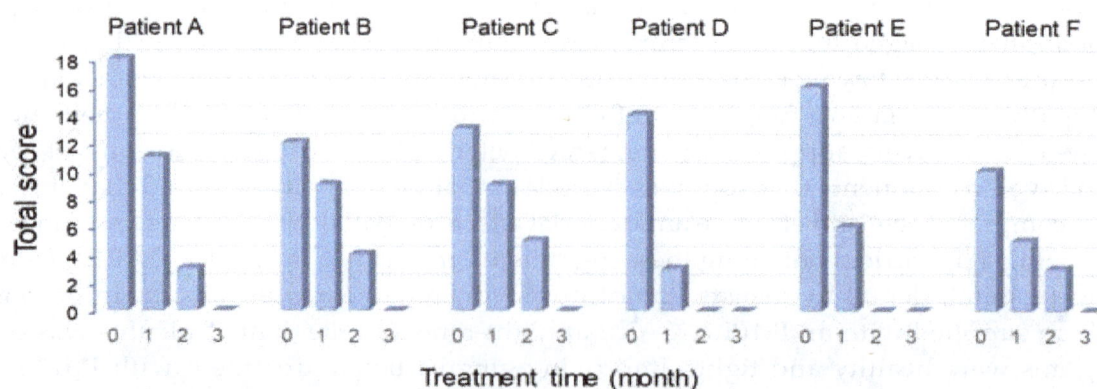

Figure 21. Effects of the IMPLA CARE. (Watanabe S, unpublished data)

Table 10. Scores showing the progress of periodontal disease.

	Examination Criteria						
Score	Swollen Pus	Redness	Bleeding	Pus Discharge	Gingival Colour	Mobility	Patient's Opinion
5	Papilla and adhering to gingiva	Extending to the papilla and gingival gums	Naturally bleeding	Naturally draining	Dark red purple	Upper and lower lip and tongue immobile	No change
3	Papilla and extending to the gingival margin	Papilla and tooth inflammation	Bleeding by acupressure	Acupressure-induced draining	Dark red	Strongly immobile	Improved a little
1	Part of the papilla	Part of the papilla	Slight bleeding with acupressure	Slight draining with acupressure	Brilliant	Slightly immobile	Tightened
0	None at all	No redness	None at all	No discharge at all	Light pink	Within a physiological range	Improved a lot

Table 11. Improvement of periodontal disease after administration of the IMPLA CARE. (Watanabe S, unpublished data).

Examination Items	Patient A				Patient B				Patient C				Patient D				Patient E				Patient F			
Scores at 0, 1, 2 or 3 Months Later	0	1	2	3	0	1	2	3	0	1	2	3	0	1	2	3	0	1	2	3	0	1	2	3
Swollen pus	1	0	0	0	1	0	0	0	3	2	1	0	3	0	0	0	5	3	0	0	1	1	0	0
Redness	5	3	1	0	3	2	1	0	3	2	1	0	3	0	0	0	3	1	0	0	3	1	1	0
Bleeding	5	3	1	0	3	2	1	0	2	1	1	0	2	0	0	0	3	0	0	0	1	0	0	0
Pus discharge	1	0	0	0	1	0	0	0	3	2	1	0	3	0	0	0	1	0	0	0	1	0	0	0
Gingival colour	3	1	0	0	3	2	1	0	2	1	1	0	2	3	0	0	3	1	0	0	3	1	1	0
Mobility	3	1	0	0	1	0	0	0	0	0	0	0	0	0	0	0	1	0	0	0	1	1	1	0
Patient's opinion		3	1	0		3	1	0		1	0	0		0	0	0		1	1	0		1	0	0
Total score	18	11	3	0	12	9	4	0	13	9	5	0	14	3	0	0	16	6	0	0	10	5	3	0

We evaluated patients who were not examined by dentists and found a self-reported improvement (Figure 22). Patient satisfaction also increased, which suggests that IMPLA CARE can be used as a primary care tool after treatment.

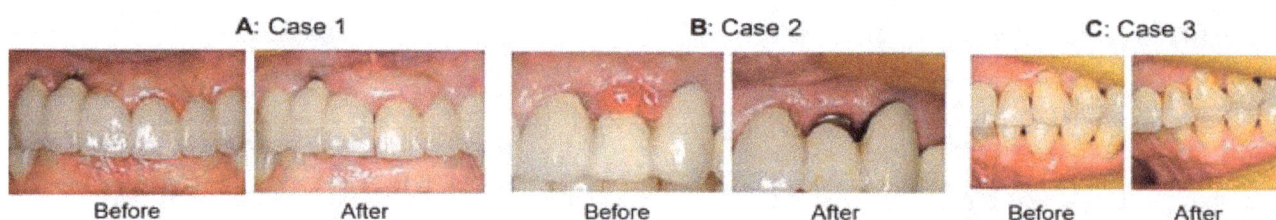

Figure 22. Case 1: A patient who was developing diabetes and hypertension (**A**), Case 2: A patient with peri-implantitis (**B**), Case3: A patient with an ulcer from sleep deprivation and work stress (**C**). (Suzuki M, unpublished data)

Case 1: A patient who was developing diabetes and hypertension. The patient had an implant in the anterior teeth of the maxilla and had teeth cleaned regularly at a dental clinic but gingivitis persisted. The doctor instructed the patient to use the IMPLA CARE before going to bed every night. Gingivitis improved gradually (Figure 22A).

Case 2: A patient with peri-implantitis. After insertion of an implant at 65 years old, a secondary operation was performed but peri-implantitis developed after the second operation. The doctor instructed the patient to use the IMPLA CARE himself before going to bed every night. Conditions gradually improved and a superstructure was formed after one month (Figure 22B).

Case3: A patient with an ulcer from sleep deprivation and work stress. A patient developed an ulcer from work stress and sleep deprivation. An IMPLA CARE was used daily in the morning and evening and improvements were observed with a week, which suggests that the IMPLA CARE containing traditional Chinese medicines did not cause gingival recession (Figure 22C).

8. Conclusions and Future Studies

Kampo is a historic traditional medicine that has been adjusted to Japanese culture. The concept of Kampo emphasizes the relationship between the human body and its social and natural environments [2]. Our experiments concluded that Kampo (JTX and *Jixueteng*) reduce a great effect on oral bacteria and inhibited the bacteria-induced alveolar bone loss. Kampo also suppressed the osteoclast differentiation. Furthermore, Kampo improved the inflammatory response in the periodontal tissues of patients. These findings suggest that Kampo is an effective agent for the prevention of dental caries and periodontitis. The administration of Kampo may ameliorate to infected oral tissue environment.

Oral health is related to life-style such as diet in many ways. The development of dental caries requires high sugar intakes [62]. On the other hand, the high consumptions of smoking and alcohol and the loss of vitamin D affects metabolic functions of periodontal tissue and induce periodontitis. Previous review has been reported that psychological stress reduces human immune system and promotes chronic inflammation in periodontal tissue [63]. Our result demonstrated that JTX affected the correlation between restraint stress and bacteria-induced periodontal destruction [6,14]. Recently, psychological stress is a risk factor of toothache, especially non-odontogenic pain [64]. Odontogenic pain is generally derived from pulpal or periodontal tissue. However, non-odontogenic pain is not often originated from the orofacial regions. The characteristics of non-odontogenic pain indicate various types of symptoms; very mild, intermittent and severe, sharp pain and continuous. The general dentists are difficult to be specified the pain regions, that confuse the exact pain control in any case. In the clinical suggestion of effective pain control, the use of Kampo is expected to reduce the non-odontogenic pain [65]. In the future, the mixed concept of Western medicine and Kampo medicine will contribute in the treatment and prevention of several oral diseases.

Supplementation of alkaline extract of *Sasa sp.* leaves (SE), which can alleviate the deoxorubicin-induced keratinocyte cytotoxicity [66] and paclitaxel-induced neurotoxicity [67] by promoting hermetic cell growth. and have anti-HIV activity [68], may enhance the potential of mastic gel tooth paste (Figure 23).

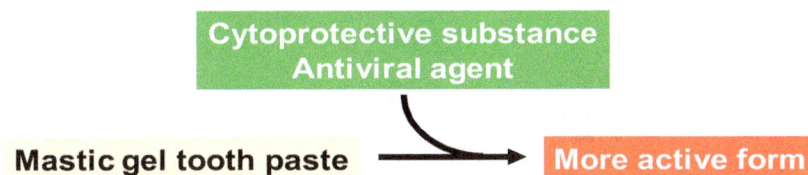

Cytoprotective substance
Antiviral agent

Mastic gel tooth paste ⟶ **More active form**

Figure 23. Manufacturing of advanced mastic gel tooth paste.

Author Contributions: S.W., N.H. and H.S. writing the paper; T.T., T.S., M.S. and A.M. collecting the data.

Acknowledgments: The authors acknowledge Tsumura Co. Ltd for the supply of Kampo and Katsushi Tamaki and Atsushi Shimada of the Division of Prosthodontic dentistry function of TMJ and Occlusion, Kanagawa Dental University and Atsushi Ishige and Jing Yu of Herbal medicine biology laboratory, Chinese herbal medicine department, Yokohama College of Pharmacy for the support for the research.

Abbreviations

ABC	alveolar bone crest
CC_{50}	50% cytotoxic concentrations
CEJ	cemento-enamel junction
CFU	colony forming unit
CMC	carboxymethylcellulose
COX	cyclooxygenase
CYP	cytochrome P450
EC_{50}	50% effective concentration
FBS	foetal bovine serum
GC/M	gas chromatography-mass spectrometry
GRS	goreisan
HGF	human gingival fibroblast
HIV	human immunodeficiency virus
HPC	human pulp cell
HPLF	human periodontal ligament fibroblast
HSV	herpes simplex virus
IC_{50}	50% inhibitory concentration
kD	kilo dalton
LPS	lipopolysaccharide
MIC	minimum inhibitory concentration
NO	nitric oxide
PGE_2	prostaglandin E_2
RANKL	receptor activator of NF-κB ligand
RCB	red complex bacteria
SI	selectivity index, determined by the ratio of CC_{50}/EC_{50}
TNF	tumour necrosis factor
TRAP	tartrate-resistant acid phosphatase
TS	tumour specificity, determined by ratio of CC_{50} for normal cells to CC_{50} for tumour cells

Appendix A

Table A1. Kampo terminology.

Byo-ja	Pathogen, disease inducing factor
Ei-ki	Ying energy, *Ki* which operates the blood flows in the blood vessels. Without *ki*, blood does not circulate
Honchi	Systemic meridian treatment for systemic route cause of the disease
Hyo	Superficies, Surface of the body
Hyochi	Local and symptomatic treatment for symptoms derived by the rout cause
Hyo-sho	Pathological condition which appears on the surface of the boy
In	*Yin*, the state opposite of *Yang*, including *ri, kan, kyo, shuren* (convergence) and *yukei* (tangible)
In-Yo	*Yin-Yang*, Bipolar nature of all phenomena or viewing the phenomena from bipolar aspect
Ja	Stress/pathogenic factor, disease-inducing factor that is harmful to the body; endogenous factor, exogenous factor, neither endogenous or exogenous factor
Jitsu	Excess of required substance of body being a disease inducing factor or its pathological condition
Jitsu-kan	Sthenic chill; *Kan-ja* inhibits *yang-ki* (heat energy) in body and deteriorates body functions
Jitsu-netsu	Sthenic heat/excess heat, affected by the exogenous cause of heat; or heat from dental stress and intemperance
Jitsu-sho	Robust/excess constitution, condition or characteristics of over-reaction caused by *byo-ja*
Kan	Chill, symptom showing coldness
Kan-netsu	Chills and fever, pathological condition of chill and heat
Kan-sho	*Kan-sho*, pathological condition showing chilly feeling
Kekkyo	*Ketsu-kyo*, pathological condition of *ketsu* insufficiency
Ketsu-netsu	Blood-heat, *ketsu* (blood) affected by heat-ja and shows *kyo-netsu*
Ki	Vital energy that operates body functions
Ki-gyaku	Pathological condition of *ki* regression
Ki-kyo	*Ki* deficiency, state of insufficient or deficient *ki*
Ki-kyo	*Ki* deficiency, state of insufficient or deficient *ki*
Ki-tai	*Ki* stagnation, pathological condition of *ki* stagnation
Ko-kan	Xerostomia, feeling mouth dryness but not wanting to drink water; tends to occur with mental strain
Ko-katsu	Mouth dryness, feeling thirst and wanting to drink water
Kyo	Deficiency/asthenia, insufficiency of functions or physiological substance that physical body requires
Kyo-kan	Asthenia-cold, *kyo-sho* symptom and belongs to Kan; insufficient *yang-ki* (heat) to warm up the body
Kyo-netsu	Asthenic heat-syndrome, where *yin-eki* is insufficient and relatively *yang* becomes overactive feeling feverish
Kyo-sho	asthenia constitution; Pathological condition of insufficiency of fundamental substances that operate body functions
Nai-netsu	Internal heat-syndrome, generated as a relative result of the imbalance of *yin-yang*; *jitsu-netsu, kyo-netsu*
Okets	Blood stagnation, symptom caused by the stagnation of the blood flow
Ri	Interior of the entire body
Sansho	a passage that controls the flow of air, blood and water, called "triple heater "

Table A1. *Cont.*

Shin-eki	Bodily transparent fluid which constitutes the human body
Shitsu	Dampness of morbidly sustained fluid in the body as a disease inducing factor
Sho	Kampo diagnosis, set of holistic pattern of a patient's pathological symptoms that cause disease
Shoko	Kampo medical conditions, symptoms in Western medical terms
Tan	phlegm, sticky fluid locally pooled due to poor water metabolism
Tan-in	Diseases due to pathological accumulation of fluids in the body
Tongue coating	Mossy substance covering the surface of the tongue
yang	Chinese term for Yo
Yin	Chinese term for In
Yin-eki	Fluid consisting of human body and composed of transparent shin-eki and red blood
Yang	Yin-deficiency Symptom of heat due to insufficient Yin-eki
Yo	Yang, the state opposite of Yin, including hyo, netsu, jitsu, hassan (divergence) and mukei (intangible)
Yo-kyo	Yang-deficiency, pathological condition that chill of ki-kyo is worsened
Yo-sho	Yang-sho, condition that has characteristics of excitement, activity and warm-heat
Shokan-ron	A treatise on Shang han, a form of an acute infectious disease

References

1. Motoo, Y.; Arai, I.; Tsutani, K. Use of Kampo diagnosis in randomized controlled trials of Kampo products in Japan: A systematic review. *PLoS ONE* **2014**, *9*, e104422. [CrossRef] [PubMed]
2. Yu, F.; Takahashi, T.; Moriya, J.; Kawaura, K.; Yamakawa, J.; Kusaka, K.; Itoh, T.; Morimoto, S.; Yamaguchi, N.; Kanda, T. Traditional Chinese medicine and Kampo: A review from the distant past for the future. *J. Int. Med. Res.* **2006**, *34*, 231–239. [CrossRef] [PubMed]
3. Yakubo, S.; Ito, M.; Ueda, Y.; Okamoto, H.; Kimura, Y.; Amano, Y.; Togo, T.; Adachi, H.; Mitsuma, T.; Watanabe, K. Pattern classification in kampo medicine. *Evid. Based Complement. Alternat. Med.* **2014**, *2014*, 535146. [CrossRef] [PubMed]
4. Katayama, K.; Yoshino, T.; Munakata, K.; Yamaguchi, R.; Imoto, S.; Miyano, S.; Watanabe, K. Prescription of kampo drugs in the Japanese health care insurance program. *Evid. Based Complement. Alternat. Med.* **2013**, *2013*, 576973. [CrossRef] [PubMed]
5. Wang, P.L.; Sunagawa, M.; Yamaguchi, K.; Kameyama, A.; Kaneko, A. EBM of Kampo medicine in oral surgery. *Oral Ther. Pharmacol.* **2015**, *34*, 23–30. (In Japanese)
6. Wang, PL.; Kaneko, A. Introduction to Kampo medicine for dental treatment—Oral pharmacotherapy that utilizes the advantages of Western and Kampo medicines. *Jpn. Dent. Sci. Rev.* **2018**, *54*, 197–204. [CrossRef] [PubMed]
7. Dong, J. The Relationship between Traditional Chinese Medicine and Modern Medicine. *Evid. Based Complement. Alternat. Med.* **2013**, *2013*, 153148. [CrossRef] [PubMed]
8. Terasawa, K. Evidence-based Reconstruction of Kampo Medicine: Part II-The Concept of Sho. *Evid. Based Complement. Alternat. Med.* **2004**, *1*, 119–123. [CrossRef] [PubMed]
9. Miyata, T. Prescription of Chinese medicine in clinical dentistry. Introduction of tongue diagnostics for dental physician and dental hygienist. In *The Nippon Dental Review*; Hyoron Publishers, Inc.: Tokyo, Japan, 2001; pp. 145–151. (In Japanese)
10. Al Jehani, Y.A. Risk factors of periodontal disease: Review of the literature. *Int. J. Dent.* **2014**, *2014*, 182513.
11. Warren, K.R.; Postolache, T.T.; Groer, M.E.; Pinjari, O.; Kelly, DL.; Reynolds, M.A. Role of chronic stress and depression in periodontal diseases. *Periodontology 2000* **2014**, *64*, 127–138. [CrossRef] [PubMed]

12. Stoeken, J.E.; Paraskevas, S.; van der Weijden, G.A. The long-term effect of a mouthrinse containing essential oils on dental plaque and gingivitis: A systematic review. *J. Periodontol.* **2007**, *78*, 1218–1228. [CrossRef] [PubMed]

13. Watanabe, S.; Imanishi, J.; Satoh, M.; Ozasa, K. Unique place of Kampo (Japanese traditional medicine) in complementary and alternative medicine: A survey of doctors belonging to the regional medical association in Japan. *Tohoku J. Exp. Med.* **2001**, *194*, 55–63. [CrossRef] [PubMed]

14. Takeda, O.; Toyama, T.; Watanabe, K.; Sato, T.; Sasaguri, K.; Akimoto, S.; Sato, S.; Kawata, T.; Hamada, N. Ameliorating effects of *Juzentaihoto* on restraint stress and *P. gingivalis*-induced alveolar bone loss. *Arch. Oral Biol.* **2014**, *59*, 1130–1138. [CrossRef] [PubMed]

15. Tan, B.K.; Vanitha, J. Immunomodulatory and antimicrobial effects of some traditional Chinese medicinal herbs: A review. *Curr. Med. Chem.* **2004**, *11*, 1423–1430. [CrossRef] [PubMed]

16. Gafner, S.; Bergeron, C.; Villinski, J.R.; Godejohann, M.; Kessler, P.; Cardellina, J.H.; Ferreira, D.; Feghali, K.; Grenier, D. Isoflavonoids and coumarins from Glycyrrhiza uralensis: Antibacterial activity against oral pathogens and conversion of isoflavans into isoflavan-quinones during purification. *J. Nat. Prod.* **2011**, *74*, 2514–2519. [CrossRef] [PubMed]

17. Kil, J.S.; Kim, M.G.; Choi, H.M.; Lim, J.P.; Boo, Y.; Kim, E.H.; Kim, J.B.; Kim, H.K.; Leem, K.H. Inhibitory effects of Angelicae Gigantis Radix on osteoclast formation. *Phytother. Res.* **2008**, *22*, 472–476. [CrossRef] [PubMed]

18. Huang, K.C. *The Pharmacology of Chinese Herbs*; CRC Press: Boca Raton, FL, USA, 1993; p. 146.

19. Yoon, J.S.; Sung, S.H.; Park, J.H.; Kim, Y.C. Flavonoids from *Spatholobus suberectus. Arch. Pharm. Res.* **2004**, *27*, 589–592. [CrossRef] [PubMed]

20. Farhadi, F.; Khameneh, B.; Iranshahi, M.; Iranshahy, M. Antibacterial activity of flavonoids and their structure-activity relationship: An update review. *Phytother. Res.* **2019**, *33*, 13–40. [CrossRef] [PubMed]

21. Saxena, M.; Saxena, J.; Pradhan, A. Flavonoids and phenolic acids as antioxidants in plants and human health. *Int. J. Pharm. Sci. Rev. Res.* **2012**, *16*, 130–134.

22. Toyama, T.; Wada-Takahashi, S.; Takamichi, M.; Watanabe, K.; Yoshida, A.; Yoshino, F.; Miyamoto, C.; Maehata, Y.; Sugiyama, S.; Takahashi, S.S.; et al. Reactive oxygen species scavenging activity of *Jixueteng* evaluated by electron spin resonance (ESR) and photon emission. *Nat. Prod. Commun.* **2014**, *9*, 1755–1759. [PubMed]

23. Toyama, T.; Sawada, T.; Takahashi, Y.; Todoki, K.; Lee, M.C.; Hamada, N. Bactericidal activities of the *Jixueteng* against cariogenic and periodontal pathigens. *Oral Therap. Pharmacol.* **2011**, *30*, 51–56. (In Japanese)

24. Ximénez-Fyvie, L.A.; Haffajee, A.D.; Socransky, S.S. Comparison of the microbiota of supra- and subgingival plaque in health and periodontitis. *J. Clin. Periodontol.* **2000**, *27*, 648–657. [CrossRef] [PubMed]

25. Takayanagi, H.; Kim, S.; Taniguchi, T. Signaling crosstalk between RANKL and interferons in osteoclast differentiation. *Arthritis Res.* **2002**, *4* (Suppl. 3), S227–S232. [CrossRef] [PubMed]

26. Toyama, T.; Todoki, K.; Takahashi, Y.; Watanabe, K.; Takahashi, S.S.; Sugiyama, S.; Lee, M.C.; Hamada, N. Inhibitory effects of *Jixueteng* on *P. gingivalis*-induced bone loss and osteoclast differentiation. *Arch. Oral Biol.* **2012**, *57*, 1529–1536. [CrossRef] [PubMed]

27. Weaver, C.M.; Alekel, D.L.; Ward, W.E.; Ronis, M.J. Flavonoid intake and bone health. *J. Nutr. Gerontol. Geriatr.* **2012**, *31*, 239–253. [CrossRef] [PubMed]

28. Suzuki, M.; Toyama, T.; Watanabe, K.; Sasaki, H.; Sugiyama, S.; Yoshino, F.; Yoshida, A.; Takahashi, S.S.; Wada-Takahashi, S.; Matsuo, M.; et al. Ameliorating effects of *Jixueteng* in a mouse model of *Porphyromonas gingivalis*-induced periodontitis: Analysis based on gingival microcirculatory system. *Nat. Prod. Commun.* **2018**, in press.

29. Bostanci, N.; Belibasakis, G.N. *Porphyromonas gingivalis*: An invasive and evasive opportunistic oral pathogen. *FEMS Microbiol. Lett.* **2012**, *333*, 1–9. [CrossRef] [PubMed]

30. Hajishengallis, G. *Porphyromonas gingivalis*-host interactions: Open war or intelligent guerilla tactics? *Microb. Infect.* **2009**, *11*, 637–645. [CrossRef] [PubMed]

31. Kim, J.; Amar, S. Periodontal disease and systemic conditions: A bidirectional relationship. *Odontology* **2006**, *94*, 10–21. [CrossRef] [PubMed]

32. Buriani, A.; Fortinguerra, S.; Sorrenti, V.; Dall'Acqua, S.; Innocenti, G.; Montopoli, M.; Gabbia, D.; Carrara, M. Human adenocarcinoma cell line sensitivity to essential oil phytocomplexes from pistacia species: A multivariate approach. *Molecules* **2017**, *22*, 1336. [CrossRef]

33. Sakagami, H.; Kishino, K.; Kobayashi, M.; Hashimoto, K.; Iida, S.; Shimetani, A.; Nakamura, Y.; Takahashi, K.; Ikarashi, T.; Fukamachi, H.; et al. Selective antibacterial and apoptosis-modulating activities of mastic. *In Vivo* **2009**, *23*, 215–223.

34. Suzuki, R.; Sakagami, H.; Amano, S.; Fukuchi, K.; Sunaga, K.; Kanamoto, T.; Terakubo, S.; Nakashima, H.; Shirataki, Y.; Tomomura, M.; et al. Evaluation of Biological Activity of Mastic Extracts Based on Chemotherapeutic Indices. *In Vivo* **2017**, *31*, 591–598. [PubMed]

35. Sharifi, M.S.; Ebrahimi, D.; Hibbert, D.B.; Hook, J.; Hazell, S.L. Bio-activity of natural polymers from the genus Pistacia: A validated model for their antimicrobial action. *Glob. J. Health Sci.* **2011**, *4*, 149–161. [CrossRef] [PubMed]

36. Aksoy, A.; Duran, N.; Toroglu, S.; Koksal, F. Short-term effect of mastic gum on salivary concentrations of cariogenic bacteria in orthodontic patients. *Angle Orthod.* **2007**, *77*, 124–128. [CrossRef] [PubMed]

37. Dimas, K.; Hatziantoniou, S.; Wyche, J.H.; Pantazis, P. A mastic gum extract induces suppression of growth of human colorectal tumor xenografts in immunodeficient mice. *In Vivo* **2009**, *23*, 63–68. [PubMed]

38. Rahman, H.S. Phytochemical analysis and antioxidant and anticancer activities of mastic gum resin from Pistacia atlantica subspecies kurdica. *Onco Targets Ther.* **2018**, *11*, 4559–4572. [CrossRef] [PubMed]

39. Seifaddinipour, M.; Farghadani, R.; Namvar, F.; Mohamad, J.; Abdul Kadir, H. Cytotoxic effects and anti-angiogenesis potential of pistachio (*Pistacia vera* L.) hulls against MCF-7 human breast cancer cells. *Molecules* **2018**, *23*, 110. [CrossRef] [PubMed]

40. Glei, M.; Ludwig, D.; Lamberty, J.; Fischer, S.; Lorkowski, S.; Schlörmann, W. Chemopreventive potential of raw and roasted pistachios regarding colon carcinogenesis. *Nutrients* **2017**, *9*, 1368. [CrossRef]

41. Catalani, S.; Palma, F.; Battistelli, S.; Benedetti, S. Oxidative stress and apoptosis induction in human thyroid carcinoma cells exposed to the essential oil from *Pistacia lentiscus* aerial parts. *PLoS ONE* **2017**, *12*, e0172138. [CrossRef] [PubMed]

42. Piccolella, S.; Nocera, P.; Carillo, P.; Woodrow, P.; Greco, V.; Manti, L.; Fiorentino, A.; Pacifico, S. An apolar *Pistacia lentiscus* L. leaf extract: GC-MS metabolic profiling and evaluation of cytotoxicity and apoptosis inducing effects on SH-SY5Y and SK-N-BE(2)C cell lines. *Food Chem. Toxicol.* **2016**, *95*, 64–74. [CrossRef] [PubMed]

43. Li, S.; Cha, I.H.; Nam, W. Chios mastic gum extracts as a potent antitumor agent that inhibits growth and induces apoptosis of oral cancer cells. *Asian Pac. J. Cancer Prev.* **2011**, *12*, 1877–1880. [PubMed]

44. Smeriglio, A.; Denaro, M.; Barreca, D.; Calderaro, A.; Bisignano, C.; Ginestra, G.; Bellocco, E.; Trombetta, D. In vitro evaluation of the antioxidant, cytoprotective, and antimicrobial properties of essential oil from *Pistacia vera* L. Variety Bronte Hull. *Int. J. Mol. Sci.* **2017**, *18*, 1212. [CrossRef] [PubMed]

45. Zhou, L.; Satoh, K.; Takahashi, K.; Watanabe, S.; Nakamura, W.; Maki, J.; Hatano, H.; Takekawa, F.; Shimada, C.; Sakagami, H. Re-evaluation of anti-inflammatory activity of mastic using activated macrophages. *In Vivo* **2009**, *23*, 583–589. [PubMed]

46. Attoub, S.; Karam, S.M.; Nemmar, A.; Arafat, K.; John, A.; Al-Dhaheri, W.; Al Sultan, M.A.; Raza, H. Short-term effects of oral administration of *Pistacia lentiscus* oil on tissue-specific toxicity and drug metabolizing enzymes in mice. *Cell Physiol. Biochem.* **2014**, *33*, 1400–1410. [CrossRef] [PubMed]

47. Paster, B.J.; Olsen, I.; Aas, J.A.; Dewhirst, F.E. The breadth of bacterial diversity in the human periodontal pocket and other oral sites. *Periodontology 2000* **2006**, *42*, 80–87. [CrossRef] [PubMed]

48. Socransky, S.S.; Haffajee, A.D.; Cugini, M.A.; Smith, C.; Kent, R.L., Jr. Microbial complexesin subgingival plaque. *J. Clin. Periodontol.* **1998**, *25*, 134–144. [CrossRef] [PubMed]

49. Holt, S.C.; Ebersole, J.L. *Porphyromonas gingivalis*, *Treponema denticola*, and *Tannerella forsythia*: The "red complex", a prototype polybacterial pathogenic consortium in periodontitis. *Periodontology 2000* **2005**, *38*, 72–122. [CrossRef] [PubMed]

50. Watanabe, S. Study and development of the prevention of the periodontal diseases using Kampo mouth wash. In *Shika Iryo*; Dai-ichi Shika Shuppan Publications: Tokyo, Japan, 2003; Volume Spring, pp. 87–97. (In Japanese)

51. Watanabe, S. Study and development of the prevention of the periodontal diseases using Kampo mouth wash. In *Shika Iryo*; Dai-ichi Shika Shuppan Publications: Tokyo, Japan, 2003; Volume Summer, pp. 61–67. (In Japanese)

52. Watanabe, S. Study and development of the prevention of the periodontal diseases using Kampo mouth wash. In *Shika Iryo*; Dai-ichi Shika Shuppan Publications: Tokyo, Japan, 2004; Volume Winter. (In Japanese)

53. Baumgartner, J.C.; Khemaleelakul, S.U.; Xia, T. Identi fication of spirochetes (treponemes) in endodontic infections. *J. Endod.* **2003**, *29*, 794–797. [CrossRef] [PubMed]

54. Foschi, F.; Cavrini, F.; Montebugnoli, L.; Stashenko, P.; Sambri, V.; Prati, C. Detection of bacteria in endodontic samples by polymerase chain reaction assays and association with defined clinical signs in Italian patients. *Oral Microbiol. Immunol.* **2005**, *20*, 289–295. [CrossRef] [PubMed]

55. Zambon, J.J. Periodontal diseases: Microbial factors. *Ann. Periodontol.* **1996**, *1*, 879–925. [CrossRef] [PubMed]

56. Lamont, R.J.; Jenkinson, H.F. Life below the gum line: Pathogenic mechanisms of *Porphyromonas gingivalis*. *Microbiol. Mol. Biol. Rev.* **1998**, *62*, 1244–1263. [PubMed]

57. Landi, L.; Amar, S.; Polins, A.S.; Van, D.T. Host mechanisms in the pathogenesis of periodontal disease. *Curr. Opin. Periodontol.* **1997**, *4*, 3–10. [PubMed]

58. Li, R.W.; David Lin, G.; Myers, S.P.; Leach, D.N. Anti-inflammatory activity of Chinese medicinal vine plants. *J. Ethnopharmacol.* **2003**, *85*, 61–67. [CrossRef]

59. Wang, D.X.; Liu, P.; Chen, Y.H.; Chen, R.Y.; Guo, D.H.; Ren, H.Y.; Chen, M.L. Stimulating effect of catechin, an active component of *Spatholobus suberectus* Dunn, on bioactivity of hematopoietic growth factor. *Chi-Med. J.* **2008**, *121*, 752–755. [CrossRef]

60. Freidovich, I. Fundamental aspects of reactive oxygen species, or what's the matter with oxygen? *Ann. N. Y. Acad. Sci.* **1999**, *893*, 13–18. [CrossRef]

61. Fang, Y.Z.; Yang, S.; Wu, G. Free radicals, antioxidants, and nutrition. *Nutrition* **2002**, *18*, 872–879. [CrossRef]

62. Moynihan, P.; Petersen, P.E. Diet, nutrition and the prevention of dental diseases. *Public Health Nutr.* **2004**, *7*, 201–226. [CrossRef] [PubMed]

63. Genco, R.J.; Borgnakke, W.S. Risk factors for periodontal disease. *Periodontology 2000* **2013**, *62*, 59–94. [CrossRef] [PubMed]

64. Sajjanhar, I.; Goel, A.; Tikku, A.P.; Chandra, A. Odontogenic pain of non-odontogenic origin: A review. *Int. J. Appl. Dent. Sci.* **2017**, *3*, 1–4.

65. Japanese Society of Orofacial Pain. *Clinical Practice Guideline for Nonodontogenic Toothache*; Japan Dental Association: Tokyo, Japan, 2011.

66. Sakagami, H.; Okudaira, N.; Masuda, Y.; Amano, O.; Yokose, S.; Kanda, Y.; Suguro, M.; Natori, T.; Oizumi, H.; Oizumi, T. Induction of apoptosis in human oral keratinocyte by doxorubicin. *Anticancer Res.* **2017**, *37*, 1023–1029. [PubMed]

67. Sakagami, H.; Shi, H.; Bandow, K.; Tomomura, M.; Tomomura, A.; Horiuchi, M.; Fujisawa, T.; Oizumi, T. Search of neuroprotective polyphenols using the "overlay" isolation method. *Molecules* **2018**, *23*, 1840. [CrossRef] [PubMed]

68. Sakagami, H.; Watanabe, T.; Hoshino, T.; Suda, N.; Mori, K.; Yasui, T.; Yamauchi, N.; Kashiwagi, H.; Gomi, T.; Oizumi, T.; et al. Recent progress of basic studies of natural products and their dental application. *Medicines* **2018**, *6*, 4. [CrossRef] [PubMed]

13

The Pathogenic Factors from Oral Streptococci for Systemic Diseases

Hiromichi Yumoto [1,*], Katsuhiko Hirota [2], Kouji Hirao [3], Masami Ninomiya [1], Keiji Murakami [4], Hideki Fujii [4] and Yoichiro Miyake [5]

[1]   Department of Periodontology and Endodontology, Institute of Biomedical Sciences, Tokushima University Graduate School, Tokushima 770-8504, Japan; masami.ninomiya@tokushima-u.ac.jp
[2]   Department of Medical Hygiene, Dental Hygiene Course, Kochi Gakuen College, Kochi 780-0955, Japan; khirota@kochi-gc.ac.jp
[3]   Department of Conservative Dentistry, Institute of Biomedical Sciences, Tokushima University Graduate School, Tokushima 770-8504, Japan; koujihirao@tokushima-u.ac.jp
[4]   Department of Oral Microbiology, Institute of Biomedical Sciences, Tokushima University Graduate School, Tokushima 770-8504, Japan; kmurakami@tokushima-u.ac.jp (K.M.); hfujii@tokushima-u.ac.jp (H.F.)
[5]   Department of Oral Health Sciences, Faculty of Health and Welfare, Tokushima Bunri University, Tokushima, Tokushima 770-8514, Japan; miyake@tks.bunri-u.ac.jp
*   Correspondence: yumoto@tokushima-u.ac.jp

Abstract: The oral cavity is suggested as the reservoir of bacterial infection, and the oral and pharyngeal biofilms formed by oral bacterial flora, which is comprised of over 700 microbial species, have been found to be associated with systemic conditions. Almost all oral microorganisms are non-pathogenic opportunistic commensals to maintain oral health condition and defend against pathogenic microorganisms. However, oral Streptococci, the first microorganisms to colonize oral surfaces and the dominant microorganisms in the human mouth, has recently gained attention as the pathogens of various systemic diseases, such as infective endocarditis, purulent infections, brain hemorrhage, intestinal inflammation, and autoimmune diseases, as well as bacteremia. As pathogenic factors from oral Streptococci, extracellular polymeric substances, toxins, proteins and nucleic acids as well as vesicles, which secrete these components outside of bacterial cells in biofilm, have been reported. Therefore, it is necessary to consider that the relevance of these pathogenic factors to systemic diseases and also vaccine candidates to protect infectious diseases caused by Streptococci. This review article focuses on the mechanistic links among pathogenic factors from oral Streptococci, inflammation, and systemic diseases to provide the current understanding of oral biofilm infections based on biofilm and widespread systemic diseases.

Keywords: Streptococci; Biofilm; Pathogenic factor; Oral infection; Systemic Diseases

1. Introduction

The human oral microbiome is comprised of over 700 microbial species, as characterized by both cultivation and culture-independent molecular approaches such as the 16S rRNA gene-based method [1]. Almost all oral microorganisms are non-pathogenic opportunistic commensals to maintain oral health condition and defend against pathogenic microorganisms [2]. The most remarkable feature of oral microflora is that numerous oral bacteria form a biofilm, so called dental plaque, which is defined as microbial communities embedded in a self-produced matrix of extracellular polymeric substances and a dynamic metabolically structure, on tooth surface and oral mucosa [3,4]. Within biofilm formed in oral niche, the polymicrobial interactions between interspecies, such as recombination and horizontal gene transfer, are caused and then specialized clones are selected [5]. Several pressures by bacterial communities and the host as well as the change in oral environment caused by the administration of antibiotics also affect the selection of bacterial species and the characterizations of their virulence. Once this homeostasis of oral microflora is disturbed by changing the local environments as well as the metabolic and physiological activities of bacteria in biofilm, oral infectious diseases such as dental caries and periodontitis, which are major two prevalent chronic diseases in oral cavity, are caused. Moreover, in the last two decades, numerous studies regarding the association between oral biofilm infectious diseases and various systemic diseases, such as cardiovascular diseases, atherosclerosis, diabetes mellitus, aspiration pneumonia, and autoimmune diseases, have been reported. To date, it has been considered that there are two major pathways by which oral bacterial infectious diseases affect systemic diseases (Figure 1). Bacteremia as direct pathway, oral bacteria residing in the oral cavity invade blood vessels in dental pulp and periodontal tissues, and then reach not only the heart but also the large blood vessels and various organs to cause systemic diseases. Another direct pathway involving aspiration, which often occurs in elderly people, involves oral bacteria reaching a respiratory organ, such as the lung via a pharynx and airway route, and causing respiratory diseases. Several bacterial products, such as endotoxin (lipopolysaccharide: LPS) and heat shock protein (HSP), as well as antigens, also involved in various systemic diseases due to the indirect causes of triggering immune responses. Therefore, the oral cavity is recognized as a source or reservoir of microbial infection and the establishment of methods to prevent oral infections is one of the most important and urgent issues in dentistry. From the viewpoint of oral biofilm infection, understanding the roles of oral microorganisms and their pathogenic factors and elucidating various systemic diseases and their onset mechanisms related to oral infections would lead to the development of novel preventive measures.

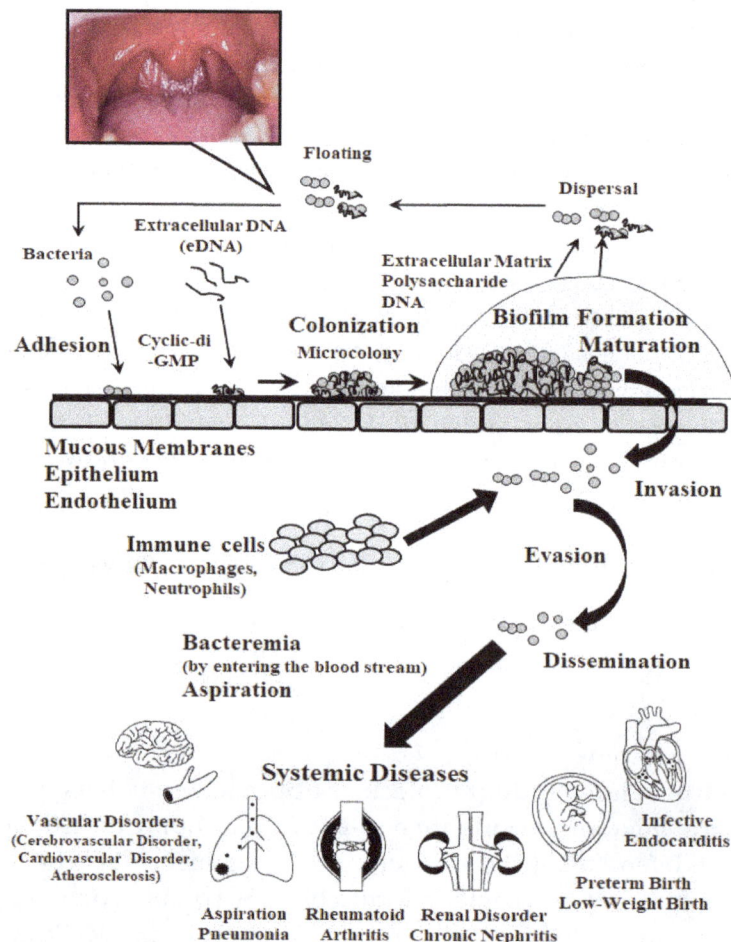

Figure 1. Life style of biofilm and the conceptual pathogenic mechanisms of oral bacterial infection leading to various systemic diseases.

Among oral bacterial species, over 100 identified oral Streptococci, which can colonize shortly after birth and play important roles in the formation of oral physiological microflora, are the predominant commensal and opportunistic inhabitants in the oral cavity and upper respiratory tract in humans, and cause opportunistic infections at sites distant from the oral cavity as well as oral infections, especially in immunocompromised patients and elderly people [6]. Pathogenic Streptococci are identified as sources of invasive infections in humans and their infections are still one of the most serious diseases in modern medical world [7]. Table 1 shows systemic diseases affected and caused by oral Streptococcal infections. Therefore, it has been recently considered that the genus Streptococci severely impacts on human health by carrying a significant number of worldwide human infections, and has been separated into following 8 distinct groups: mitis, sanguinis, anginosus, salivalius, downei, mutans, pyogenic, and bovis using gene clustering, as well as phylogenetic and gene gain/loss analyses (Figure 2) [8]. The distribution of oral Streptococcal species in the oral cavity has been also reported [9,10]. The mitis and sanguinis groups, such as *S. sanguinis*, *S. mitis*, *S. gordonii*, and *S. oralis* are common commensals, primarily involved in initial dental plaque formation as the first colonizers of the tooth surface, but are also associated with an increased risk of systemic diseases and invasive infections, including infective endocarditis, by entering the bloodstream through transient bacteremia after daily activities such as brushing and flossing, as well as invasive dental procedures such as tooth extraction. A recent descriptive epidemiological study has reported the distribution of Streptococci causing infective endocarditis [11]. Figure 3 shows one clinical case of infective endocarditis mainly caused by oral *S. sanguinis*. We encountered the patient with infective endocarditis caused by oral Streptococci, who had severe systemic conditions such as mitral and tricuspid regurgitations and a continuous fever over 37 °C, and who was urgently hospitalized in our university hospital. This case was rigorously diagnosed by the detection of oral *Streptococcus sanguinis*, as well as the examination of chest radiograph and echocardiogram at the time of the onset of infective endocarditis. Therefore, as the presentative case of infective endocarditis, the detailed therapeutic course following the guideline is described below and in Figure 3. The guideline for systemic complications, such as infective endocarditis, shows that bactericidal antibiotics are selected based on the results from microbiological examination, such as blood culture, and long-term antibiotic treatment is performed at high doses in order to kill the causative bacteria and to prevent recurrence. It is also very important to identify the causative bacteria in order to suppress side effects as much as possible. Following this guideline, the patient received viccilin (ampicillin sodium: 6000 mg/day) and gentamicin (a type of aminoglycoside: 60 mg/day) after microbiological examination. Afterwards, the symptoms were improved and no bacteria were detected by blood culture. It has been recognized that *S. mutans* playing important roles in the initiation and progression of dental caries is inversely associated with oral health [12]. The *S. anginosus* group is detected as part of the oropharyngeal microflora and is commonly associated with a variety of purulent infections and abscess formations in the brain, meninx, heart, liver, lung, and spleen. It is caused by bacteremia, as well as periapical odontogenic lesions [13–17]. In particular, *S. intermedius* and *S. constellatus* found in dental plaque has been associated with the development of periodontal diseases [18]. In contrast, *S. salivarius* group, in which *S. salivarius* is predominant in the saliva and on the surface of oral mucosa, is related to oral health rather than disease by producing bacteriocins targeting cariogenic *S. mutans* in addition to some enzymes such as dextranase and urease, which can inhibit the accumulation of dental plaque and acidification, respectively. A previous probiotic study reported that *S. salivarius* provides potential oral benefits to children [19].

Table 1. Systemic diseases affected by oral Streptococcal infections.

Bacteremia and Sepsis
Infective Endocarditis, Pericarditis
Heart Valve Disease
Aortic Aneurysm

Table 1. *Cont.*

| Deep-seated purulent Abscess (Brain, Tonsillar, Abdominal, Spleen or Liver Abscess) |
| Pleural Empyema |
| Meningitis |
| Cerebrovascular Disease (Cerebral Hemorrhage etc.) |
| Gastrointestinal Diseases (Exacerbation and Chronicity of Enteritis) |
| Kidney Diseases (IgA Nephropathy) |
| Pneumonia |
| Pharyngitis, Tonsillitis |
| Sinusitis |
| Premature Birth, Neonatal Infections, Puerperal Sepsis |
| Urinary Tract Infection |
| Central Nerve System Infections |
| Arthritis, Necrotizing Fasciitis |
| Pyarthrosis |
| Toxic Shock Syndrome |
| Osteomyelitis |
| Vulvovaginitis |
| Peritonitis |
| Impetigo, Cellulitis, Pyoderma |
| Otitis Media |
| Conjunctivitis |
| Scarlet Fever |

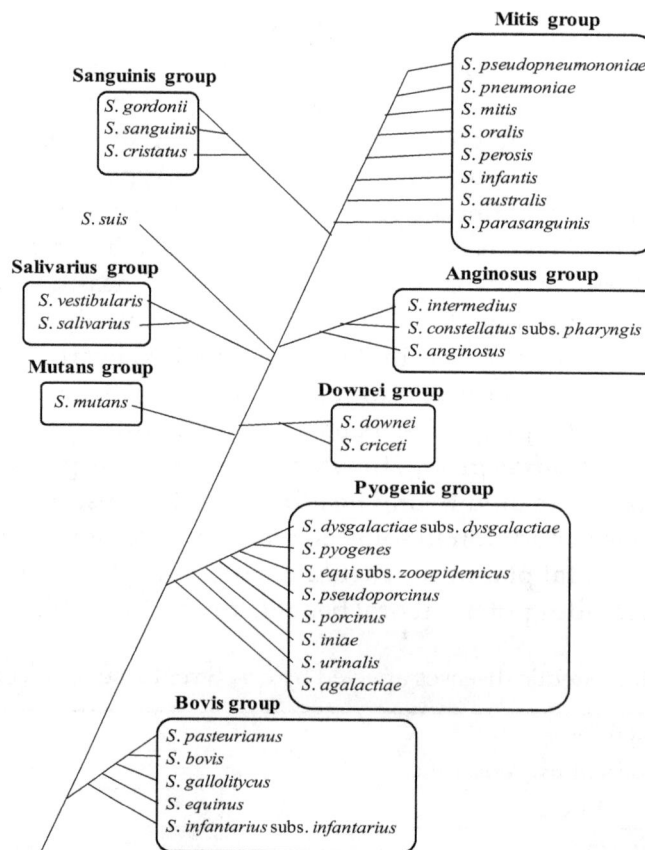

Figure 2. The phylogenetic relationship among 8 major groups of human Streptococcal species.

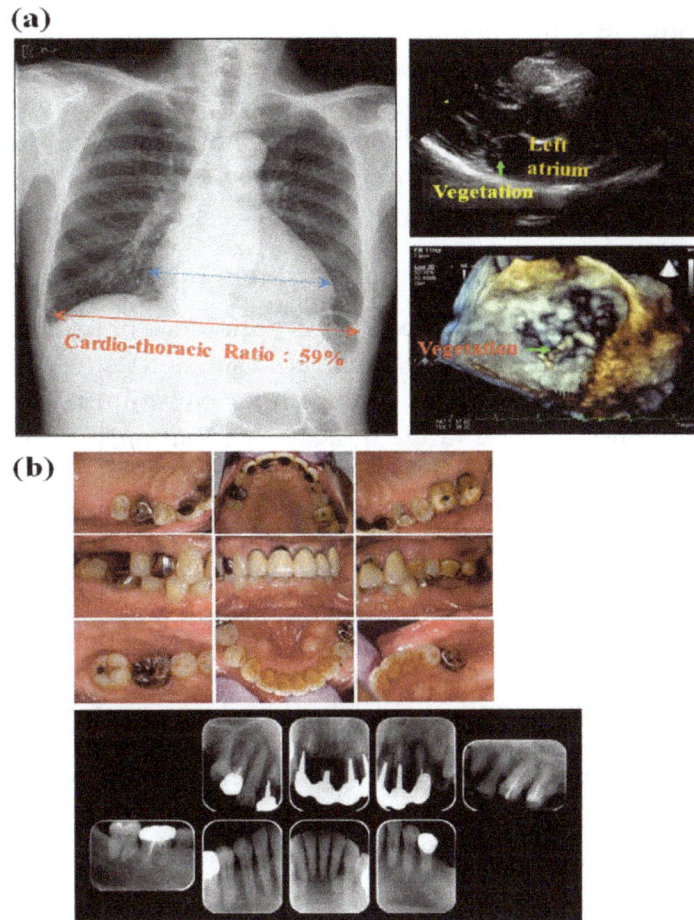

Figure 3. A clinical case of infective endocarditis caused by oral *Streptococcus sanguinis*. A 72 years-old male patient with mitral and tricuspid regurgitations was urgently hospitalized for continuous fever over 37 °C and diagnosed as infective endocarditis by detection of oral Streptococcus, *S. sanguinis*. During the hospitalization for 1 month, patient received viccilin (ampicillin sodium: 6000 mg/day) and gentamicin (a type of aminoglycoside: 60 mg/day). After the improvement of symptoms and no bacterial detection by blood culture, patient underwent artificial valve replacement and tricuspid ring annuloplasty, and then was discharged from hospital due to the stabilization of symptoms. The patient came to our dental department for the prevention of recurrence with a referral from the medical doctor. (**a**) Chest radiograph and echocardiogram at the time of the onset of infective endocarditis. Cardiac hypertrophy (Cardio-thoracic Ratio: CTR: ≥ 50%) was observed due to abnormalities in the mitral valve, and the left atrium was enlarged markedly. Vegetation (green arrow) was observed in the mitral valve. (**b**) Oral and X-ray photographs of patient with infective endocarditis. Gingival redness and slight swelling were observed in full mouth, and dental calculus deposition were observed on mandibular anterior teeth and upper left molars. Mobility of upper anterior teeth and left premolars was also observed. From dental X-ray radiographs, root fractures of upper right central and lateral incisors, and a endodontic-periodontal combined lesion of the upper left incisor and canines were found. Severe alveolar bone loss around the upper anterior teeth and left premolars as well as root caries on the upper lateral incisor and 1st premolar was also observed. The number of total Streptococci in 10 μL of saliva was 1.0×10^7 copies and various periodontal pathogens, such as *Porphyromonas gingivalis*, *Aggregatibacter actinomycetemcomitans*, *Tannerella forsythia*, *Treponema denticola* and *Fusobacterium nucleatum*, were also detected at significantly high level.

Streptococci have an array of virulence factors, which include surface proteins for adhesion, invasion/internalization, extracellular enzymatic proteases, and toxins delivered to cell surface as well as extracellular environments, which are associated with their colonization at various sites in the human body, dissemination, evasion from immune system for survival, destruction of host tissues, and modulation of the host immune function [20,21]. Some vaccine candidates are currently being considered to protect against infectious diseases caused by SStreptococci. This review article focuses on the mechanistic links among crucial pathogenic factors from oral Streptococci, inflammation, and systemic diseases to provide the current understanding of oral infections and widespread systemic diseases. In particular, our recent findings regarding the roles of histone-like DNA binding protein and extracellular DNA in biofilm formation and systemic diseases are also summarized.

2. Pathogenic Factors Involved in Adhesion, Colonization, Internalization and Invasion

In general, the first step on bacterial infections is adherence of bacterial cells with host tissues via the interaction between bacterial adhesion factor, adhesin, and its receptor. This step is extremely important for bacterial survival in bacterial multicellular communities and the establishment of infections. Streptococci express a wide range of adhesins that are specific for the surface of host tissues to colonize, grow, and form biofilm (Table 2). These adhesion and colonization factors of oral Streptococci also play pivotal roles in resistant to antimicrobial peptides and protection against host innate immune defense system. Among the numerous adhesion factors, representative molecules are described below.

Table 2. The pathogenic factors expressed in oral Streptococci for colonization, inflammation, infection causing systemic diseases.

Pathogenic Factors	References
Factors for adhesion, colonization, and evasion from host immune defense	
Antigen I/II	[22–24]
Fibronectin-binding proteins	[23,25–27]
Collagen-binding proteins	[20,28]
Laminin-binding proteins	
Fibrinogen-binding proteins	
Platelet-binding proteins	
Serine-rich repeat proteins	[23,29,30]
Pili	[20,23,31–37]
Major surface adhesins (M protein)	[38–41]
Enolase	[23,42,43]
Proteases	
SpeB	[44–47]
C5a peptidase	[26,48–51]
Capsule	
Lipoteichoic acid as pathogen-associated molecular pattern (PAMP)	

2.1. Cell Wall-Anchored Polypeptides

Among the cell wall-anchored polypeptides produced by oral Streptococci, antigen I/II acts as a mediator on the adherence of Streptococci to salivary glycoproteins called pellicles coated on the surfaces of teeth as well as collagen, fibronectin and laminin in the tissues, and is also engaged in biofilm formation by interacting with other oral microorganisms, such as *Actinomyces naeslundii*, *Porphyromonas gingivalis*, and *Candida albicans*, platelet aggregation, and tissue invasion [22,23]. Antigen I/II is conserved in oral Streptococcus species including *S. pyogenes*, *S. suis* and *S. agalactiae*. Spy1325, a member of the antigen I/II family and cell surface-anchored molecule produced by oral Streptococci, is very well conserved in group A Streptococcus (GAS) strains. Interestingly, the immunization of mice with recombinant Spy1325 fragments conferred protection against GAS-mediated mortality, suggesting that Spy1325 may represent a shared virulence factor among GAS, GBS, and oral Streptococci [24]. Therefore, these adhesion factors are considered as a candidate molecule for preventive and therapeutic measures against Streptococcal infections, including dental caries.

Fibronectin-binding protein expressed in all Streptococci plays the role of providing a bridge between Streptococci and host cells by attachment to the extracellular matrix, fibronectin [23,25]. Fibronectin binding proteins can be divided into two types: one type contains fibronectin binding repeats and another type has no repeats [26,27]. This kind of adhesion is different between the binding activity and structure. Some can bind soluble fibronectin and others attach to immobilized fibronectin expressed on the surface of host cells. Moreover, most of these adhesins are anchored to the bacterial cell wall, but some are not. In addition to the role of adhesins mediating attachment, fibronectin-binding protein has been identified as invasins invading epithelial and endothelial cells, which have contributed to evasion from host's innate immune defense mechanisms, such as the complement system and phagocytosis [27].

As another cell wall-anchored protein, collagen binding proteins adhere to collagen-rich tissues for colonization of oral and extra-oral tissues [28] and also bind complement C1 recognition protein, C1q, as inhibitors of the classical complement defense. Therefore, this function confers the ability of immune evasion on oral Streptococci [20].

Serine-rich repeat glycoproteins expressed in wide range of oral Streptococci has multiple serine-rich repeats, which are estimated as an approximately 75% of this protein [23]. After invading into bloodstream, oral Streptococci can bind to human platelets through this adhesion and are disseminated systemically [29]. Binding to platelets leads to form a thrombus, by which oral Streptococci can evade the host immune defense and antibiotics circulated in blood, and then cause infective endocarditis [30]. Therefore, this adhesin is considered as a major virulence factor of endocarditis.

Pili are filamentous apparatus typically extending 1–3 mm from the bacterial cell surface, and the genes encoding pili are identified in discrete loci called pilus islands flanked by mobile genetic elements [20,23]. Pili as virulent factors adhere to various host epithelial cells as well as extracellular matrix proteins such as collagen and fibrinogen, and then promotes Streptococcal colonization and biofilm formation on various sites in the host as well as non-biological surfaces [31]. In addition to adhesion, pili can facilitate bacterial invasion into human epithelial and endothelial cells and lead to Streptococcal dissemination in the host during the critical infection steps [32,33]. Moreover, pili have immunomodulatory abilities to evoke inflammatory cytokine responses and thwart the host innate immune defenses of resist phagocyte killing [34–36]. Therefore, pili have gotten much attention as potential vaccine candidates because of animal studies showing conferred protective immunity against Streptococcal infection [37].

M proteins expressed on a bacterial cell surface, α-helical coiled-coil dimers extending as hair like projections, bind host proteins such as immunoglobulins, fibronectin, and fibrinogen, complement factors such as albumin, and adhere to epithelial cells [38]. Interestingly, antigenically variable M proteins are considered as major virulence factors and immunogens in Streptococci by inducing pro-inflammatory responses and inhibiting phagocytic activities to assist Streptococci in evading host innate immune defenses [39,40]. Soluble M1 protein secreted from Streptococci has been also considered as a novel Streptococcal superantigen because it contributes to excess T cell activation and inflammatory response, such as the induction of T-cell proliferation and Th1 type cytokines production, during invasive Streptococcal infections [41]. Therefore, M proteins may be promising vaccine immunogens [39].

2.2. Cell Wall-Anchorless Polypeptides

Enolase, cell wall-anchorless adhesin and cytoplasmic glycolytic enzyme, is well conserved structurally in Streptococci [23,42]. α-enolase functionally binds to plasmin and plasminogen as well as laminin, fibronectin, and collagens, and also enhances plasminogen activation [43]. Plasmin cleaved from plasminogen by plasminogen activators can degrade extracellular matrix, in turn breakdown epithelial barriers and finally lead to bacterial invasion and infection. Therefore, this anchorless cell surface protein has been considered in promising vaccine candidates for the prevention of Streptococcal infection [42].

2.3. Proteases

Some proteases secreted from Streptococci have associated with their virulence. In addition to the role of adhesin to glycoprotein and laminin, Streptococcal pyrogenic exotoxin B (SpeB), predominant cysteine protease, has relatively indiscriminant specificity to degrade the extracellular matrix proteins, including fibronectin, cytokines, chemokines, compliment components, immunoglobulins, immune system components such as the antimicrobial peptide cathelicidin LL-37, and serum protease inhibitors. It also activates interleukin-1β [44,45]. This protease also degrades some proteins targeted by autophagy in the host cell cytosol, which is an important innate immune defense, and this proteolytic activity helps Streptococci to evade autophagy, to replicate in the cytoplasm of host cells, to colonize deep-seated tissues, and finally to lead to tissue destruction [46]. Moreover, SpeB increases the production of proapoptotic molecules, such as tumor necrosis factor (TNF)-α and Fas ligand, by activation of matrix metalloproteinase (MMP)- 9 and -2 and then induces apoptosis of host cells [45]. Based on the significant roles of SpeB as critical virulence factor, SpeB combined with inactive SpeA, Streptococcal pyrogenic endotoxin, has been considered as a potential vaccine candidate, which can produce neutralizing antibodies to prevent Streptococcal infection [47].

C5a peptidase, also called SCPA, is a cell wall-anchored immunogenic 125-kDa protein and a well-conserved antigen in Streptococci, and enzymatically cleaves the compliment component C5a to specifically inactivate [48–50]. As an adhesin, C5a peptidase binds directly integrin by the Arg-Gly-Asp (RGD) motifs and the extracellular matrix, fibronectin, with high affinity as well to epithelial cells [51]. This peptidase also inhibits neutrophil chemotaxis and the recruitment of phagocytes to the site of Streptococcal infection by cleavage of C5a and promotes invasion and colonization on damaged epithelium as invasin [26,51]. Therefore, C5a peptidase plays roles as a virulence factor through its multifunctional activities and is considered to be a promising vaccine candidate.

3. Pathogenic Factors Associated with Biofilm Formation

The characteristics of biofilm include high resistance to antibiotics and host immunity, as described above. Therefore, the Center for Disease Control (CDC) has warned that biofilm is involved in over 65% of human bacterial infections which are difficult to prevent, and that the emergence of multidrug-resistant bacteria and delays in biofilm measures is a serious problem in the entire medical field. Biofilm formed in the microbial immediate environment after their colonization creates a self-produced matrix consisting of extracellular polymeric substances (EPS), which are composed of polysaccharides, proteins, nucleic acids, and lipids [52]. EPS confers the adhesion ability and mechanical stability of biofilm, as well as embedded bacterial cells. Regarding the roles of biofilm in the etiology of systemic infectious diseases, the characteristic of resistance against abuse of a wider spectrum of antibiotics for biofilm infections has been focused on, and it has been considered that the ineffectiveness of the antimicrobial agent as a major feature of biofilm is greatly involved in the emergences of multidrug-resistant bacteria and higher toxic pathogens [7]. It has been also reported that the transformation is caused by frequent horizontal gene transfer, which occurs between bacteria in dental plaque biofilm. This leads to the acquisition of new resistance genes and high antibiotic resistance [53]. Moreover, microorganisms in biofilm share their metabolites and have an intercellular communication (cell-cell interaction) mechanism called quorum sensing (QS) that senses the cell density showing numbers of self and different species and synchronously regulates the expression of specific genes encoding virulent factors, such as enzymes and toxins. Therefore, solving these antibiotics-dependent problems requires the development of novel therapeutic methods to effectively suppress the biofilm formation without selective pressure, not using selective microorganisms based on the conventional antimicrobial sensitivity or the mechanism of antimicrobial action. Biofilm forms and matures through several stages (Figure 1). At each stage in the life style of biofilm, focusing on molecules common in bacteria involved in biofilm formation may lead to develop novel therapeutic agents. The first step of biofilm formation is that floating bacteria attaching to the biological surfaces, and this adhesion process is involved in various bacterial products and adhesins, including pili and surface proteins as described in the previous section.

3.1. Bis-(3′-5′)-Cyclic Dimeric Guanosine Monophosphate (Cyclic di-GMP) as a Bacterial Second Messenger

The attached bacteria grow and increase their number to form a microcolony, and subsequently produce extracellular matrix components consisting of polysaccharides, DNA, and proteins which connect the bacterial cells and strengthen the adhesion to the biological surface. The extracellular matrix of mature biofilm protects bacterial cells from the stresses, such as phagocytosis by host cells and oxidation, and bacterial communication in biofilm is more highly activated by the accumulation of signal substances and metabolites involved in QS. Some dispersal bacteria detached from the mature biofilm attach themselves to the new biological surface and then cause the infection to spread. Recently, it has been shown that an intracellular second messenger called bis-(3′-5′)-cyclic dimeric guanosine monophosphate (cyclic-di-GMP) plays an important role in the transition from reversible attachment to irreversible attachment and also regulates various genes expression through transcriptional factors [54]. With regard to the transition from the floating state to the biofilm state and vice versa, it has been reported that the change in the concentration of cyclic-di-GMP, the intracellular second messenger in bacterial cells, regulates the bacterial virulence, motility, the cell cycle and the synthesis of extracellular matrix, as well as biofilm formation [55]. Most cyclic-di-GMP-dependent signaling pathways also regulate the ability of bacteria to interact with other bacterial and eukaryotic cells. Therefore, cyclic di-GMP plays important roles in biofilm lifestyle including the multicellular bacterial biofilm development. Regarding these abilities, the modulation of bacterial cyclic-di-GMP signaling pathways might be a novel potential way to control biofilm formation in the medical area, and cyclic-di-GMP is considered to be a possible candidate for a vaccine adjuvant [56].

3.2. Extracellular DNA (eDNA)

In addition to polysaccharides and proteins, the extracellular matrix components in biofilm contain not only bacteria but also DNA derived from the host, and the interaction of eDNA in biofilm with other extracellular matrix components is also considered in terms of pathogenic factors in biofilm (Table 3). The roles of these eDNAs in the formation of biofilm have been also focused on as a target to replace or complement the use of antibiotics [57]. A previous study reported that the addition of DNase I suppresses biofilm formation and also degrades the mature biofilm, suggesting that eDNA is essential for biofilm formation and maturation as well as for its structural maintenance properties [58]. Therefore, it has been considered that enzymatic degradation of eDNA can prevent biofilm formation or sensitize biofilm to antimicrobials. Regarding oral bacterial biofilm, evidence showing eDNA plays a number of important roles in biofilm formation and maturation on oral soft and hard tissues and in its structural integrity has been accumulated [59]. The concentration of eDNA in Streptococcal biofilm is also involved in strength and rigidity of biofilm structure as well as biofilm formation and maturation. When the concentration of eDNA in Streptococcal biofilm is extremely high, biofilm maturation is suppressed and the bacteria in biofilm tends to detach [60]. This suggests that a high concentration of eDNA in formed or matured biofilm makes its structure fragile and makes bacteria easily disperse. In other words, when the concentration of eDNA in biofilm is increased and its concentration reaches a certain level, some bacteria in biofilm are detached and then attach to new sites to form biofilm, resulting in the spread of infection. Intriguingly, DNA derived from different bacteria, such as *Escherichia coli*, *Staphylococcus aureus*, and *Pseudomonas aeruginosa* in humans have also shown similar characteristics [60]. A recent interesting study has reported that calcium ion-regulated autolysin AtlA maturation mediates the release of eDNA by *S. mutans*, which contributes to its biofilm formation in infective endocarditis [61]. Therefore, all eDNAs present in biofilm, regardless of their origin, have been shown to be involved in biofilm formation, maturation, and structure, and an eDNA-targeting novel strategy may be applicable to novel treatments for bacterial biofilm-related infectious diseases.

Table 3. Interaction of eDNA with other pathogenic factors present in the extracellular matrix of biofilm.

Pathogenic Factors	Roles
1. DNA binding proteins	Binding to eDNA strand Present in the biofilm matrix and on the surface of bacterial cells Involvement in transformation ability
2. Toxins	Cross-linked with eDNA Secreted virulence factor Insoluble nuclear-protein complex formation
3. Pili	Binding to eDNA Involvement in motility Involvement in the structure of biofilm
4. Polysaccharides	Co-localization with eDNA
5. Membrane Vesicles	Interaction with eDNA Involvement in the secretion and transport of DNA, toxins and cell membrane components such as lipoproteins to outside of bacterial cells

3.3. DNA Binding Protein

The eukaryotic cell has a protein called histone, which plays a role of compactly housing its chromosomal DNA in the nucleus. Prokaryotes, such as bacteria, also have histone-like DNA binding protein (HLP) to compactly house their chromosomal DNA in small bacterial cells. The bacterial HLP equivalent to eukaryotic histone goes beyond the concept of the nucleoid-related protein which forms a DNA-protein complex, and involves itself in various intracellular processes, including the binding ability to DNA and mRNA, regulation of gene transcription and translation, replication, and rearrangement. To clarify the pathogenicity and roles of HLP in biofilm, we cloned the *hlp* gene of *S. intermedius* (*Si-hlp*) and sequenced its DNA. Through the homology analysis of the amino acid sequence predicted from its DNA sequence, it has been revealed that HLP has high homology (89–94%) at an amino acid sequence level and is structurally highly conserved in Streptococci [62,63]. Further functional analysis showed that *Si*-HLP forms homodimers outside of the cells and co-stimulation of *Si*-HLP with pathogen-associated molecular patterns (PAMPs) produced by bacteria synergistically or additively induces pro-inflammatory cytokines production in human monocytes, indicating that HLP itself has a possible role in causing inflammation at the site of bacterial infection [62]. Moreover, the knockdown of HLP expression with the antisense RNA expression system inhibits the growth of *S. intermedius* and suppresses its biofilm formation, suggesting that HLP is an essential protein for the viability and growth of *S. intermedius* as well as biofilm formation [63]. The knockdown of HLP reduced the hydrophobicity of the cell surface and suppressed the expression of its cytolytic toxin, intermedilysin, which is the main pathogenic factor of *S. intermedius*, suggesting that HLP also affects the regulation of pathogenic factors expression in addition to bacterial adhesion and aggregation [63]. As a bacterial pathogenic factor, HLP is not only involved in bacterial survival, growth, biofilm formation, and maturation, but also has the ability to directly induce pro-inflammatory responses in host cells and therefore HLP has huge roles in bacterial infection. Interestingly, fluorescence microscopic observation showed that eDNA and *Si*-HLP in biofilm were co-localized and uniformly distributed in biofilm (Figure 4). These findings suggest that HLP in addition to eDNA may also be a target as a novel treatment for biofilm infection control.

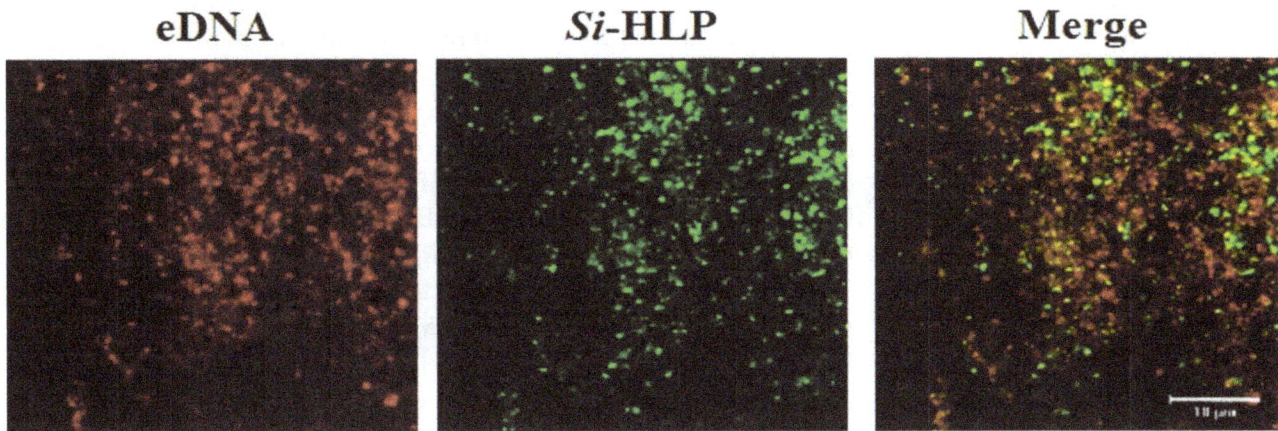

Figure 4. Co-localization and distribution of eDNA and *Si*-HLP in *S. intermedius* biofilm. eDNA in the formed *S. intermedius* biofilm was stained with propidium iodide (PI; red fluorescence), and *Si*-HLP was stained with anti-*Si*-HLP antibody and Alexafluor 488 (green fluorescence). Fluorescence microscopic observation showed that eDNA and HLP are co-localized (yellow fluorescence) and uniformly distributed in biofilm.

3.4. Membrane Vesicle

Membrane vesicles released from lots of bacterial species extracellularly contain proteins, nucleic acids such as DNA and RNA, and toxins. Lipoproteins, one of PAMPs, are also included as the cell membrane components of the surface of vesicles and released from the vesicles. Released PAMPs induce pro-inflammatory cytokines production after binding to the pattern recognition receptors (PRRs) expressed in host cells, suggesting that vesicles are involved in the exacerbation of inflammation [64]. Studies on membrane vesicles has been studied mainly using Gram-negative bacteria for a long time, but many research results on membrane vesicles of Gram-positive bacteria have been also shown increasingly in the last 10 years [65]. Membrane vesicles contained in the extracellular matrix of biofilm have various biological functions, such as intercellular communication, transport of toxins in vesicles, and horizontal gene transfer. Moreover, due to the similarity to liposomes, membrane vesicles is being tried in applications as drug delivery systems and vaccines using nanobiotechnology in the medical field [66].

As the second step following this bacterial adherence and biofilm formation, bacteria, which evaded antimicrobial peptides and host defense systems such as neutrophils and internalization by macrophages, invade the susceptible tissues to stimulate host cellular responses using capsule and PAMPs, such as lipoteichoic acid (LTA), in Streptococci. Neutrophils, key response cells recruited to the infectious site, release granule proteins and chromatin that together form extracellular fibers that bind bacteria. These neutrophil extracellular traps (NETs) are a form of innate response that binds microorganisms, prevents them from spreading, and degrade virulence factors and kill bacteria [67]. A recent intriguing study has shown that a nuclease, DeoC, in *S. mutans* degrades NETs and contributes to the escape of *S. mutans* from neutrophil killing and to the spread of *S. mutans* through biofilm dispersal [68]. After invasion into host cells and blood vessels of bacteria evaded from host innate defense system, bacteria are disseminated to tissues around the infection site and dispersed to colonize new sites through the blood stream.

4. Effects of Oral Streptococci on Systemic Diseases

The Viridans Group Streptococci is one of the most predominant bacterial groups in the oral bacterial flora, and has long been considered to be pathogens of severe infections such as infective endocarditis, sepsis, and meningitis (Table 1) [69]. In recent years, among the pathogenic factors possessed by the cariogenic bacterium *S. mutans*, a collagen binding protein (CBP, coding gene; *cnm*) has been focused for being associated with various systemic diseases. *S. mutans* expressing a CBP invade blood vessels, damage vascular endothelial cells, bind to collagen in the vascular endothelium to suppress platelet aggregation, and induce the expression of MMP-9, finally leading to the exacerbation of cerebral hemorrhage [70]. The epidemiological research also showed that the correlation between the occurrence of brain microbleeding and the high detection rate of CBP-positive *S. mutans* strains, suggesting that CBP-positive *S. mutans* is an independent risk for the onset and progression of cerebrovascular diseases [71]. Moreover, *S. mutans* expressing a CBP invade blood vessels, reach the liver and are then taken up into hepatic parenchymal cells to induce the production of cytokines such as interferon (IFN)-γ in the liver. It has also been reported that the imbalance of immune reactions and immune mechanisms caused by the infection of *cnm*-positive *S. mutans* leads to aggravation and deterioration of enteritis and ulcerative colitis in the digestive tracts [72]. Furthermore, the relationship between high DMFT (decayed, missing, and filled teeth) index and high urinary protein levels in patients with *cnm*-positive *S. mutans* has been shown and also suggests the association of its infection with renal diseases such as IgA nephropathy [73]. Recent study has reported that a 190-kDa protein antigen (PA), known as SpaP, P1 and antigen 1/2, of *S. mutans* affects the interaction with human serum, and the heart valves extirpated from rat infected with CBP-positive/PA-negative *S. mutans* strain showed prominent bacterial mass formation using in vivo infective endocarditis model, suggesting that CBP-positive/PA-negative *S. mutans* strain contribute to the pathogenicity in infective endocarditis [74].

5. Relationship Between Oral Streptococci and Autoimmune Diseases

Autoimmune diseases are types of chronic inflammation that occur in target organs as a result of the failure of immune tolerance to self-antigens and cellular immune responses by antibodies produced against self-antigens. In recent years, in addition to the reaction to the microorganisms which caused some types of infections, "molecular mimic" which cross-reacts with self-antigens has been considered to play roles in the mechanisms of onset and progression of autoimmune diseases. From this point of view, since the oral cavity is inhabited by lots of bacteria, it is always exposed to antigens derived from various bacteria, suggesting an association between the sensitization to antigens from resident bacteria and the onset of autoimmune diseases.

Regarding the association between oral bacteria, especially Gram-positive bacteria, and autoimmune diseases, some studies have focused on primary biliary cirrhosis (PBC) as autoimmune diseases. PBC is an autoimmune disease of unknown pathogenesis that often occurs in postmenopausal middle-aged women and its lesion is mainly composed of non-suppurative inflammation (chronic non-suppurative destructive cholangitis) around the intrahepatic small bile ducts. With progression of PBC to liver failure from liver cirrhosis, liver transplantation is the only way to treat the disease, and therefore it has been considered that PBC is an intractable disease. Laboratory findings of patients with PBC show that elevated biliary tract enzymes and high levels of IgM, and positive results for many autoantibodies, such as anti-mitochondrial antibody and anti-gp210, nuclear membrane protein, at a high rate (> 90%). Previous reports showed that LTA, a cell wall component of Gram-positive bacteria, was detected in the cytoplasm of lymphocytes and plasma cells infiltrating the site of chronic non-suppurative inflammation around interlobular bile ducts and in the serum of PBC patients, and it has been also reported that the levels of anti-LTA antibodies of IgM and IgA classes in PBC patients are higher than compared to those in healthy subjects and in patients with chronic hepatitis C, indicating that some Gram-positive bacteria might be involved in the onset and progression of PBC [75,76]. Moreover, the results of ELISA using whole cells of several Gram-positive Streptococci showed that the sera of PBC patients are highly reactive with these Streptococcal bacteria, especially *S. intermedius* and *Si*-HLP, compared to those of healthy subjects and patients with chronic hepatitis C, and HLP was detected in the lesion of PBC by immunohistochemical staining [77]. These results suggest that Streptococci and HLP may play important roles in the onset and progression of PBC. The administration of either live or heat-killed several Streptococci including *S. intermedius* twice a week for 8 weeks to the gingiva of BALB/c mice cause chronic non-suppurative inflammation around portal vein and the liver small bile ducts closely resembling PBC. Moreover, PBC-like clinical condition is observed even 20 months after the last administration and immunohistochemical staining showed that HLP was also detected in the non-suppurative inflammation area around the small bile duct of the liver, and inflammation was observed in the renal tubules [78]. Interestingly, although no bacteria were detected in the infected focal area, the depositions of LTA and HLP were observed around the small bile ducts similar to tissues from PBC patients, and the transplantation with the splenocytes (T cells) of this mouse into RAG2$^{-/-}$ immunodeficient mice caused similar chronic non-suppurative inflammation around the small bile ducts [79]. These findings also suggest the relationship between oral biofilm infection and autoimmune diseases. In patients with PBC, anti-gp210 autoantibodies are positive, and these positive patients progress to cirrhosis at a high rate compared to negative patients, and therefore anti-gp210 antibody levels are treated as a prognostic factor and are suggested to be deeply involved in the progression of PBC. More interestingly, a previous study reported that the epitope of gp210 was also found within the HLP sequence and the anti-HLP antibody cross-reacted with gp210 in mouse, indicating the sharing of the epitope [78]. Taken together, it has been suggested that Streptococci, especially dominant resident bacteria in the oral cavity and LTA, are strongly associated with the onset and progression of PBC.

6. Conclusions

The oral cavity is suggested as the reservoir of bacterial infection, and the oral and pharyngeal biofilms formed by oral bacterial flora have been found to be associated with various systemic diseases such as cardiovascular disease, arteriosclerosis, and diabetes. With the increasingly aging society, the rate of the elderly people with compromised immune function that are susceptible to infection is high and the onset and spread of infectious diseases among elderly people in nursing homes have become a major social problem. Therefore, the establishment of more effective prevention and treatment methods to reduce or minimize bacterial biofilm-related infectious diseases and their systemic complications is desired. However, even now, it has been pointed out that abuse of antibiotics for biofilm infections leads to the acquisition of antibiotic resistance and the emergence of higher toxic pathogens, such as emergence of multidrug resistant bacteria. In order to solve these problems, the development of therapeutic methods to effectively suppress the bacterial attachment, colonization, and biofilm formation without selective pressure, not for selective measures based on the conventional antimicrobial sensitivity or the mechanism of antimicrobial action, is expected. Regarding biofilm, which is the cause of bacterial infections, and considering its life cycle and its pathogenic factors, nucleic acids, such as DNAs that are commonly possessed by microorganisms, DNA binding proteins widely structurally conserved among microorganisms, and cyclic-di-GMP, intracellular second messenger involved in bacterial virulence and biofilm formation, may possibly be considered as target molecules to prevent and treat biofilm infections. Nucleic acids and their receptors are attracting attention as targets for the development of therapeutics not only for infectious diseases but also for other systemic diseases, such as autoimmune diseases and cancer. Therefore, the development of further research is expected.

Abbreviations

LPS	Lipopolysaccharide
HSP	heat shock protein
GAS	group A Streptococcus
SpeB	Streptococcal pyrogenic exotoxin B
TNF	tumor necrosis factor
MMP	matrix metalloproteinase
RGD	Arg-Gly-Asp

EPS	extracellular polymeric substances
QS	quorum sensing
cyclic-di-GMP	bis-(3'-5')-cyclic dimeric guanosine monophosphate
HLP	histone-like DNA binding protein
PAMPs	pathogen-associated molecular patterns
PRRs	pattern recognition receptors
LTA	lipoteichoic acid
NETs	neutrophil extracellular traps
CBP	collagen binding protein
DMFT	decayed, missing, and filled teeth
PA	190-kDa protein antigen
PBC	primary biliary cirrhosis

References

1. Dewhirst, F.E.; Chen, T.; Izard, J.; Paster, B.J.; Tanner, A.C.; Yu, W.H.; Lakshmanan, A.; Wade, W.G. The human oral microbiome. *J. Bacteriol.* **2010**, *192*, 5002–5017. [CrossRef] [PubMed]

2. Zbinden, A.; Bostanci, N.; Belibasakis, G.N. The novel species streptococcus tigurinus and its association with oral infection. *Virulence* **2015**, *6*, 177–182. [CrossRef] [PubMed]

3. Flemming, H.C.; Wingender, J.; Szewzyk, U.; Steinberg, P.; Rice, S.A.; Kjelleberg, S. Biofilms: An emergent form of bacterial life. *Nat. Rev. Microbiol.* **2016**, *14*, 563–575. [CrossRef] [PubMed]

4. Struzycka, I. The oral microbiome in dental caries. *Pol. J. Microbiol.* **2014**, *63*, 127–135. [PubMed]

5. Sitkiewicz, I. How to become a killer, or is it all accidental? Virulence strategies in oral streptococci. *Mol. Oral Microbiol.* **2018**, *33*, 1–12. [CrossRef] [PubMed]

6. Whiley, R.A.; Beighton, D. Current classification of the oral streptococci. *Oral Microbiol. Immunol.* **1998**, *13*, 195–216. [CrossRef] [PubMed]

7. Krzysciak, W.; Pluskwa, K.K.; Jurczak, A.; Koscielniak, D. The pathogenicity of the streptococcus genus. *Eur. J. Clin. Microbiol. Infect. Dis.* **2013**, *32*, 1361–1376. [CrossRef] [PubMed]

8. Richards, V.P.; Palmer, S.R.; Pavinski Bitar, P.D.; Qin, X.; Weinstock, G.M.; Highlander, S.K.; Town, C.D.; Burne, R.A.; Stanhope, M.J. Phylogenomics and the dynamic genome evolution of the genus streptococcus. *Genome Biol. Evol.* **2014**, *6*, 741–753. [CrossRef] [PubMed]

9. Frandsen, E.V.; Pedrazzoli, V.; Kilian, M. Ecology of viridans streptococci in the oral cavity and pharynx. *Oral Microbiol. Immunol.* **1991**, *6*, 129–133. [CrossRef] [PubMed]

10. Abranches, J.; Zeng, L.; Kajfasz, J.K.; Palmer, S.R.; Chakraborty, B.; Wen, Z.T.; Richards, V.P.; Brady, L.J.; Lemos, J.A. Biology of oral streptococci. *Microbiol. Spectr.* **2018**, *6*. [CrossRef]

11. Kim, S.L.; Gordon, S.M.; Shrestha, N.K. Distribution of streptococcal groups causing infective endocarditis: A descriptive study. *Diagn Microbiol. Infect. Dis.* **2018**, *91*, 269–272. [CrossRef] [PubMed]

12. Smith, E.G.; Spatafora, G.A. Gene regulation in s. Mutans: Complex control in a complex environment. *J. Dent. Res.* **2012**, *91*, 133–141. [CrossRef] [PubMed]

13. Ng, K.W.; Mukhopadhyay, A. Streptococcus constellatus bacteremia causing septic shock following tooth extraction: A case report. *Cases J.* **2009**, *2*, 6493. [CrossRef] [PubMed]

14. Tran, M.P.; Caldwell-McMillan, M.; Khalife, W.; Young, V.B. Streptococcus intermedius causing infective endocarditis and abscesses: A report of three cases and review of the literature. *BMC Infect. Dis.* **2008**, *8*, 154. [CrossRef] [PubMed]

15. Neumayr, A.; Kubitz, R.; Bode, J.G.; Bilk, B.; Haussinger, D. Multiple liver abscesses with isolation of streptococcus intermedius related to a pyogenic dental infection in an immuno-competent patient. *Eur J. Med. Res.* **2010**, *15*, 319–322. [CrossRef] [PubMed]

16. Whiley, R.A.; Beighton, D.; Winstanley, T.G.; Fraser, H.Y.; Hardie, J.M. Streptococcus intermedius, streptococcus constellatus, and streptococcus anginosus (the streptococcus milleri group): Association with different body sites and clinical infections. *J. Clin. Microbiol.* **1992**, *30*, 243–244.

17. Fisher, L.E.; Russell, R.R. The isolation and characterization of milleri group streptococci from dental periapical abscesses. *J. Dent. Res.* **1993**, *72*, 1191–1193. [CrossRef]

18. Socransky, S.S.; Haffajee, A.D.; Cugini, M.A.; Smith, C.; Kent, R.L., Jr. Microbial complexes in subgingival plaque. *J. Clin. Periodontol* **1998**, *25*, 134–144. [CrossRef]

19. Burton, J.P.; Drummond, B.K.; Chilcott, C.N.; Tagg, J.R.; Thomson, W.M.; Hale, J.D.; Wescombe, P.A. Influence of the probiotic streptococcus salivarius strain m18 on indices of dental health in children: A randomized double-blind, placebo-controlled trial. *J. Med. Microbiol.* **2013**, *62*, 875–884. [CrossRef]
20. Nobbs, A.H.; Jenkinson, H.F.; Everett, D.B. Generic determinants of streptococcus colonization and infection. *Infect. Genet. Evol.* **2015**, *33*, 361–370. [CrossRef]
21. Cunningham, M.W. Pathogenesis of group a streptococcal infections and their sequelae. *Adv. Exp. Med. Biol* **2008**, *609*, 29–42. [PubMed]
22. Brady, L.J.; Maddocks, S.E.; Larson, M.R.; Forsgren, N.; Persson, K.; Deivanayagam, C.C.; Jenkinson, H.F. The changing faces of streptococcus antigen i/ii polypeptide family adhesins. *Mol. Microbiol.* **2010**, *77*, 276–286. [CrossRef] [PubMed]
23. Nobbs, A.H.; Lamont, R.J.; Jenkinson, H.F. Streptococcus adherence and colonization. *Microbiol. Mol. Biol Rev.* **2009**, *73*, 407–450. [CrossRef] [PubMed]
24. Zhang, S.; Green, N.M.; Sitkiewicz, I.; Lefebvre, R.B.; Musser, J.M. Identification and characterization of an antigen i/ii family protein produced by group a streptococcus. *Infect. Immun.* **2006**, *74*, 4200–4213. [CrossRef] [PubMed]
25. Christie, J.; McNab, R.; Jenkinson, H.F. Expression of fibronectin-binding protein fbpa modulates adhesion in streptococcus gordonii. *Microbiology* **2002**, *148*, 1615–1625. [CrossRef] [PubMed]
26. Walker, M.J.; Barnett, T.C.; McArthur, J.D.; Cole, J.N.; Gillen, C.M.; Henningham, A.; Sriprakash, K.S.; Sanderson-Smith, M.L.; Nizet, V. Disease manifestations and pathogenic mechanisms of group a streptococcus. *Clin. Microbiol. Rev.* **2014**, *27*, 264–301. [CrossRef] [PubMed]
27. Yamaguchi, M.; Terao, Y.; Kawabata, S. Pleiotropic virulence factor-streptococcus pyogenes fibronectin-binding proteins. *Cell Microbiol.* **2013**, *15*, 503–511. [CrossRef]
28. Aviles-Reyes, A.; Miller, J.H.; Lemos, J.A.; Abranches, J. Collagen-binding proteins of streptococcus mutans and related streptococci. *Mol. Oral Microbiol.* **2017**, *32*, 89–106. [CrossRef]
29. Kahn, F.; Hurley, S.; Shannon, O. Platelets promote bacterial dissemination in a mouse model of streptococcal sepsis. *Microbes Infect.* **2013**, *15*, 669–676. [CrossRef]
30. Xiong, Y.Q.; Bensing, B.A.; Bayer, A.S.; Chambers, H.F.; Sullam, P.M. Role of the serine-rich surface glycoprotein gspb of streptococcus gordonii in the pathogenesis of infective endocarditis. *Microb. Pathog.* **2008**, *45*, 297–301. [CrossRef]
31. Kimura, K.R.; Nakata, M.; Sumitomo, T.; Kreikemeyer, B.; Podbielski, A.; Terao, Y.; Kawabata, S. Involvement of t6 pili in biofilm formation by serotype m6 streptococcus pyogenes. *J. Bacteriol.* **2012**, *194*, 804–812. [CrossRef] [PubMed]
32. Pezzicoli, A.; Santi, I.; Lauer, P.; Rosini, R.; Rinaudo, D.; Grandi, G.; Telford, J.L.; Soriani, M. Pilus backbone contributes to group b streptococcus paracellular translocation through epithelial cells. *J. Infect. Dis.* **2008**, *198*, 890–898. [CrossRef] [PubMed]
33. Maisey, H.C.; Hensler, M.; Nizet, V.; Doran, K.S. Group b streptococcal pilus proteins contribute to adherence to and invasion of brain microvascular endothelial cells. *J. Bacteriol.* **2007**, *189*, 1464–1467. [CrossRef] [PubMed]
34. Barocchi, M.A.; Ries, J.; Zogaj, X.; Hemsley, C.; Albiger, B.; Kanth, A.; Dahlberg, S.; Fernebro, J.; Moschioni, M.; Masignani, V.; et al. A pneumococcal pilus influences virulence and host inflammatory responses. *Proc. Natl. Acad. Sci. USA* **2006**, *103*, 2857–2862. [CrossRef] [PubMed]
35. Maisey, H.C.; Quach, D.; Hensler, M.E.; Liu, G.Y.; Gallo, R.L.; Nizet, V.; Doran, K.S. A group b streptococcal pilus protein promotes phagocyte resistance and systemic virulence. *FASEB J.* **2008**, *22*, 1715–1724. [CrossRef] [PubMed]
36. Jiang, S.; Park, S.E.; Yadav, P.; Paoletti, L.C.; Wessels, M.R. Regulation and function of pilus island 1 in group b streptococcus. *J. Bacteriol.* **2012**, *194*, 2479–2490. [CrossRef] [PubMed]
37. Gianfaldoni, C.; Censini, S.; Hilleringmann, M.; Moschioni, M.; Facciotti, C.; Pansegrau, W.; Masignani, V.; Covacci, A.; Rappuoli, R.; Barocchi, M.A.; et al. Streptococcus pneumoniae pilus subunits protect mice against lethal challenge. *Infect. Immun.* **2007**, *75*, 1059–1062. [CrossRef] [PubMed]
38. Nilson, B.H.; Frick, I.M.; Akesson, P.; Forsen, S.; Bjorck, L.; Akerstrom, B.; Wikstrom, M. Structure and stability of protein h and the m1 protein from streptococcus pyogenes. Implications for other surface proteins of gram-positive bacteria. *Biochemistry* **1995**, *34*, 13688–13698. [CrossRef]

39. McNamara, C.; Zinkernagel, A.S.; Macheboeuf, P.; Cunningham, M.W.; Nizet, V.; Ghosh, P. Coiled-coil irregularities and instabilities in group a streptococcus m1 are required for virulence. *Science* **2008**, *319*, 1405–1408. [CrossRef]

40. Smeesters, P.R.; McMillan, D.J.; Sriprakash, K.S. The streptococcal m protein: A highly versatile molecule. *Trends Microbiol.* **2010**, *18*, 275–282. [CrossRef]

41. Pahlman, L.I.; Olin, A.I.; Darenberg, J.; Morgelin, M.; Kotb, M.; Herwald, H.; Norrby-Teglund, A. Soluble m1 protein of streptococcus pyogenes triggers potent t cell activation. *Cell Microbiol.* **2008**, *10*, 404–414. [CrossRef] [PubMed]

42. Henningham, A.; Chiarot, E.; Gillen, C.M.; Cole, J.N.; Rohde, M.; Fulde, M.; Ramachandran, V.; Cork, A.J.; Hartas, J.; Magor, G.; et al. Conserved anchorless surface proteins as group a streptococcal vaccine candidates. *J. Mol. Med.* **2012**, *90*, 1197–1207. [CrossRef] [PubMed]

43. Antikainen, J.; Kuparinen, V.; Lahteenmaki, K.; Korhonen, T.K. Enolases from gram-positive bacterial pathogens and commensal lactobacilli share functional similarity in virulence-associated traits. *FEMS Immunol. Med. Microbiol.* **2007**, *51*, 526–534. [CrossRef] [PubMed]

44. Nelson, D.C.; Garbe, J.; Collin, M. Cysteine proteinase speb from streptococcus pyogenes-a potent modifier of immunologically important host and bacterial proteins. *Biol Chem.* **2011**, *392*, 1077–1088. [CrossRef] [PubMed]

45. Tamura, F.; Nakagawa, R.; Akuta, T.; Okamoto, S.; Hamada, S.; Maeda, H.; Kawabata, S.; Akaike, T. Proapoptotic effect of proteolytic activation of matrix metalloproteinases by streptococcus pyogenes thiol proteinase (streptococcus pyrogenic exotoxin b). *Infect. Immun.* **2004**, *72*, 4836–4847. [CrossRef] [PubMed]

46. Barnett, T.C.; Liebl, D.; Seymour, L.M.; Gillen, C.M.; Lim, J.Y.; Larock, C.N.; Davies, M.R.; Schulz, B.L.; Nizet, V.; Teasdale, R.D.; et al. The globally disseminated m1t1 clone of group a streptococcus evades autophagy for intracellular replication. *Cell Host Microbe* **2013**, *14*, 675–682. [CrossRef]

47. Morefield, G.; Touhey, G.; Lu, F.; Dunham, A.; HogenEsch, H. Development of a recombinant fusion protein vaccine formulation to protect against streptococcus pyogenes. *Vaccine* **2014**, *32*, 3810–3815. [CrossRef]

48. Brown, C.K.; Gu, Z.Y.; Matsuka, Y.V.; Purushothaman, S.S.; Winter, L.A.; Cleary, P.P.; Olmsted, S.B.; Ohlendorf, D.H.; Earhart, C.A. Structure of the streptococcal cell wall c5a peptidase. *Proc. Natl. Acad. Sci. USA* **2005**, *102*, 18391–18396. [CrossRef]

49. Sagar, V.; Bergmann, R.; Nerlich, A.; McMillan, D.J.; Nitsche Schmitz, D.P.; Chhatwal, G.S. Variability in the distribution of genes encoding virulence factors and putative extracellular proteins of streptococcus pyogenes in india, a region with high streptococcal disease burden, and implication for development of a regional multisubunit vaccine. *Clin. Vaccine Immunol.* **2012**, *19*, 1818–1825. [CrossRef]

50. Tamura, G.S.; Hull, J.R.; Oberg, M.D.; Castner, D.G. High-affinity interaction between fibronectin and the group b streptococcal c5a peptidase is unaffected by a naturally occurring four-amino-acid deletion that eliminates peptidase activity. *Infect. Immun.* **2006**, *74*, 5739–5746. [CrossRef]

51. Cheng, Q.; Stafslien, D.; Purushothaman, S.S.; Cleary, P. The group b streptococcal c5a peptidase is both a specific protease and an invasin. *Infect. Immun.* **2002**, *70*, 2408–2413. [CrossRef] [PubMed]

52. Flemming, H.C.; Wingender, J. The biofilm matrix. *Nat. Rev. Microbiol.* **2010**, *8*, 623–633. [CrossRef] [PubMed]

53. Li, Y.H.; Lau, P.C.; Lee, J.H.; Ellen, R.P.; Cvitkovitch, D.G. Natural genetic transformation of streptococcus mutans growing in biofilms. *J. Bacteriol.* **2001**, *183*, 897–908. [CrossRef] [PubMed]

54. Jakobsen, T.H.; Tolker-Nielsen, T.; Givskov, M. Bacterial biofilm control by perturbation of bacterial signaling processes. *Int J. Mol. Sci.* **2017**, *18*, 1970. [CrossRef] [PubMed]

55. McDougald, D.; Rice, S.A.; Barraud, N.; Steinberg, P.D.; Kjelleberg, S. Should we stay or should we go: Mechanisms and ecological consequences for biofilm dispersal. *Nat. Rev. Microbiol.* **2011**, *10*, 39–50. [CrossRef] [PubMed]

56. Romling, U.; Galperin, M.Y.; Gomelsky, M. Cyclic di-gmp: The first 25 years of a universal bacterial second messenger. *Microbiol. Mol. Biol Rev.* **2013**, *77*, 1–52. [CrossRef] [PubMed]

57. Okshevsky, M.; Regina, V.R.; Meyer, R.L. Extracellular DNA as a target for biofilm control. *Curr. Opin. Biotechnol.* **2015**, *33*, 73–80. [CrossRef]

58. Whitchurch, C.B.; Tolker-Nielsen, T.; Ragas, P.C.; Mattick, J.S. Extracellular DNA required for bacterial biofilm formation. *Science* **2002**, *295*, 1487. [CrossRef]

59. Jakubovics, N.S.; Burgess, J.G. Extracellular DNA in oral microbial biofilms. *Microbes Infect.* **2015**, *17*, 531–537. [CrossRef]

60. Nur, A.; Hirota, K.; Yumoto, H.; Hirao, K.; Liu, D.; Takahashi, K.; Murakami, K.; Matsuo, T.; Shu, R.; Miyake, Y. Effects of extracellular DNA and DNA-binding protein on the development of a streptococcus intermedius biofilm. *J. Appl. Microbiol.* **2013**, *115*, 260–270. [CrossRef]

61. Jung, C.J.; Hsu, R.B.; Shun, C.T.; Hsu, C.C.; Chia, J.S. Atla mediates extracellular DNA release, which contributes to streptococcus mutans biofilm formation in an experimental rat model of infective endocarditis. *Infect. Immun.* **2017**, *85*, e00252-17. [CrossRef]

62. Liu, D.; Yumoto, H.; Hirota, K.; Murakami, K.; Takahashi, K.; Hirao, K.; Matsuo, T.; Ohkura, K.; Nagamune, H.; Miyake, Y. Histone-like DNA binding protein of streptococcus intermedius induces the expression of pro-inflammatory cytokines in human monocytes via activation of erk1/2 and jnk pathways. *Cell Microbiol.* **2008**, *10*, 262–276. [CrossRef]

63. Liu, D.; Yumoto, H.; Murakami, K.; Hirota, K.; Ono, T.; Nagamune, H.; Kayama, S.; Matsuo, T.; Miyake, Y. The essentiality and involvement of streptococcus intermedius histone-like DNA-binding protein in bacterial viability and normal growth. *Mol. Microbiol.* **2008**, *68*, 1268–1282. [CrossRef] [PubMed]

64. Brown, L.; Wolf, J.M.; Prados-Rosales, R.; Casadevall, A. Through the wall: Extracellular vesicles in gram-positive bacteria, mycobacteria and fungi. *Nat. Rev. Microbiol.* **2015**, *13*, 620–630. [CrossRef] [PubMed]

65. Kim, J.H.; Lee, J.; Park, J.; Gho, Y.S. Gram-negative and gram-positive bacterial extracellular vesicles. *Semin Cell Dev. Biol* **2015**, *40*, 97–104. [CrossRef]

66. Toyofuku, M.; Tashiro, Y.; Hasegawa, Y.; Kurosawa, M.; Nomura, N. Bacterial membrane vesicles, an overlooked environmental colloid: Biology, environmental perspectives and applications. *Adv. Colloid Interface Sci.* **2015**, *226*, 65–77. [CrossRef]

67. Brinkmann, V.; Reichard, U.; Goosmann, C.; Fauler, B.; Uhlemann, Y.; Weiss, D.S.; Weinrauch, Y.; Zychlinsky, A. Neutrophil extracellular traps kill bacteria. *Science* **2004**, *303*, 1532–1535. [CrossRef] [PubMed]

68. Liu, J.; Sun, L.; Liu, W.; Guo, L.; Liu, Z.; Wei, X.; Ling, J. A nuclease from streptococcus mutans facilitates biofilm dispersal and escape from killing by neutrophil extracellular traps. *Front. Cell Infect. Microbiol.* **2017**, *7*, 97. [CrossRef] [PubMed]

69. Mitchell, T.J. The pathogenesis of streptococcal infections: From tooth decay to meningitis. *Nat. Rev. Microbiol.* **2003**, *1*, 219–230. [CrossRef] [PubMed]

70. Nakano, K.; Hokamura, K.; Taniguchi, N.; Wada, K.; Kudo, C.; Nomura, R.; Kojima, A.; Naka, S.; Muranaka, Y.; Thura, M.; et al. The collagen-binding protein of streptococcus mutans is involved in haemorrhagic stroke. *Nat. Commun* **2011**, *2*, 485. [CrossRef] [PubMed]

71. Miyatani, F.; Kuriyama, N.; Watanabe, I.; Nomura, R.; Nakano, K.; Matsui, D.; Ozaki, E.; Koyama, T.; Nishigaki, M.; Yamamoto, T.; et al. Relationship between cnm-positive streptococcus mutans and cerebral microbleeds in humans. *Oral Dis* **2015**, *21*, 886–893. [CrossRef] [PubMed]

72. Kojima, A.; Nakano, K.; Wada, K.; Takahashi, H.; Katayama, K.; Yoneda, M.; Higurashi, T.; Nomura, R.; Hokamura, K.; Muranaka, Y.; et al. Infection of specific strains of streptococcus mutans, oral bacteria, confers a risk of ulcerative colitis. *Sci. Rep.* **2012**, *2*, 332. [CrossRef] [PubMed]

73. Misaki, T.; Naka, S.; Hatakeyama, R.; Fukunaga, A.; Nomura, R.; Isozaki, T.; Nakano, K. Presence of streptococcus mutans strains harbouring the cnm gene correlates with dental caries status and iga nephropathy conditions. *Sci. Rep.* **2016**, *6*, 36455. [CrossRef] [PubMed]

74. Otsugu, M.; Nomura, R.; Matayoshi, S.; Teramoto, N.; Nakano, K. Contribution of streptococcus mutans strains with collagen-binding proteins in the presence of serum to the pathogenesis of infective endocarditis. *Infect. Immun.* **2017**, *85*, e00401-17. [CrossRef]

75. Tsuneyama, K.; Harada, K.; Kono, N.; Hiramatsu, K.; Zen, Y.; Sudo, Y.; Gershwin, M.E.; Ikemoto, M.; Arai, H.; Nakanuma, Y. Scavenger cells with gram-positive bacterial lipoteichoic acid infiltrate around the damaged interlobular bile ducts of primary biliary cirrhosis. *J. Hepatol.* **2001**, *35*, 156–163. [CrossRef]

76. Haruta, I.; Hashimoto, E.; Kato, Y.; Kikuchi, K.; Kato, H.; Yagi, J.; Uchiyama, T.; Kobayash, M.; Shiratori, K. Lipoteichoic acid may affect the pathogenesis of bile duct damage in primary biliary cirrhosis. *Autoimmunity* **2006**, *39*, 129–135. [CrossRef] [PubMed]

77. Haruta, I.; Kikuchi, K.; Hashimoto, E.; Kato, H.; Hirota, K.; Kobayashi, M.; Miyake, Y.; Uchiyama, T.; Yagi, J.; Shiratori, K. A possible role of histone-like DNA-binding protein of streptococcus intermedius in the pathogenesis of bile duct damage in primary biliary cirrhosis. *Clin. Immunol.* **2008**, *127*, 245–251. [CrossRef]

78. Haruta, I.; Kikuchi, K.; Hashimoto, E.; Nakamura, M.; Miyakawa, H.; Hirota, K.; Shibata, N.; Kato, H.; Arimura, Y.; Kato, Y.; et al. Long-term bacterial exposure can trigger nonsuppurative destructive cholangitis associated with multifocal epithelial inflammation. *Lab. Invest.* **2010**, *90*, 577–588. [CrossRef]

79. Haruta, I.; Kikuchi, K.; Nakamura, M.; Hirota, K.; Kato, H.; Miyakawa, H.; Shibata, N.; Miyake, Y.; Hashimoto, E.; Shiratori, K.; et al. Involvement of commensal bacteria may lead to dysregulated inflammatory and autoimmune responses in a mouse model for chronic nonsuppurative destructive cholangitis. *J. Clin. Immunol.* **2012**, *32*, 1026–1037. [CrossRef]

14

The Biological Efficacy of Natural Products against Acute and Chronic Inflammatory Diseases in the Oral Region

Toshiaki Ara [1]⊙, **Sachie Nakatani** [2], **Kenji Kobata** [2], **Norio Sogawa** [1] **and Chiharu Sogawa** [3],*⊙

[1] Department of Dental Pharmacology, Matsumoto Dental University, 1780 Gobara Hirooka, Shiojiri 399-0781, Japan; toshiaki.ara@mdu.ac.jp (T.A.); norio.sogawa@mdu.ac.jp (N.S.)

[2] Faculty of Pharmacy and Pharmaceutical Sciences, Josai University, 1-1 Keyakidai, Sakado, Saitama 350-0295, Japan; s-nakata@josai.ac.jp (S.N); kobata@josai.ac.jp (K.K.)

[3] Department of Dental Pharmacology, Okayama University Graduate School of Medicine, Dentistry and Pharmaceutical Sciences, 2-5-1 Shikata-cho, Okayama 700-8525, Japan

* Correspondence: caoki@md.okayama-u.ac.jp

Abstract: The oral inflammatory diseases are divided into two types: acute and chronic inflammatory diseases. In this review, we summarize the biological efficacy of herbal medicine, natural products, and their active ingredients against acute and chronic inflammatory diseases in the oral region, especially stomatitis and periodontitis. We review the effects of herbal medicines and a biscoclaurin alkaloid preparation, cepharamthin, as a therapy against stomatitis, an acute inflammatory disease. We also summarize the effects of herbal medicines and natural products against periodontitis, a chronic inflammatory disease, and one of its clinical conditions, alveolar bone resorption. Recent studies show that several herbal medicines such as kakkonto and ninjinto reduce LPS-induced PGE_2 production by human gingival fibroblasts. Among herbs constituting these herbal medicines, shokyo (*Zingiberis Rhizoma*) and kankyo (*Zingiberis Processum Rhizoma*) strongly reduce PGE_2 production. Moreover, anti-osteoclast activity has been observed in some natural products with anti-inflammatory effects used against rheumatoid arthritis such as carotenoids, flavonoids, limonoids, and polyphenols. These herbal medicines and natural products could be useful for treating oral inflammatory diseases.

Keywords: inflammatory disease; stomatitis; periodontitis; anti-osteoclast activity; cepharanthin; herbal medicine; natural product; arachidonic acid cascade

1. Introduction

Oral inflammatory disease is a general term for the inflammatory lesions developed in oral mucosa. The pathogenesis of oral inflammatory diseases is non-uniform due to the involvement of various factors—such as external and mechanical stimuli, the presence of microorganisms, and the overall physical conditions—that play a role in the onset of inflammation. There is a wide range of variations in the aspect of oral inflammatory diseases, and the aspect is unequal. Therefore, we construed the oral inflammatory diseases as a symptom of inflammation, and categorized them into acute and chronic inflammatory diseases. In the oral region, the representative example of acute inflammatory diseases is stomatitis (also named as oral mucositis), and that of chronic inflammatory diseases is periodontitis. Several Japanese herbal medicines (also known as kampo medicines) are clinically used for the treatment of inflammatory diseases. Recent reviews have summarized the therapeutic application of herbal medicines for oral diseases such as stomatitis and periodontitis [1]. For example, hangeshashinto (TJ-14) is used for inflammatory diseases such as acute or chronic gastrointestinal catarrh, nervous gastritis and stomatitis.

In this review, we aim to summarize the biological efficacy of herbal medicine, natural products, and their active ingredients against acute and chronic inflammatory diseases in the oral region, especially stomatitis and periodontitis.

2. Biological Efficacy of Natural Products against Acute Inflammatory Disease: Stomatitis

2.1. Stomatitis (Oral Mucositis)

Stomatitis is an inflammatory condition of the oral and oropharyngeal mucosa with both pain and ulcers in severe cases. The causes of stomatitis is classified into (1) bacterial or viral infection, (2) chemotherapy and/or radiation for the treatment of cancers, (3) autoimmune disease (such as lichen planus and pemphigus vulgaris), and (4) unknown (such as recurrent aphthous stomatitis). Recurrent aphthous stomatitis is a common condition characterized by the repeated formation of benign and non-contagious mouth ulcers (aphthae). However, the cause of aphthous stomatitis is still unknown.

2.2. Effect of Hangeshashinto on Stomatitis

Recently, clinical administration of herbal medicine, such as the treatment of recurrent aphthous stomatitis, has been increasing in Japan. Herbal medicines are chosen according to the patient's condition, called "sho" (pattern), for example "excess pattern" or "deficiency pattern." Among the herbal medicines, some products such as hangeshashinto (TJ-14), orengedokuto (TJ-15), orento (TJ-120), inchinkoto (TJ-135), byakkokaninjinto (TJ-34), juzentaihoto (TJ-48), and shosaikoto (TJ-9) are selected in the treatment against oral inflammatory diseases, including recurrent aphthous stomatitis, according to the patient's pattern [2]. In addition, it seems that hangeshashinto is considered effective in the treatment of stomatitis caused by anti-tumor agents and radiation therapy [2].

In a preliminary study, rinsing with hangeshashinto reduced the grade of stomatitis [by Common Terminology Criteria for Adverse Events (CTCAE) version 4.0, National Cancer Institute, Bethesda, MD] [3]. Moreover, in a double-blind, placebo-controlled, random, phase II study, the rinsing of the oral cavity with hangeshashinto showed a trend to reduce the risk of chemotherapy-induced stomatitis in patients with gastric cancer [4]. In this study, hangeshashinto reduced the risk of grade 1 stomatitis but did not reduce those of more than grade 2 [4]. In a retrospective study, rinsing and gargling with hangeshashinto prevented grade 3/4 stomatitis induced by (chemo)radiation in patients with head and neck cancers (odds ratio = 0.21, 95% CI: 0.045–0.780, hangeshashinto: $n = 27$, placebo: $n = 32$) [5]. In addition, hangeshashinto also improved the rates of the treatment of stomatitis [5].

In an animal model, free intake of diet mixed with 2% hangeshashinto prevented radiation-induced mucositis within the buccal mucosa in hamsters [6]. In addition, hangeshashinto inhibited the infiltration of neutrophils and COX-2 expression in irradiated buccal mucosa [6]. Moreover, in an in vitro study using oral keratinocytes, hangeshashinto was suggested to be effective in the treatment of chemotherapy-induced stomatitis [7]. As just described, hangeshashinto is effective for the improvement of stomatitis although there is little evidence in in vivo and in vitro studies.

2.3. Effect of Cepharanthin® on Stomatitis

A biscoclaurin alkaloid preparation, Cepharanthin® (CE), has also been used for the cure of oral mucosal disease, such as recurrent aphthous stomatitis, leukoplakia, and oral lichen planus. CE is a drug product, prepared from extracts of *Stephania cephalantha* Hayata, and has been widely used for several decades to treat a range of acute and chronic diseases in Japan [8,9]. As CE is reported to elicit an anti-inflammatory effect and increase blood stem cell count, immuno-enhancing effects, and anti-allergic properties, it has seen clinical application against inflammatory diseases as well as post-radiation-therapy leukocytopenia, pit viper bite, alopecia areata, and bronchial asthma. Nakase et al. reported that the rate of excellent or moderate efficacy was 100% for aphthous stomatitis and 25.0% for reducing the size of oral lichen planus, and its efficacy for glossodynia was 83.4% by CE treatment with gargle-internal use (15 mg/day) for two weeks [10]. Moreover, Saki et al. also reported—regarding the efficacy of CE against these oral mucosal diseases— that the improvement rate by oral administration of CE (20 mg/day) for 4 weeks or more was 83.3% for aphthous stomatitis, 87.0% for oral lichen planus, 77.8% for glossodynia, and 80.0% for leukoplakia. In this case, they evaluated the clinical response and rated according to the assessment points such as the degrees of pain, ulcer, erosion, and erythema [11]. Taken together, it is considered that CE is beneficial in the cure of aphthous stomatitis, according to previous clinical reports [12].

CE is a biscoclaurin alkaloid preparation, and the main active ingredients are four alkaloids: cepharanthine (26%), isotetrandrine (32%), berbamine (13%), and cycleanine (10%) (Figure 1). Using a mixture of these four active ingredients in CE exhibits almost an equal effect as that of CE [13,14]. Functional mechanisms of CE and its main active ingredients for inflammatory diseases have been reported in previous studies. For example, CE reduced the production of superoxide anion (O_2^-) by neutrophils [15] and by macrophages [16], and decreased the levels of several types of reactive oxygen species (O_2^-, H_2O_2, $OH^{\cdot}$) by behaving as a reactive oxygen species (ROS) scavenger [17].

cepharanthine

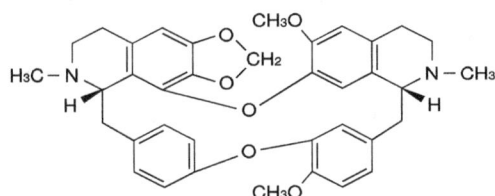

isotetrandrine

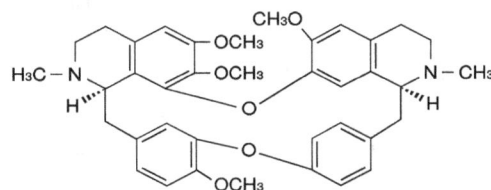

cycleanine

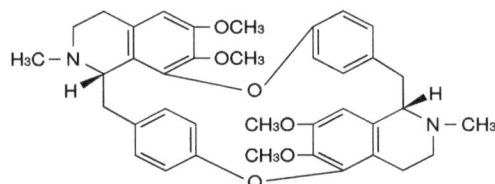

berbamine

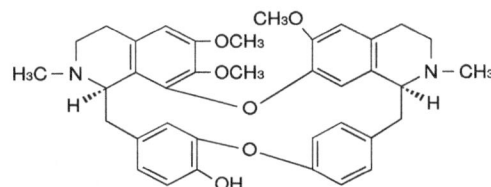

Figure 1. The structures of active ingredients in Cepharanthin®.

According to previous literatures corresponding to the application of the four main active ingredients, cepharanthine was reported to inhibit the synthesis of leukotriene B4 through the reduction of arachidonic acid release [18]. Moreover, each of the four main active ingredients reduced NO production by activated macrophages [19]. However, there was a difference in the efficacy against the O_2^- and TNF-α production among main active ingredients; the efficacy of cepharanthine and isotetrandrine seemed to be more than that of berbamine and cycleanine in the reduction of O_2^- production by neutrophils [20]. It was also reported that cepharanthine, isotetrandrine, and cycleanine, but not berbamine, significantly reduced the level of TNF-α or acute lethal toxicity induced by lipopolysaccharide (LPS) in mice [13,21]. Additionally, Matsuno et al. reported that the decreasing effect of O_2^- production through neutrophil stimulation by arachidonic acid and N-formylmethionine-leucyl-phenylalanine (FMLP) was more evident in cepharanthine than in opsonized zymogen [20]. This finding indicates the cell membrane to be a possible operating point of CE, and this hypothesis is supported in the following study by Sugiyama et al., who reported that cepharanthine could inhibit histamine release from mast cells through the stabilization of the membrane by decreasing membrane fluidity via interaction with the lipid bilayer of the cell membrane [22].

Interestingly, the pharmacological actions of CE on living bodies vary depending on the method of administration. We reported that the single injection of CE reduced the LPS-induced histidine decarboxylase (HDC) activity, although contrastingly, LPS-induced HDC activity in mice spleens increased after consecutive administration of CE [23]. Moreover, it was considered that mast cell was closely associated with this reduction of HDC activity, because LPS-induced HDC activity in mast-cell-deficient mice increased, but decreased in normal mice following a single administration of CE [23]. CE has immuno-enhancing effects as well as anti-inflammatory effects. The inhibition of mast cells may be closely related to the difference of CE action.

Conclusively, CE is considered to be an effective treatment of oral inflammatory diseases, such as recurrent aphthous stomatitis, through the reduction of various function in immunocytes closely related to inflammation.

3. Biological Efficacy of Natural Products against Chronic Inflammatory Disease; Periodontitis

3.1. Periodontitis

Periodontal disease (periodontitis) comprises a group of infections that leads to inflammation of the gingiva and destruction of periodontal tissues, and is accompanied by alveolar bone loss in severe clinical cases. The tissue destruction is the result of activation of the host's immuno-inflammatory response to virulent factors such as LPS and peptidoglycan. In inflammatory responses and tissue degradation, prostaglandin E_2 (PGE_2), interleukin (IL)-6, and IL-8 play important roles. As PGE_2 has several functions in vasodilation, the enhancement of vascular permeability and pain, and osteoclastogenesis induction, PGE_2 participates in inflammatory responses and alveolar bone resorption in periodontitis [24].

Generally, periodontitis is a chronic inflammation, and the elimination of these virulent factors by initial preparation is very important for the treatment of periodontitis. However, during the acute advanced stage, non-steroidal anti-inflammatory drugs (NSAIDs) are administrated to improve gingival inflammation. In fact, many studies have demonstrated that systemic administration of acid NSAIDs prevented gingival inflammation and alveolar bone resorption in animals and humans [25]. However, acid NSAIDs are well known to have side effects such as gastrointestinal dysfunction and bronchoconstriction. Therefore, the usage of alternative agents is necessary for patients with gastrointestinal ulcer or bronchial asthma. Previously, we suggested that several herbal medicines are effective for the improvement of periodontitis. In this review, we focused on the anti-inflammatory effects of herbal medicines on mainly periodontitis —in particular, about the effects on human gingival fibroblasts (HGFs). In addition, we summarized the effects of ingredients in herbs and their mechanism against arachidonic acid cascade.

Here, we will explain the importance of HGFs in the study of periodontitis. (1) HGFs are the most prominent cells in periodontal tissue. LPS-treated HGFs produce inflammatory chemical mediators, such as PGE_2, and inflammatory cytokines such as IL-6 and IL-8. (2) More importantly, unlike macrophages, HGFs continue to produce PGE_2 [26], IL-6, and IL-8 [27] in the presence of LPS. From these findings, the large amount of chemical mediators and cytokines derived from HGFs may be contained in periodontal tissues. Therefore, we believe that examining the effects of pharmaceuticals on HGFs is needed in the study of periodontitis.

3.2. Brief Summary of Arachidonic Acid Cascade

At first, we explain arachidonic acid cascade briefly, focusing on sites of action for herbs and ingredients. PGE_2 is produced by arachidonic acid cascade (Figure 2). Phospholipids in plasma membrane are digested by phospholipase A_2 (PLA_2), producing arachidonic acid. Cyclooxygenases (COXs) convert arachidonic acid into PGH_2, and thereafter PGE synthase converts into PGE_2.

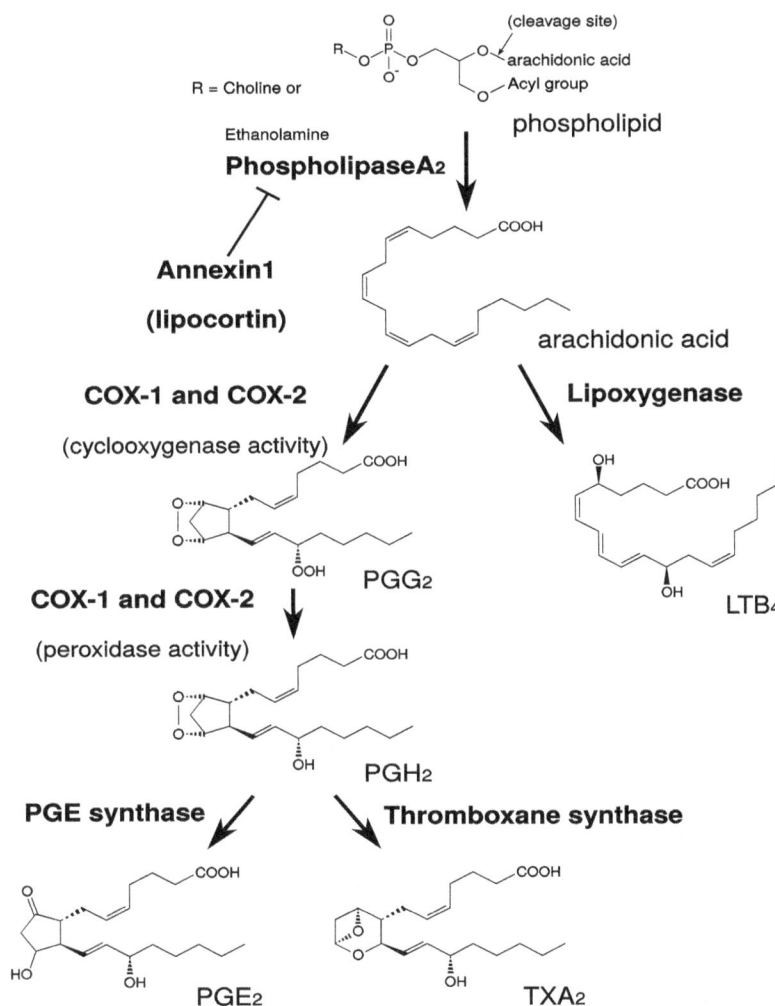

Figure 2. Simplified schema of arachidonic acid cascade.

PLA$_2$ is the most upstream enzyme in the arachidonic acid cascade and releases arachidonic acid from the plasma membrane. PLA$_2$ forms a superfamily and is classified into cytosolic PLA$_2$ (cPLA$_2$), calcium-independent PLA$_2$ (iPLA$_2$), secretory PLA$_2$ (sPLA$_2$), and others [28]. Among these isoforms, cPLA$_2$ is the primary isoform in HGFs from the results using PLA$_2$ inhibitors [29]. cPLA$_2$ activity is directly regulated by extracellular signal-regulated kinase (ERK). The active form of ERK (phosphorylated ERK) phosphorylates Ser505 of cPLA$_2$ and activates cPLA$_2$ [30–32]. Therefore, the suppression of ERK phosphorylation leads to the suppression of cPLA$_2$ activation and the reduction of PGE$_2$ production [30–32]. In contrast, annexin1, also named as lipocortin, is an anti-inflammatory mediator produced by steroidal anti-inflammatory drugs (SAIDs) that inhibits PLA$_2$ activity [33,34].

COX is classified into COX-1 and COX-2. COX-1 is constitutive expressed at low level, and is involved in normal functions such as protection of gastric mucosa. In contrast, COX-2 is induced by the various stimuli such as LPS and peptidoglycan, and involved in inflammatory response. The expression of COX-2 is upregulated by NF-κB. The reduction of PGE$_2$ by anti-inflammatory drugs is one of the important mechanisms. Acid NSAIDs inhibit both COX-1 and COX-2 activities. The inhibition of COX-2 improve inflammatory response, while the inhibition of COX-1 causes gastric irritation. SAIDs also have powerful anti-inflammatory effects, and inhibit NF-κB activity and suppress COX-2 expression.

Recently, protein kinase A (PKA) pathway is reported to regulate LPS-induce PGE$_2$ production in HGFs [35]. PKA inhibitor (H-89) reduced LPS-induced PGE$_2$ production in a concentration-dependent manner. In contrast, PKA activator (dibutyryl cAMP; dbcAMP) and drugs which increased intracellular cAMP (adrenaline and aminophylline) increased LPS-induced PGE$_2$ production in a concentration-dependent manner. However, the effects of PKA pathway on arachidonic acid cascade have not been examined in this report [35].

3.3. Effect of Herbal Medicines on Periosontal Disease

Similar to NSAIDs, several herbal medicines also reduce PGE_2 production. Examples of herbal medicine which have been reported to reduce PGE_2 production in in vitro and/or animal models are shown in Table 1. In particular, we reported that kakkonto (TJ-1), shosaikoto (TJ-9), hangeshashinto (TJ-14), shinbuto (TJ-30), ninjinto (TJ-32), and orento (TJ-120) reduced LPS-induced PGE_2 production using HGFs [36–40]. Other groups have also demonstrated that several herbal medicines reduced PGE_2 production using human periodontal ligament cells [41], human monocytes [42], mouse macrophage RAW264.7 cells [43,44], human oral keratinocytes [7], and animals [45–48].

Table 1. Japanese traditional herbal medicines which are reported to reduce PGE_2 production.

Herbal Medicine	Cells or Animal	References
kakkonto (TJ-1)	HGFs	[36]
shosaikoto (TJ-9)	HGFs	[37]
	human monocytes	[42]
	mouse	[45]
hangeshashinto (TJ-14)	HGFs	[38,41]
	human periodontal ligament cells	[41]
	human oral keratinocytes	[7]
	rat	[46–48]
shinbuto (TJ-30)	HGFs	[39]
ninjinto (TJ-32)	HGFs	[39]
rikkosan (TJ-110)	RAW264.7	[43]
saireito (TJ-114)	RAW264.7	[44]
orento (TJ-120)	HGFs	[40]

We introduce briefly the effects and mechanisms of herbal medicines on periodontitis in clinical, animal, and/or in vitro studies. Moreover, in this section, we will demonstrate the effects of herbal medicines on the reduction of PGE_2 in HGFs. From our data, the mechanisms of these herbal medicines on arachidonic acid cascade are divided into three groups as follows.

- Shosaikoto (TJ-9) inhibited COX-2 activity and suppressed COX-2 expression, but did not alter $cPLA_2$ expression (the effects on annexin1 expression and ERK phosphorylation were not examined) [37]. Hangeshashinto (TJ-14) inhibited both COX-1 and COX-2 activities, and suppressed $cPLA_2$ and COX-2 expressions and ERK phosphorylation [38]. Therefore, these herbal medicines are suggested to inhibit arachidonic acid cascade at multiple points.

- Shinbuto (TJ-30) and ninjinto (TJ-32) enhanced annexin1 expression, but did not alter ERK phosphorylation and COX activity [39]. However, the contribution of enhancement of annexin1 expression is considered to be small because shokyo, which is the main herb in shinbuto to reduce PGE_2 production, did not affect annexin1 expression.

- Kakkonto (TJ-1) suppressed ERK phosphorylation, but neither inhibited COXs activities nor suppressed the expression of molecules in arachidonic acid cascade [36]. In addition, orento (TJ-120) suppressed ERK phosphorylation, but neither inhibited COXs activities nor suppressed the expression of molecules in arachidonic acid cascade, but rather increased COX-2 expression [40]. However, its contribution in the suppression of ERK phosphorylation is considered to be small as described at keihi (*Cinnamomi Cortex*). Indeed, we did not examine the direct effect of herbal medicines on $cPLA_2$ activity. Nevertheless, we consider that these herbal medicines inhibit $cPLA_2$ activity and that this effect is due to shokyo (*Zingiberis Rhizoma*) and kankyo (*Zingiberis Processum Rhizoma*) as described below.

3.4. Effect of Herbs on Arachidonic Acid Cascade

Next, we will demonstrate the experimental results at the herb level. The ingredients in the formula of herbal medicines that were used are shown in Tables 2–7. In our experiments at the herb level, shokyo (*Zingiberis Rhizoma*), kankyo (*Zingiberis Processum Rhizoma*), kanzo (*Glycyrrhizae Radix*), and keihi (*Cinnamomi Cortex*) reduced PGE$_2$ production (Figures 3 and 4) [29,39]. We summarized major ingredients in herbs and their mechanism against arachidonic acid cascade in Table 8. In addition to these four herbs, ogon (*Scutellariae Radix*), and oren (*Coptidis Rhizoma*) are shown in Table 8 because ogon (included in shosaikoto and hangeshashinto) and oren (included in hangeshashinto and orento) also have several bioactive ingredients such as flavonoids, saponin, and chalcones. We will describe the effects and mechanisms of these herbs, particularly shokyo and kankyo, on arachidonic cascade.

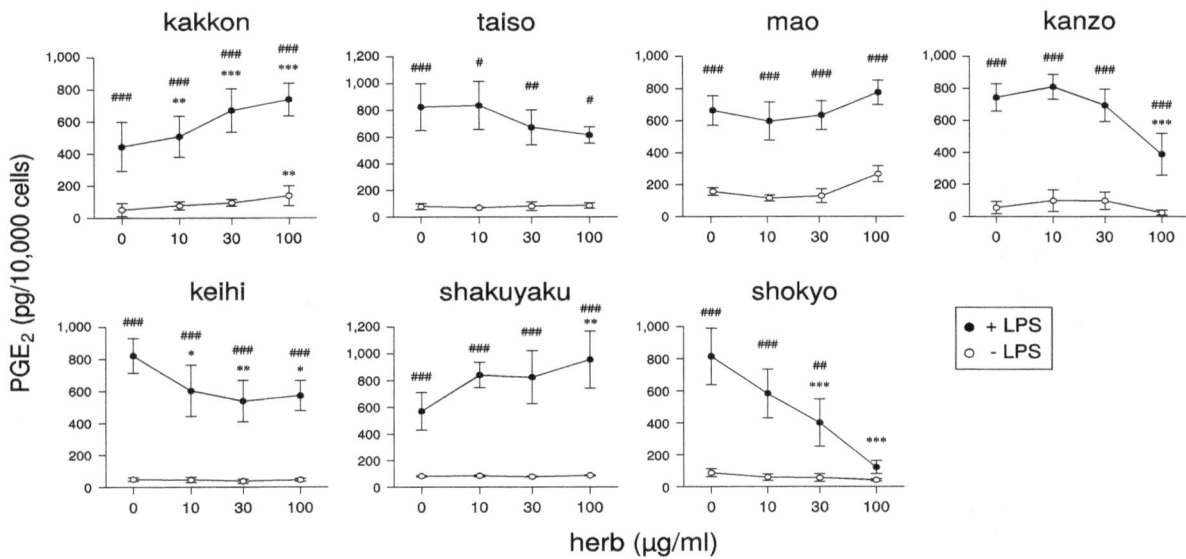

Figure 3. The effect of herbs in kakkonto (TJ-1) on PGE$_2$ production: This figure is cited from Ara and Sogawa [29] (CC-BY-4.0) and modified for this review.

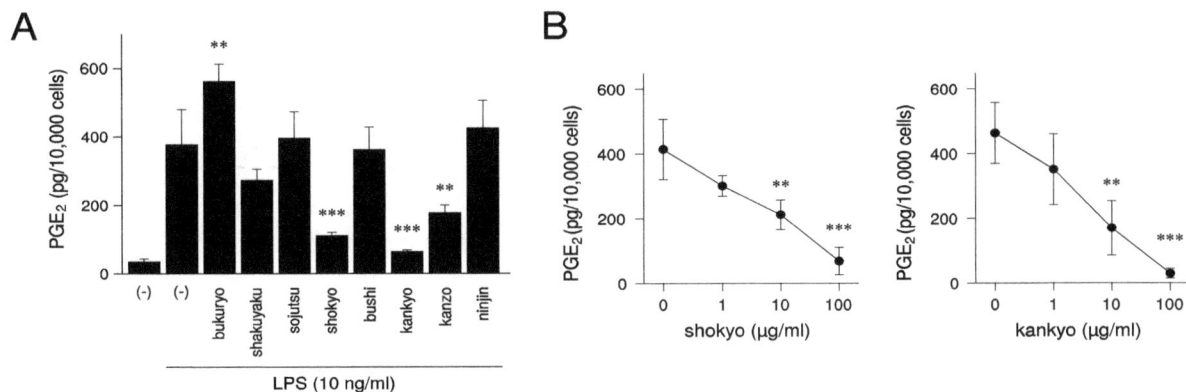

Figure 4. The effect of herbs in shinbuto (TJ-30) and ninjinto (TJ-32) on PGE$_2$ production: This figure is cited from Ara and Sogawa [39] (CC-BY-4.0) and modified for this review. (**A**): Effect of each herb, (**B**): Concentration-dependent effects of shokyo and kankyo.

Table 2. The ingredients in the kakkonto (TJ-1) formula.

Japanese Name (Latin Name)	Scientific Name	Amount (g)	Amount * (g/g of Product)
kakkon (*Puerariae Radix*)	*Pueraria lobata* Ohwi	4.0	0.111
taiso (*Zizyphi Fructus*)	*Ziziphus jujuba* Miller var. *inermis* Rehder	3.0	0.083
mao (*Ephedrae Herba*)	*Ephedra sinica* Stapf *Ephedra intermedia* Schrenk et C.A.Meyer *Ephedra equisetina* Bunge	3.0	0.083
kanzo (*Glycyrrhizae Radix*)	*Glycyrrhiza uralensis* Fischer *Glycyrrhiza glabra* Linné	2.0	0.056
keihi (*Cinnamomi Cortex*)	*Cinnamomum cassia* Blume	2.0	0.056
shyakuyaku (*Paeoniae Radix*)	*Paeonia lactiflora* Pallas	2.0	0.056
shokyo (*Zingiberis Rhizoma*)	*Zingiber officinale* Roscoe	2.0	0.056
total		18.0	0.500

* 7.5 g of kakkonto product contains 3.75 g of a dried extract of the mixed crude drugs.

Table 3. The ingredients in the shosaikoto (TJ-9) formula.

Japanese Name (Latin Name)	Scientific Name	Amount (g)	Amount * (g/g of Product)
saiko (*Bupleuri Radix*)	*Bupleurum falcatum* Linné	7.0	0.175
hange (*Pinelliae tuber*)	*Pinellia ternata* Breitenbach	5.0	0.125
ogon (*Scutellariae radix*)	*Scutellaria baicalensis* Georgi	3.0	0.075
taiso (*Zizyphi Fructus*)	*Ziziphus jujuba* Miller var. *inermis* Rehder	3.0	0.075
ninjin (*Ginseng Radix*)	*Panax ginseng* C.A. Meyer	3.0	0.075
kanzo (*Glycyrrhizae Radix*)	*Glycyrrhiza uralensis* Fischer *Glycyrrhiza glabra* Linné	2.0	0.050
shokyo (*Zingiberis Rhizoma*)	*Zingiber officinale* Roscoe	1.0	0.025
total		24.0	0.600

* 7.5 g of shosaikoto product contains 4.5 g of a dried extract of the mixed crude drugs.

Table 4. The ingredients in the hangeshashinto (TJ-14) formula.

Japanese Name (Latin Name)	Scientific Name	Amount (g)	Amount * (g/g of Product)
hange (*Pinelliae tuber*)	*Pinellia ternata* Breitenbach	5.0	0.162
ogon (*Scutellariae radix*)	*Scutellaria baicalensis* Georgi	2.5	0.081
kankyo (*Zingiberis Processum Rhizoma*)	*Zingiber officinale* Roscoe	2.5	0.081
kanzo (*Glycyrrhizae Radix*)	*Glycyrrhiza uralensis* Fischer *Glycyrrhiza glabra* Linné	2.5	0.081
taiso (*Zizyphi Fructus*)	*Ziziphus jujuba* Miller var. *inermis* Rehder	2.5	0.081
ninjin (*Ginseng Radix*)	*Panax ginseng* C.A. Meyer	2.5	0.081
oren (*Coptidis rhizoma*)	*Coptis japonica* Makino *Coptis chinensis* Franchet *Coptis deltoidea* C. Y. Cheng et Hsiao *Coptis teeta* Wallich	1.0	0.032
total		18.5	0.600

* 7.5 g of hangeshashinto product contains 4.5 g of a dried extract of the mixed crude drugs.

Table 5. The ingredients in the shinbuto (TJ-30) formula.

Japanese Name (Latin Name)	Scientific Name	Amount (g)	Amount * (g/g of Product)
bukuryo (*Poria Sclerotium*)	*Wolfiporia cocos* Ryvarden et Gilbertson (*Poria cocos* Wolf)	4.0	0.089
shakuyaku (*Paeoniae Radix*)	*Paeonia lactiflora* Pallas	3.0	0.067
sojutsu (*Atractylodis Lanceae Rhizoma*)	*Atractylodes lancea* De Candolle *Atractylodes schinensis* Koidzumi	3.0	0.067
shokyo (*Zingiberis Rhizoma*)	*Zingiber officinale* Roscoe	1.5	0.033
bushi (*Processi Aconiti Radix*)	*Aconitum carmichaeli* Debeaux *Aconitum japonicum* Thunberg	0.5	0.011
total		12.0	0.267

* 7.5 g of shinbuto product contains 2.0 g of a dried extract of the mixed crude drugs.

Table 6. The ingredients in the ninjinto (TJ-32) formula.

Japanese Name (Latin Name)	Scientific Name	Amount (g)	Amount * (g/g of Product)
kankyo (*Zingiberis Processum Rhizoma*)	*Zingiber officinale* Roscoe	3.0	0.083
kanzo (*Glycyrrhizae Radix*)	*Glycyrrhiza uralensis* Fischer *Glycyrrhiza glabra* Linné	3.0	0.083
sojutsu (*Atractylodis Lanceae Rhizoma*)	*Atractylodes lancea* De Candolle *Atractylodes schinensis* Koidzumi	3.0	0.083
ninjin (*Ginseng Radix*)	*Panax ginseng* C.A. Meyer	3.0	0.083
total		12.0	0.333

* 7.5 g of ninjinto product contains 2.5 g of a dried extract of the mixed crude drugs.

Table 7. The ingredients in the orento (TJ-120) formula.

Japanese Name (Latin Name)	Scientific Name	Amount (g)	Amount * (g/g of Product)
hange (*Pinelliae tuber*)	*Pinellia ternata* Breitenbach	6.0	0.133
oren (*Coptidis rhizoma*)	*Coptis japonica* Makino *Coptis chinensis* Franchet *Coptis deltoidea* C. Y. Cheng et Hsiao *Coptis teeta* Wallich	3.0	0.067
kankyo (*Zingiberis Processum Rhizoma*)	*Zingiber officinale* Roscoe	3.0	0.067
kanzo (*Glycyrrhizae Radix*)	*Glycyrrhiza uralensis* Fischer *Glycyrrhiza glabra* Linné	3.0	0.067
keihi (*Cinnamomi Cortex*)	*Cinnamomum cassia* Blume	3.0	0.067
taiso (*Zizyphi Fructus*)	*Ziziphus jujuba* Miller var. *inermis* Rehder	3.0	0.067
ninjin (*Ginseng Radix*)	*Panax ginseng* C.A. Meyer	3.0	0.067
total		24.0	0.533

* 7.5 g of orento product contains 4.0 g of a dried extract of the mixed crude drugs.

Table 8. Major ingredients in herbs and their mechanism against arachidonic acid cascade.

Herb	Ingredients	Mechanisms	References
shokyo/kankyo	gingerol, shogaol	inhibition of COX-2 activity	[49,50]
		suppression of COX-2 expression	[7,51–54]
		suppression of NF-κB activation	[52–56]
		inhibition of PLA_2 activity	[57]
kanzo	glycyrrhizin	suppression of COX-2 expression	[58–60]
		suppression of NF-κB activation	[61]
		inhibition of TLR4 homodimerization	[62]
	isoliquiritigenin	suppression of COX-2 expression	[58,63,64]
		suppression of NF-κB activation	[64]
		inhibition of TLR4 homodimerization	[62]
	liquiritin	suppression of COX-2 expression	[58]
keihi	cinnamic aldehyde	suppression of COX-2 expression	[65,66]
		suppression of NF-κB activation	[67]
		inhibition of COX-activity	[68]
		inhibition of TLR4 oligomerization	[69]
ogon	baicalin	suppression of COX-2 expression	[7,70]
		suppression of NF-κB activation	[70]
	baicalein	suppression of COX-2 expression	[7,71]
		suppression of NF-κB activation	[72]
	wogonin	suppression of COX-2 expression	[7,73,74]
		suppression of MAPK [a] phosphorylation	[7]
oren	berberin	suppression of COX-2 expression	[75]
		suppression of NF-κB activation	[75]
		suppression of MAPK [a] phosphorylation	[76–79]
		enhancement of AMPK [b]	[76–78]

[a] MAP kinases; [b] AMP-activated protein kinase.

3.4.1. Shokyo (*Zingiberis Rhizoma*)/Kankyo (*Zingiberis Processum Rhizoma*)

Shokyo is the powdered rhizome of *Zingiber offinale* Roscoe (ginger), and kankyo is the steamed and powdered rhizome of ginger. Both shokyo and kankyo are the aqueous extracts of ginger. Among the herbal medicines shown in Table 1, shokyo is included in kakkonto (TJ-1), shosaikoto (TJ-9), shinbuto (TJ-30), saireito (TJ-114), and orento (TJ-120), and kankyo is included in hangeshashinto (TJ-14) and ninjinto (TJ-32). Many reports have demonstrated that ginger possesses anti-inflammatory effects in human [80,81] and animal models [82–84], and in vitro [85]. Ginger has been widely used in diet and as a treatment for rheumatoid arthritis, fever, emesis, nausea, and migraine headache [80]. A recent systematic review shows that the extracts of ginger including turmeric, ginger, Javanese ginger, and galangal are clinically effective as hypoanalgesic agents [81]. In an animal model, the aqueous extract of ginger significantly reduced serum PGE_2 level by oral or intraperitoneal administration in rats [82]. Moreover, crude hydroalcoholic extract of ginger reduced the serum level of PGE_2, and improved tracheal hyperreactivity and lung inflammation induced by LPS in rats [83]. Ethanol extract of ginger reduced the tissue level of PGE_2, and improved acetic acid-induced ulcerative colitis in rats [84].

Gingerols and shogaols are the major ingredients in ginger. Their structures are indicated in Figure 5. With prolonged storage or heat-treatment of ginger, gingerols are converted to shogaols, which are the dehydrated form of the gingerols [80] (Figure 5). Therefore, kankyo contains a larger amount of shogaols than shokyo although both shokyo and kankyo contain gingerols and shogaols. In in vitro models, gingerols and shogaols have been reported to reduce PGE_2 production by several mechanisms. The effects of gingerols and shogaols on arachidonic acid cascade are briefly summarized in Table 8.

1. Gingerols and shogaols inhibit COX-2 activity. Their IC_{50} values were μM order: 6-gingerol (>50 μM), 8-gingerol (10.0 μM), 10-gingerol (3.7 μM), 6-shogaol (2.1 μM), and 8-shogaol (7.2 μM) in human lung adenocarcinoma A549 cells [49], and 10-gingerol (32.0 μM), 8-shogaol (17.5 μM), 10-shogaol (7.5 μM) in a cell-free assay [50].

2. Gingerols and shogaols suppress COX-2 expression. For example, 6-, 8-, and 10-gingerol suppressed COX-2 expression in LPS-treated human leukemic monocyte lymphoma U937 cells [51]. Similarly, 6-gingerol and 6-shogaol suppressed LPS-induced COX-2 expression in mouse macrophage RAW264.7 cells [52], mouse microglial BV-2 cells [53], and primary rat astrocytes [86]. 6-Gingerol suppressed COX-2 expression in TPA-treated mouse skin in vivo [54].

3. As aforementioned, the expression of COX-2 is regulated by NF-κB. Gingerols and shogaols are reported to suppress NF-κB activation, and to downregulate COX-2 expression. For example, 6-shogaol suppressed LPS-induced NF-κB activation in RAW264.7 cells [52], mouse primary cultured microglia cells [53], and human breast cancer MDA-MB-231 cells [56]. 6-Shogaol suppressed TPA-induced NF-κB activation in mouse skin [54]. Similarly, 6-gingerol suppressed *Vibrio cholerae*-induced NF-κB activation in human intestinal epithelial cells [55]. These results suggest that gingerols and shogaols suppress NF-κB activation directly or indirectly, leading to the inhibition of COX-2 expression.

4. Gingerols and shogaols inhibit PLA_2 activities [57]. In more detail, $iPLA_2$ activity was inhibited by 6-, 8-, and 10-gingerol and 6-, 8-, and 10-shogaol, whereas $cPLA_2$ activity was inhibited by 6-gingerol and 6-, 8-, and 10-shogaol. In particular, IC_{50} values of 10-shogaol against $iPLA_2$ and $cPLA_2$ were 0.7 μM and 3 μM, respectively, in U937 cells.

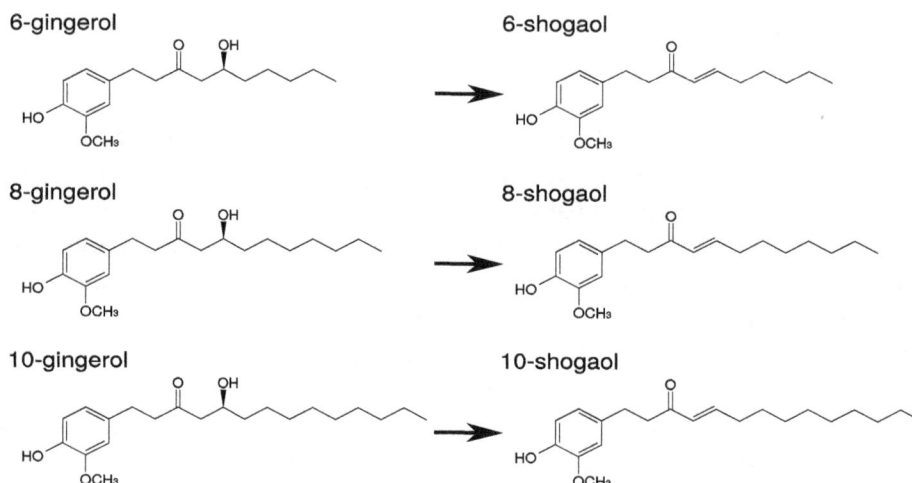

Figure 5. The structures of ingredients in shokyo (*Zingiberis Rhizoma*) and kankyo (*Zingiberis Processum Rhizoma*).

As aforementioned, many reports have examined the effects of ginger. However, there is little report using ginger as "shokyo" and "kankyo." For this reason, we examined the mechanism of the actions of shokyo and kankyo on the reduction of PGE_2 production in HGFs. Shokyo and kankyo concentration-dependently reduced LPS-induced PGE_2 production by HGFs, and the effects of kankyo were slightly stronger than those of shokyo (Figure 4) [39]. The effects of shokyo and kankyo on arachidonic cascade in HGFs are described as follows.

- Both shokyo and kankyo only slightly increased $cPLA_2$ expression, and did not alter annexin1 expression [39].
- Shokyo did not alter LPS-induced ERK phosphorylation in HGFs [29] (but we have not examined the effect of kankyo). Therefore, shokyo (and perhaps kankyo) may have little to no effect on $cPLA_2$ activation, and the subsequent arachidonic acid production.
- Both shokyo and kankyo did not inhibit COX-2 and PGE synthase activities, and did not alter LPS-induced COX-2 expression in HGFs [29,39]. These findings suggest shokyo and kankyo primarily inhibit $cPLA_2$ activity in HGFs. Although we have no direct data to show that shokyo and kankyo inhibit $cPLA_2$ activity, this assumption is consistent with the results that ginger (and gingerols/shogaols) inhibits both $iPLA_2$ and $cPLA_2$ activities [57].

As described above, our data that shokyo did not alter COX-2 activity and COX-2 expression are different from those of gingerols and shogaols in Table 8. Although there is no obvious evidence, the reason may be the preparation method of shokyo and kankyo. Gingerols and shogaols are extremely hydrophobic by their structures. These ingredients were extracted from hydrophobic phase, whereas shokyo and kankyo were prepared by decoction. Therefore, hydrophobic ingredients such as gingerol and shogaol are unlikely to be extracted, and their concentration might be lower than those in previous reports. Quantification of these ingredients is needed to explain these discrepancies.

3.4.2. Kanzo (*Glycyrrhizae Radix*)

Kanzo is the powdered root or stolon of *Glycyrrhiza uralensis* Fischer (licorice). Among the herbal medicines shown in Table 1, kanzo is included in kakkonto (TJ-1), shosaikoto (TJ-9), hangeshashinto (TJ-14), ninjinto (TJ-32), rikkosan (TJ-110), saireito (TJ-114), and orento (TJ-120). Licorice is also known to have anti-inflammatory effects [87] such as inhibition of COX-2 activity [46].

Licorice contains triperpene saponin such as glycyrrhizin (glycyrrhizin acid), and chalcones such as liquiritin and isoliquiritigenin. Their structures are indicated in Figure 6. Glycyrrhizin, liquiritin, and isoliquiritigenin are reported to reduce PGE_2 production. The effects of these ingredients on arachidonic acid cascade are briefly summarized in Table 8.

1. Glycyrrhizin suppressed COX-2 expression in LPS-treated mouse microglial BV2 cells [58] and uterus of ovariectominezed mice [59]. Moreover, orally administrated glycyrrhizin suppressed COX-2 expression in the cerebral cortex of LPS-treated mice [60]. Liquiritin and isoliquiritigenin also suppressed LPS-induced COX-2 expression in RAW264.7 cells [63] and BV2 cells [58].

2. Glycyrrhizin suppressed TNF-α or IL-1β-induced NF-κB activation in human lung epithelial A549 cells [61]. Isoliquiritigenin also suppressed NF-κB activity and suppressed LPS-induced COX-2 expression in RAW264.7 cells [64].

3. Glycyrrhizin and isoliquiritigenin inhibited TLR4 (receptor of LPS) homodimerization and downstream signal pathway [62], resulting in the suppression of COX-2 expression.

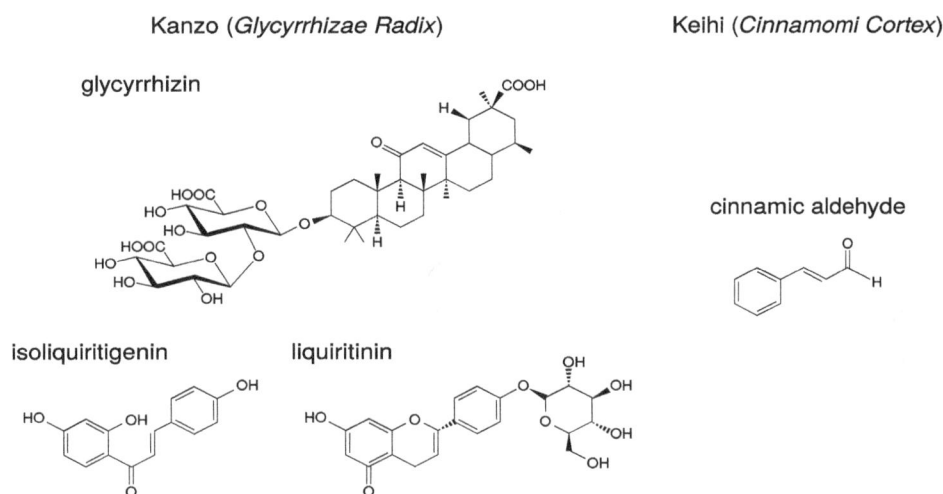

Figure 6. The structures of ingredients in kanzo (*Glycyrrhizae Radix*) and keihi (*Cinnamomi Cortex*).

Indeed, although glycyrrhizin has anti-inflammatory effects, glycyrrhizin is known to show a serious adverse effect, pseudohyperaldosteronism. Excessive dietary intake of licorice can cause a syndrome mimicking hypermineralocorticoidism, characterized by hypertension, hypokalemia, alkalosis, and reduced plasma renin [88–91]. Glycyrrhizin inhibits 11β-hydroxysteroid dehydrogenase type 2 (11β-HSD2), which converts active glucocorticoid cortisol to inactive cortisone [92]. This inhibition results in the activation of renal mineralocorticoid receptors by cortisol, inducing Na$^+$ reabsorption, K$^+$ excretion, hypertension, hypokalemia, and metabolic alkalosis. These phenotypes are similar to that of apparent mineralocorticoid excess syndrome. [91,93].

We examined the mechanism of the action of kanzo on the reduction of PGE$_2$ production in HGFs. However, the effects of kanzo on arachidonic acid cascade in HGFs cannot be explained by those of glycyrrhizin, liquiritin, and isoliquiritigenin.

• As reported previously [46], kanzo inhibited COX-2 activity because kanzo decreased LPS-induced PGE$_2$ production when arachidonic acid was added [29]. In contrast, kanzo did not inhibit PGE synthase activity because kanzo did not alter LPS-induced PGE$_2$ production when PGH$_2$ was added [29].

• Kanzo increased both cPLA$_2$ and annexin1 expressions [29], thus leaving the effect of kanzo on PLA$_2$ unconcluded.

• Kanzo increased LPS-induced COX-2 expression [29] although glycyrrhizin, liquiritin, and isoliquiritigenin suppressed COX-2 expression [58–60,63,64].
    This result is the same as those observed using orento [40] and saireito [44], which contain kanzo.

Therefore, these effects of kanzo were different from those of glycyrrhizin, liquiritin, and isoliquiritigenin, suggesting that other ingredients may contribute to our findings. In addition, not all herbal medicines which contain kanzo increased annexin1 as kakkonto, hangeshashinto, and orento did not alter annexin1 expression.

3.4.3. Keihi (*Cinnamomi Cortex*)

Keihi is the powdered bark of *Cinnamomum cassia* (cinnamon). Among the herbal medicines shown in Table 1, keihi is included in kakkonto (TJ-1), saireito (TJ-114), and orento (TJ-120). Cinnamon has been widely used for the treatment of fever and inflammation [28]. Cinnamon improves nephritis, purulent dermatitis, and hypertension, and it also enhances wound healing. Cinnamon extracts have been used for the improvement or prevention of common cold, diarrhea, and pain [28]. Ethanol-extract of *C. cassia* reduced LPS-induced PGE_2 production by RAW264.7 cells, and it suppressed NF-κB activity and the following COX-2 expression [66].

Keihi contains the ingredients such as cinnamic aldehyde, cinnamic alcohol, cinnamic acid, and coumarin. The structure of cinnamic aldehyde is indicated in Figure 6. Cinnamic aldehyde is reported to reduce PGE_2 production. The effects of cinnamic aldehyde on arachidonic acid cascade are briefly summarized in Table 8.

1. Cinnamic aldehyde suppressed carrageenan-induced COX-2 expression and improved footpad edema in mice [65]. Cinnamic aldehyde, but not others, suppressed LPS-induced COX-2 expression and decreased PGE_2 production by RAW264.7 cells [65,66].
2. Cinnamic aldehyde suppressed LPS-induced NF-κB activity in RAW264.7 cells and TLR4-expressing HEK293 cells [67].
3. Cinnamic aldehyde inhibited IL-1β-induced COX-2 activity in rat cerebral microvascular endothelial cells although its effect is weak [68].
4. Cinnamic aldehyde inhibited TLR4 oligomerization and downstream signal pathway, which include NF-κB. Sulfhydryl modification is suggested to be an important contributing factor for the regulation of TLR4 activation [69].

We examined the mechanism of action of keihi on the reduction of PGE_2 production in HGFs. However, the effects of keihi on arachidonic acid cascade in HGFs cannot be explained by that of cinnamic aldehyde.

*   Keihi inhibited COX-2 activity because keihi decreased LPS-induced PGE_2 production when arachidonic acid is added [29]. This mechanism is accounted for by that of cinnamic aldehyde. In contrast, keihi did not inhibit PGE synthase activity as well as kanzo.
*   As well as kakkonto [81] and orento [40], keihi suppressed ERK phosphorylation in LPS-treated HGFs [29], leading to inhibit $cPLA_2$ activation. However, the contribution of suppression of ERK phosphorylation is considered to be small because the ability of keihi to decrease LPS-induced PGE_2 production was weak (Figure 3).
*   Keihi increased LPS-induced COX-2 expression.

Therefore, these effects of keihi are different from that of cinnamic aldehyde, suggesting that other ingredients may contribute to our findings.

3.4.4. Ogon (*Scutellariae Radix*)

Ogon is the powdered root of *Scutellaria baicalensis* Georgi. Among the herbal medicines shown in Table 1, ogon is included in shosaikoto (TJ-9), hangeshashinto (TJ-14), and saireito (TJ-114). Among the herbs constituting saireito, ogon is reported to reduce PGE_2 production by LPS-treated RAW264.7 cells [44].

The major ingredients of ogon are flavonoids such as baicalin, baicalein, and wogonin. Their structures are indicated in Figure 7. Baicalin is the glucuronide of baicalein and is an inactive form. Administered baicalein is metabolized to baicalin, which is an active form. Baicalin, baicalein, and wogonin reduce PGE_2 production in human oral keratinocytes [7] and RAW264.7 cells [94].

1. Wogonin suppressed LPS-induced COX-2 expression in RAW264.7 cells [73,74], whereas baicalin and baicalein did not [73]. Other group demonstrated that baicalein (but not baicalin) suppressed

LPS-induced COX-2 expression in RAW264.7 cells [71]. This discrepancy may be due to the concentrations of LPS and flavonoids among these reports. Moreover, baicalein and wogonin suppressed COX-2 expression in human oral keratinocytes [7].

2.   Baicalin [70], baicalein [72], and wogonin [7] suppressed NF-κB activity.
3.   Baicalin, baicalein, and wogonin did not inhibit COX-2 activity in RAW264.7 cells [73].

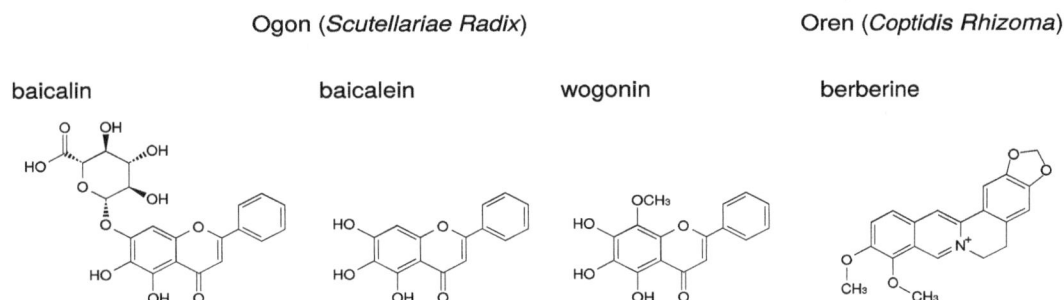

Figure 7. The structures of ingredients in ogon (*Scutellariae Radix*) and oren (*Coptidis Rhizoma*).

Our data indicate that shosaikoto and hangeshashinto, which include ogon, suppressed LPS-induced COX-2 expression in HGFs [37,38]. This mechanism is accounted for by those of baicalin, baicalein, and wogonin.

3.4.5. Oren (*Coptidis Rhizoma*)

Oren is the powdered rhizome of *Coptis japonica* Makino, *Coptis chinensis* Franchet, *Coptis deltoidea* C. Y. Cheng et Hsiao, or *Coptis teeta* Wallich (Ranunculaceae). Among the herbal medicines shown in Table 1, oren is included in hangeshashinto (TJ-14) and orento (TJ-120).

Berberine, one of benzylisoquinoline alkaloid, is the major ingredient of oren. The structure of berberine is indicated in Figure 7. Berberine is reported to reduce PGE_2 production. The effects of berberine on arachidonic acid cascade are briefly summarized in Table 8.

1.   Berberine suppressed NF-κB activation and COX-2 expression in human leukemia Jurkat cells [75] and oral cancer OC2 and KB cells [95,96].
2.   Berberine suppressed MAP kinases phosphorylation (including ERK) and activated AMP-activated protein kinase (AMPK) in peritoneal macrophages and RAW 264.7 cells [76], BV-2 cells [77], and melanoma cells [78]. Therefore, berberine is considered to inhibit $cPLA_2$ activation through suppression of ERK phosphorylation. In addition, because AMPK is reported to suppress NF-κB activation [97], berberine suppressed COX-2 expression due to activation of AMPK.

3.5. Conclusion about Herbal Medicines and Herbs

We have described the effects of herbal medicines, herbs, and their ingredients on arachidonic acid cascade in this review. Several herbal medicines show reduced LPS-induced PGE_2 production by HGFs. These results suggest that these herbal medicines may be effective in the improvement of the inflammatory symptoms in periodontitis. Herbal medicines must be properly selected by the patterns of each patient —excess patterns, medium patterns, or deficiency patterns. Among the herbal medicines in our studies, kakkonto (TJ-1) and orento (TJ-120) are used for the patients with excess patterns. Shosaikoto (TJ-9), hangeshashinto (TJ-14), and orento are used for the patients with medium patterns. Shinbuto (TJ-30) and ninjinto (TJ-32) are used for the patients with deficiency patterns. Therefore, it may be possible to use appropriate herbal medicines to patients with any pattern.

As shown in the above-mentioned descriptions, not all effects of herbal medicines are explainable by the effects of herbs constituting herbal medicines. Similarly, not all effects of herbs are explainable by the effects of ingredients contained in herbs. Experiments using "herbal medicines" or "herbs" themselves may be important rather than those using ingredients. The concentrations of these hydrophobic ingredients may also be low because the herbs that we used are water-soluble fractions. Therefore, it is considered that the concentrations of their ingredients need to be measured. Moreover, the unanalyzed ingredients other than those explained in this review are likely to be present. It is to be desired that further analyses reveal the novel ingredients and their action of mechanisms.

4. Anti-Osteoclastogenic Effects of Natural Products

Like periodontitis (PD), rheumatoid arthritis (RA) is a disease associated with inflammation and bone destruction. Although therapeutics of RA have recently advanced with the development of antibody drugs, natural substances displaying anti-inflammatory and anti-osteoclast characteristics against RA are still being used as widely as they have been in the past.

Some studies have revealed a relationship between PD and RA. RA prevalence is increased in patients with PD [98,99]. The presence of PD may contribute to the progression of RA; that is, RA patients with PD receiving non-surgical periodontal treatment resulted in a noteworthy improvement in the clinical outcome for RA [100]. From the aspect of the clinical marker, RA and PD are similar in cytokines and mediators involved in inflammation and bone destruction [101]. For example, TNF-α, receptor activator of nuclear factor-κB ligand (RANKL), and matrix metalloproteinase (MMP) family increase in production in RA and PD [102–106]. Due to these similarities, natural products used for RA are probably effective for PD.

The structures of natural products described in this review are indicated in Figure 8.

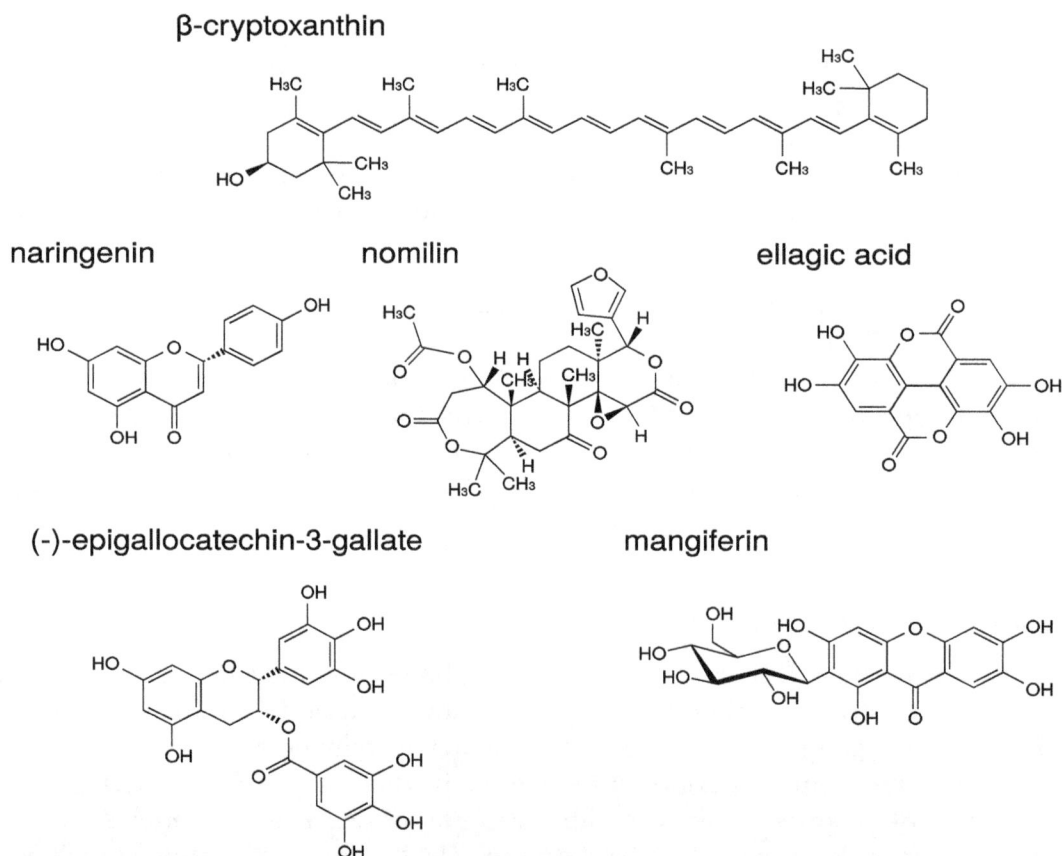

Figure 8. The structures of natural products.

Epidemiological studies have revealed a positive correlation between bone health and increased consumption of fruits and vegetables [107,108]. Some fruits and vegetables contain components that inhibit both inflammation and osteoclast activity.

β-Cryptoxanthin is a carotenoid present in a wide range of citrus fruits and in *Diospyros kaki* Thunb., *Physalis alkekengi* L., etc. β-Cryptoxanthin has a potent inhibitory effect on osteoclast-like cell formation in mouse marrow culture [109]. Moreover, in a mouse model of PD, β-cryptoxanthin suppressed bone resorption in the mandibular alveolar bone in vitro and restored alveolar bone loss induced by LPS in vivo [110].

Naringenin is a flavonoid contained in citrus fruits such as oranges and grapefruits. Accumulating evidence has suggested that naringenin modulates chronic inflammation [111]. In a murine model of collagen-induced arthritis, naringenin inhibited pro-inflammatory cytokine production by decreasing MAPK and NF-κB signaling activation [112]. La et al. showed naringenin thus holds promise as a therapeutic and preventive agent for bone-related diseases such as PD [113]. Thus, there are cases in which components demonstrating anti-osteoclast behavior are demonstrated to be effective against PD. In addition to naringenin, citrus fruits contain components that suppress osteoclast activity via MAPK. Nomilin, a limonoid present in citrus fruits, displays inhibitory effects on osteoclastic differentiation through the suppression of MAPK signaling pathways [114].

Ellagic acid is a polyphenol contained in berries, pomegranates, nuts, etc. Ellagic acid has an anti-inflammatory effect in various organs such as the liver, stomach, small intestine, and skin [115–118]. Moreover, ellagic acid has anti-osteoclast activity and significantly reduced serum levels of pro-inflammatory cytokines, TNF-α, IL-1β, and IL-17 in RA model mice [119]. A recent study supported the traditional use of *Geum urbanum* L. root contained ellagic acid derivatives in cavity inflammation including mucositis, gingivitis, and PD [120].

Additional useful components against both RA and PD have been found in tea. (-)-Epigallocatechin-3-gallate (EGCG) is a major catechin derivative present in green tea. Previous studies have also suggested that EGCG decreases MMP-1, MMP-2, and MMP-3 production by RA synovial fibroblasts, thereby preventing further cartilage and bone destruction [121,122]. Moreover, it has been reported that EGCG selectively inhibited IL-1β-induced IL-6 synthesis in RA synovial fibroblasts and suppressed IL-6 trans-signaling via upregulation of an endogenous inhibitor, a soluble gp130 [123]. Clinical study of EGCG suggested that local drug delivery utilizing green tea extract could be used as an adjunct in the treatment of chronic PD [124].

Traditional medicine in Ayurveda also presents useful teas against RA and PD. *Salacia reticulata* Wight is a plant native to Sri Lanka that has been used for the prevention of RA, gonorrhea, and skin disease. We previously reported that leaf of *S. reticulata* alleviates collagen antibody-induced arthritis in RA model mice [125]. *S. reticulata* contains a polyphenol known as mangiferin that inhibits osteoclastic bone resorption by promoting ERβ mRNA expression in mouse bone marrow macrophage cells [126].

In conclusion, natural products displaying both anti-inflammation and anti-osteoclast characteristics are suggested to be useful for the prevention and treatment of PD.

Author Contributions: C.S. conceived, designed, proved, and edited the whole review manuscript. N.S. and C.S. wrote "Introduction" and the topic of "Biological Efficacy of Natural Products against Acute Inflammatory Disease: Stomatitis", T.A. wrote the topic of "Biological Efficacy of Natural Products against Chronic Inflammatory Disease: Periodontitis", S.N. and K.K. wrote a second half part of the topic "Anti-Osteoclastogenic Effects of Natural Products".

Acknowledgments: We would like to thank also to the stuffs of Matsumoto Dental University, Josai University, and Okayama University Graduate School for technical support.

References

1. Veilleux, M.; Moriyama, S.; Yoshioka, M.; Hinode, D.; Grenier, D. A Review of Evidence for a Therapeutic Application of Traditional Japanese Kampo Medicine for Oral Diseases/Disorders. *Medicines* **2018**, *5*, 35. [CrossRef] [PubMed]

2. Wang, P. Kampo medicines for oral disease. *Oral Ther. Pharmacol.* **2012**, *31*, 67–82.

3. Kono, T.; Satomi, M.; Chisato, N.; Ebisawa, Y.; Suno, M.; Asama, T.; Karasaki, H.; Matsubara, K.; Furukawa, H. Topical Application of Hangeshashinto (TJ-14) in the Treatment of Chemotherapy-Induced Oral Mucositis. *World J. Oncol.* **2010**, *1*, 232–235. [PubMed]

4. Aoyama, T.; Nishikawa, K.; Takiguchi, N.; Tanabe, K.; Imano, M.; Fukushima, R.; Sakamoto, J.; Oba, M.; Morita, S.; Kono, T.; et al. Double-blind, placebo-controlled, randomized phase II study of TJ-14 (hangeshashinto) for gastric cancer chemotherapy-induced oral mucositis. *Cancer Chemother. Pharmacol.* **2014**, *73*, 1047–1054. [CrossRef] [PubMed]

5. Yamashita, T.; Araki, K.; Tomifuji, M.; Kamide, D.; Tanaka, Y.; Shiotani, A. A traditional Japanese medicine– Hangeshashinto (TJ-14)–alleviates chemoradiation-induced mucositis and improves rates of treatment completion. *Support Care Cancer* **2015**, *23*, 29–35. [CrossRef] [PubMed]

6. Kamide, D.; Yamashita, T.; Araki, K.; Tomifuji, M.; Shiotani, A. Hangeshashinto (TJ-14) prevents radiation-induced mucositis by suppressing cyclooxygenase-2 expression and chemotaxis of inflammatory cells. *Clin. Transl. Oncol.* **2017**, *19*, 1329–1336. [CrossRef] [PubMed]

7. Kono, T.; Kaneko, A.; Matsumoto, C.; Miyagi, C.; Ohbuchi, K.; Mizuhara, Y.; Miyano, K.; Uezono, Y. Multitargeted effects of hangeshashinto for treatment of chemotherapy-induced oral mucositis on inducible prostaglandin E2 production in human oral keratinocytes. *Integr. Cancer Ther.* **2014**, *13*, 435–445. [CrossRef] [PubMed]

8. Furusawa, S.; Wu, J. The effects of biscoclaurine alkaloid cepharanthine on mammalian cells: Implications for cancer, shock, and inflammatory diseases. *Life Sci.* **2007**, *80*, 1073–1079. [CrossRef] [PubMed]

9. Rogosnitzky, M.; Danks, R. Therapeutic potential of the biscoclaurine alkaloid, cepharanthine. *Pharmacol. Rep.* **2011**, *63*, 337–347. [CrossRef]

10. Nakase, M.; Nomura, J.; Inui, M.; Murata, T.; Kawarada, Y.; Tagawa, T.; Ohsugi, H. Evaluation of clinical efficacy of Cepharanthin® (gargle-internal use) treatment for oral mucosal lesions. *J. Jpn. Oral Muco. Membr.* **1997**, *3*, 76–81. [CrossRef]

11. Saki, H.; Ichihara, H.; Kato, Y.; Ando, M.; Abe, K.; Win, K.; Inoue, T.; Fujitsuka, H.; Hyodo, I.; Sugiyama, T.; et al. Evaluation of clinical efficiency of Cepharanthin® for the treatment of oral mucosal lesions and glossodynia. *J. Jpn. Stomatol. Soc.* **1994**, *43*, 84–89.

12. Saito, Y.; Ikeda, M.; Tanaka, H.; Iijima, J.; Sakata, K. A literatue study of oral therapeutics and pharmacology Report 1; Evidence of off-label use of cepharanthin. *Oral. Ther. Pharmacol.* **2001**, *20*, 110–116.

13. Sogawa, N.; Sogawa, C.; Nakano, M.; Fukuoka, R.; Furuta, H. Effects of propargylglycine on endotoxin-induced acute lethal toxicity and defensive effect of cepharanthin on this toxicity. *J. Okayama Dent. Soc.* **1998**, *17*, 251–259.

14. Sogawa, N.; Sogawa, C.; Furuta, H. A study of active ingredients in Cepharanthin® on enhancement of lipopolysaccharide-induced histidine decarboxylase activities in mice spleens. *Med. Biol.* **2000**, *140*, 69–72.

15. Yokota, T.; Yokota, K.; Matsuura, T.; Shiwa, M. Suppressive effects of Cepharanthin® on the production of superoxide anion by neutrophils during hemodialysis. *J. Jpn. Soc. Dial. Ther.* **1993**, *26*, 1703–1708. [CrossRef]

16. Sawamura, D.; Sato, S.; Suzuki, M.; Nomura, K.; Hanada, K.; Hashimoto, I. Effect of cepharanthin on superoxide anion (O_2^-) production by macrophages. *J. Dermatol.* **1988**, *15*, 304–307. [CrossRef] [PubMed]

17. Akamatsu, H.; Komura, J.; Asada, Y.; Niwa, Y. Effects of cepharanthin on neutrophil chemotaxis, phagocytosis, and reactive oxygen species generation. *J. Dermatol.* **1991**, *18*, 643–648. [CrossRef] [PubMed]

18. Kawada, N.; Mizoguchi, Y.; Kondo, H.; Seki, S.; Kobayashi, K.; Yamamoto, S.; Morisawa, S. Effect of cepharanthine on metabolism of arachidonic acid from rat peritoneal exudate cells. *Jpn. J. Inflamm.* **1988**, *8*, 347–349.

19. Kondo, Y.; Takano, F.; Hojo, H. Inhibitory effect of bisbenzylisoquinoline alkaloids on nitric oxide production in activated macrophages. *Biochem. Pharmacol.* **1993**, *46*, 1887–1892. [CrossRef]

20. Matsuno, T.; Okazoe, Y.; kobayashi, S.; Obuchi, H.; Sato, E.; Edashige, K.; Utsumi, K. Measurement of active oxygen of neutrophils by means of luminol chemiluminescence and their inhibition by biscoclaurine alkaloids. *Igaku Yakugaku* **1989**, *21*, 889–894.

21. Kondo, Y.; Takano, F.; Hojo, H. Suppression of lipopolysaccharide-induced fulminant hepatitis and tumor necrosis factor production by bisbenzylisoquinoline alkaloids in bacillus Calmette-Guerin-treated mice. *Biochem. Pharmacol.* **1993**, *46*, 1861–1863. [CrossRef]

22. Sugiyama, K.; Sasaki, J.; Utsumi, K.; Miyahara, M. Inhibition by cepharanthine of histamine release from rat peritoneal mast cells. *Allergy* **1976**, *25*, 685–690.

23. Sogawa, N.; Aoki-Sogawa, C.; Iwata-Abuku, E.; Inoue, T.; Oda, N.; Kishi, K.; Furuta, H. Opposing pharmacological actions of cepharanthin on lipopolysaccharide-induced histidine decarboxylase activity in mice spleens. *Life Sci.* **2001**, *68*, 1395–1403. [CrossRef]

24. Noguchi, K.; Ishikawa, I. The roles of cyclooxygenase-2 and prostaglandin E_2 in periodontal disease. *Periodontology 2000* **2007**, *43*, 85–101. [CrossRef] [PubMed]

25. Salvi, G.; Lang, N. Host response modulation in the management of periodontal diseases. *J. Clin. Periodontol.* **2005**, *32* (Suppl. 6), 108–129. [CrossRef] [PubMed]

26. Ara, T.; Fujinami, Y.; Imamura, Y.; Wang, P. Lipopolysaccharide-treated human gingival fibroblasts continuously produce PGE_2. *J. Hard Tissue Biol.* **2008**, *17*, 121–124. [CrossRef]

27. Ara, T.; Kurata, K.; Hirai, K.; Uchihashi, T.; Uematsu, T.; Imamura, Y.; Furusawa, K.; Kurihara, S.; Wang, P. Human gingival fibroblasts are critical in sustaining inflammation in periodontal disease. *J. Periodontal. Res.* **2009**, *44*, 21–27. [CrossRef] [PubMed]

28. Burke, J.; Dennis, E. phospholipase A_2 biochemistry. *Cardiovasc Drugs Ther.* **2009**, *23*, 49–59. [CrossRef] [PubMed]

29. Ara, T.; Sogawa, N. Studies on shokyo, kanzo, and keihi in kakkonto medicine on prostaglandin E_2 production in lipopolysaccharide-treated human gingival fibroblasts. *Int. Sch. Res. Notices* **2016**, *2016*, 9351787. [CrossRef] [PubMed]

30. Nemenoff, R.; Winitz, S.; Qian, N.; Van Putten, V.; Johnson, G.; Heasley, L. Phosphorylation and activation of a high molecular weight form of phospholipase A_2 by p42 microtubule-associated protein 2 kinase and protein kinase C. *J. Biol. Chem.* **1993**, *268*, 1960–1964. [PubMed]

31. Lin, L.; Wartmann, M.; Lin, A.; Knopf, J.; Seth, A.; Davis, R. $cPLA_2$ is phosphorylated and activated by MAP kinase. *Cell* **1993**, *72*, 269–278. [CrossRef]

32. Gijón, M.; Spencer, D.; Kaiser, A.; Leslie, C. Role of phosphorylation sites and the C2 domain in regulation of cytosolic phospholipase A_2. *J. Cell. Biol.* **1999**, *145*, 1219–1232. [CrossRef] [PubMed]

33. Gupta, C.; Katsumata, M.; Goldman, A.; Herold, R.; Piddington, R. Glucocorticoid-induced phospholipase A_2-inhibitory proteins mediate glucocorticoid teratogenicity in vitro. *Proc. Natl. Acad. Sci. USA* **1984**, *81*, 1140–1143. [CrossRef] [PubMed]

34. Wallner, B.; Mattaliano, R.; Hession, C.; Cate, R.; Tizard, R.; Sinclair, L.; Foeller, C.; Chow, E.; Browing, J.; Ramachandran, K.; et al. Cloning and expression of human lipocortin, a phospholipase A_2 inhibitor with potential anti-inflammatory activity. *Nature* **1986**, *320*, 77–81. [CrossRef] [PubMed]

35. Ara, T.; Fujinami, Y.; Urano, H.; Hirai, K.; Hattori, T.; Miyazawa, H. Protein kinase A enhances lipopolysaccharide-induced IL-6, IL-8, and PGE_2 production by human gingival fibroblasts. *J. Negat. Results Biomed.* **2012**, *11*, 10. [CrossRef] [PubMed]

36. Kitamura, H.; Urano, H.; Ara, T. Preventive effects of a kampo medicine, kakkonto, on inflammatory responses via the suppression of extracellular signal-regulated kinase phosphorylation in lipopolysaccharide-treated human gingival fibroblasts. *ISRN Pharmacol.* **2014**, *2014*, 784019. [CrossRef] [PubMed]

37. Ara, T.; Maeda, Y.; Fujinami, Y.; Imamura, Y.; Hattori, T.; Wang, P. Preventive effects of a Kampo medicine, Shosaikoto, on inflammatory responses in LPS-treated human gingival fibroblasts. *Biol. Pharm. Bull.* **2008**, *31*, 1141–1144. [CrossRef] [PubMed]

38. Nakazono, Y.; Ara, T.; Fujinami, Y.; Hattori, T.; Wang, P. Preventive effects of a kampo medicine, hangeshashinto on inflammatory responses in lipopolysaccharide-treated human gingival fibroblasts. *J. Hard Tissue Biol.* **2010**, *19*, 43–50. [CrossRef]

39. Ara, T.; Sogawa, N. Effects of shinbuto and ninjinto on prostaglandin E_2 production in lipopolysaccharide-treated human gingival fibroblasts. *PeerJ* **2017**, *5*, e4120. [CrossRef] [PubMed]

40. Ara, T.; Honjo, K.; Fujinami, Y.; Hattori, T.; Imamura, Y.; Wang, P. Preventive effects of a kampo medicine, orento on inflammatory responses in lipopolysaccharide treated human gingival fibroblasts. *Biol. Pharm. Bull.* **2010**, *33*, 611–616. [CrossRef] [PubMed]

41. Kato, T.; Segami, N.; Sakagami, H. Anti-inflammatory activity of hangeshashinto in IL-1β-stimulated gingival and periodontal ligament fibroblasts. *In Vivo* **2016**, *30*, 257–263. [PubMed]

42. Miyamoto, K.; Lange, M.; McKinley, G.; Stavropoulos, C.; Moriya, S.; Matsumoto, H.; Inada, Y. Effects of sho-saiko-to on production of prostaglandin E_2 (PGE_2), leukotriene B_4 (LTB_4) and superoxide from peripheral monocytes and polymorphonuclear cells isolated from HIV infected individuals. *Am. J. Chin. Med.* **1996**, *24*, 1–10. [CrossRef] [PubMed]

43. Horie, N.; Hashimoto, K.; Kato, T.; Shimoyama, T.; Kaneko, T.; Kusama, K.; Sakagami, H. COX-2 as possible target for the inhibition of PGE_2 production by Rikko-san in activated macrophage. *In Vivo* **2008**, *22*, 333–336. [PubMed]

44. Kaneko, T.; Chiba, H.; Horie, N.; Kato, T.; Hashimoto, K.; Kusama, K.; Sakagami, H. Effect of Sairei-to and its ingredients on prostaglandin E_2 production by mouse macrophage-like cells. *In Vivo* **2008**, *22*, 571–575. [PubMed]

45. Inoue, M.; Shen, Y.; Ogihara, Y. Shosaikoto (kampo medicine) protects macrophage function from suppression by hypercholesterolemia. *Biol. Pharm. Bull.* **1996**, *19*, 652–654. [CrossRef] [PubMed]

46. Kase, Y.; Saitoh, K.; Ishige, A.; Komatsu, Y. Mechanisms by which Hange-shashin-to reduces prostaglandin E2 levels. *Biol. Pharm. Bull.* **1998**, *21*, 1277–1281. [CrossRef] [PubMed]

47. Kase, Y.; Hayakawa, T.; Ishige, A.; Aburada, M.; Komatsu, Y. The effects of *Hange-shashin-to* on the content of prostaglandin E_2 and water absorption in the large intestine of rats. *Biol. Pharm. Bull.* **1997**, *20*, 954–957. [CrossRef] [PubMed]

48. Kase, Y.; Saitoh, K.; Yuzurihara, M.; Ishige, A.; Komatsu, Y. Effects of *Hange-shashin-to* on cholera toxin-induced fluid secretion in the small intestine of rats. *Biol. Pharm. Bull.* **1998**, *21*, 117–120. [CrossRef] [PubMed]

49. Tjendraputra, E.; Tran, V.; Liu-Brennan, D.; Roufogalis, B.; Duke, C. Effect of ginger constituents and synthetic analogues on cyclooxygenase-2 enzyme in intact cells. *Bioorg. Chem.* **2001**, *29*, 156–163. [CrossRef] [PubMed]

50. van Breemen, R.; Tao, Y.; Li, W. Cyclooxygenase-2 inhibitors in ginger (*Zingiber officinale*). *Fitoterapia* **2011**, *82*, 38–43. [CrossRef] [PubMed]

51. Lantz, R.; Chen, G.; Sarihan, M.; Solyom, A.; Jolad, S.; Timmermann, B. The effect of extracts from ginger rhizome on inflammatory mediator production. *Phytomedicine* **2007**, *14*, 123–128. [CrossRef] [PubMed]

52. Pan, M.; Hsieh, M.; Hsu, P.; Ho, S.; Lai, C.; Wu, H.; Sang, S.; Ho, C. 6-Shogaol suppressed lipopolysaccharide-induced up-expression of iNOS and COX-2 in murine macrophages. *Mol. Nutr. Food Res.* **2008**, *52*, 1467–1477. [CrossRef] [PubMed]

53. Ha, S.; Moon, E.; Ju, M.; Kim, D.; Ryu, J.; Oh, M.; Kim, S. 6-Shogaol, a ginger product, modulates neuroinflammation: A new approach to neuroprotection. *Neuropharmacology* **2012**, *63*, 211–223. [CrossRef] [PubMed]

54. Kim, S.; Kundu, J.; Shin, Y.; Park, J.; Cho, M.; Kim, T.; Surh, Y. [6]-Gingerol inhibits COX-2 expression by blocking the activation of p38 MAP kinase and NF-κB in phorbol ester-stimulated mouse skin. *Oncogene* **2005**, *24*, 2558–2567. [CrossRef] [PubMed]

55. Saha, P.; Katarkar, A.; Das, B.; Bhattacharyya, A.; Chaudhuri, K. 6-Gingerol inhibits *Vibrio cholerae*-induced proinflammatory cytokines in intestinal epithelial cells via modulation of NF-κB. *Pharm. Biol.* **2016**, *54*, 1606–1615. [CrossRef] [PubMed]

56. Ling, H.; Yang, H.; Tan, S.; Chui, W.; Chew, E. 6-Shogaol, an active constituent of ginger, inhibits breast cancer cell invasion by reducing matrix metalloproteinase-9 expression via blockade of nuclear factor-κB activation. *Br. J. Pharmacol.* **2010**, *161*, 1763–1777. [CrossRef] [PubMed]

57. Nievergelt, A.; Marazzi, J.; Schoop, R.; Altmann, K.; Gertsch, J. Ginger phenylpropanoids inhibit IL-1β and prostanoid secretion and disrupt arachidonate-phospholipid remodeling by targeting phospholipases A_2. *J. Immunol.* **2011**, *187*, 4140–4150. [CrossRef] [PubMed]

58. Yu, J.; Ha, J.; Kim, K.; Jung, Y.; Jung, J.; Oh, S. Anti-inflammatory activities of licorice extract and its active compounds, glycyrrhizic acid, liquiritin and liquiritigenin, in BV2 cells and mice liver. *Molecules* **2015**, *20*, 13041–13054. [CrossRef] [PubMed]

59. Niwa, K.; Lian, Z.; Onogi, K.; Yun, W.; Tang, L.; Mori, H.; Tamaya, T. Preventive effects of glycyrrhizin on estrogen-related endometrial carcinogenesis in mice. *Oncol. Rep.* **2007**, *17*, 617–622. [CrossRef] [PubMed]

60. Song, J.; Lee, J.; Shim, B.; Lee, C.; Choi, S.; Kang, C.; Sohn, N.; Shin, J. Glycyrrhizin alleviates neuroinflammation and memory deficit induced by systemic lipopolysaccharide treatment in mice. *Molecules* **2013**, *18*, 15788–15803. [CrossRef] [PubMed]

61. Takei, H.; Baba, Y.; Hisatsune, A.; Katsuki, H.; Miyata, T.; Yokomizo, K.; Isohama, Y. Glycyrrhizin inhibits interleukin-8 production and nuclear factor-κB activity in lung epithelial cells, but not through glucocorticoid receptors. *J. Pharmacol. Sci.* **2008**, *106*, 460–468. [CrossRef] [PubMed]

62. Honda, H.; Nagai, Y.; Matsunaga, T.; Saitoh, S.; Akashi-Takamura, S.; Hayashi, H.; Fujii, I.; Miyake, K.; Muraguchi, A.; Takatsu, K. Glycyrrhizin and isoliquiritigenin suppress the LPS sensor toll-like receptor 4/MD-2 complex signaling in a different manner. *J. Leukoc. Biol.* **2012**, *91*, 967–976. [CrossRef] [PubMed]

63. Takahashi, T.; Takasuka, N.; Iigo, M.; Baba, M.; Nishino, H.; Tsuda, H.; Okuyama, T. Isoliquiritigenin, a flavonoid from licorice, reduces prostaglandin E$_2$ and nitric oxide, causes apoptosis, and suppresses aberrant crypt foci development. *Cancer Sci.* **2004**, *95*, 448–453. [CrossRef] [PubMed]

64. Kim, J.; Park, S.; Yun, K.; Cho, Y.; Park, H.; Lee, K. Isoliquiritigenin isolated from the roots of *Glycyrrhiza uralensis* inhibitsLPS-induced iNOS and COX-2 expression via the attenuation of NF-κB in RAW 264.7 macrophages. *Eur. J. Pharmacol.* **2008**, *584*, 175–184. [CrossRef] [PubMed]

65. Liao, J.; Deng, J.; Chiu, C.; Hou, W.; Huang, S.; Shie, P.; Huang, G. Anti-inflammatory activities of *Cinnamomum cassia* constituents in vitro and in vivo. *Evid. Based Complement. Alternat. Med.* **2012**, *2012*, 429320. [CrossRef] [PubMed]

66. Yu, T.; Lee, S.; Yang, W.; Jang, H.; Lee, Y.; Kim, T.; Kim, S.; Lee, J.; Cho, J. The ability of an ethanol extract of *Cinnamomum cassia* to inhibit Src and spleen tyrosine kinase activity contributes to its anti-inflammatory action. *J. Ethnopharmacol.* **2012**, *139*, 566–573. [CrossRef] [PubMed]

67. Kim, B.; Lee, Y.; Lee, J.; Lee, J.; Cho, J. Regulatory effect of cinnamaldehyde on monocyte/macrophage-mediated inflammatory responses. *Mediators Inflamm.* **2010**, *2010*, 529359. [CrossRef] [PubMed]

68. Guo, J.; Huo, H.; Zhao, B.; Liu, H.; Li, L.; Ma, Y.; Guo, S.; Jiang, T. Cinnamaldehyde reduces IL-1β-induced cyclooxygenase-2 activity in rat cerebral microvascular endothelial cells. *Eur. J. Pharmacol.* **2006**, *537*, 174–180. [CrossRef] [PubMed]

69. Youn, H.; Lee, J.; Choi, Y.; Saitoh, S.; Miyake, K.; Hwang, D.; Lee, J. Cinnamaldehyde suppresses toll-like receptor 4 activation mediated through the inhibition of receptor oligomerization. *Biochem. Pharmacol.* **2008**, *75*, 494–502. [CrossRef] [PubMed]

70. Altavilla, D.; Squadrito, F.; Bitto, A.; Polito, F.; Burnett, B.; Di Stefano, V.; Minutoli, L. Flavocoxid, a dual inhibitor of cyclooxygenase and 5-lipoxygenase, blunts pro-inflammatory phenotype activation in endotoxin-stimulated macrophages. *Br. J. Pharmacol.* **2009**, *157*, 1410–1418. [CrossRef] [PubMed]

71. Woo, K.; Lim, J.; Suh, S.; Kwon, Y.; Shin, S.; Kim, S.; Choi, Y.; Park, J.; Kwon, T. Differential inhibitory effects of baicalein and baicalin on LPS-induced cyclooxygenase-2 expression through inhibition of C/EBPβ DNA-binding activity. *Immunobiology* **2006**, *211*, 359–368. [CrossRef] [PubMed]

72. Seo, M.; Lee, S.; Jeon, Y.; Im, J. Inhibition of p65 nuclear translocation by baicalein. *Toxicol. Res.* **2011**, *27*, 71–76. [CrossRef] [PubMed]

73. Chen, Y.; Shen, S.; Chen, L.; Lee, T.; Yang, L. Wogonin, baicalin, and baicalein inhibition of inducible nitric oxide synthase and cyclooxygenase-2 gene expressions induced by nitric oxide synthase inhibitors and lipopolysaccharide. *Biochem. Pharmacol.* **2001**, *61*, 1417–1427. [CrossRef]

74. Pan, M.; Lai, C.; Wang, Y.; Ho, C. Acacetin suppressed LPS-induced up-expression of iNOS and COX-2 in murine macrophages and TPA-induced tumor promotion in mice. *Biochem. Pharmacol.* **2006**, *72*, 1293–1303. [CrossRef] [PubMed]

75. Pandey, M.; Sung, B.; Kunnumakkara, A.; Sethi, G.; Chaturvedi, M.; Aggarwal, B. Berberine modifies cysteine 179 of IκBα kinase, suppresses nuclear factor-κB-regulated antiapoptotic gene products, and potentiates apoptosis. *Cancer Res.* **2008**, *68*, 5370–5379. [CrossRef] [PubMed]

76. Jeong, H.; Hsu, K.; Lee, J.; Ham, M.; Huh, J.; Shin, H.; Kim, W.; Kim, J. Berberine suppresses proinflammatory responses through AMPK activation in macrophages. *Am. J. Physiol. Endocrinol. Metab.* **2009**, *296*, E955–E964. [CrossRef] [PubMed]

77. Lu, D.; Tang, C.; Chen, Y.; Wei, I. Berberine suppresses neuroinflammatory responses through AMP-activated protein kinase activation in BV-2 microglia. *J. Cell. Biochem.* **2010**, *110*, 697–705. [CrossRef] [PubMed]

78. Kim, H.; Kim, M.; Kim, E.; Yang, Y.; Lee, M.; Lim, J. Berberine-induced AMPK activation inhibits the metastatic potential of melanoma cells via reduction of ERK activity and COX-2 protein expression. *Biochem. Pharmacol.* **2012**, *83*, 385–394. [CrossRef] [PubMed]

79. Liang, K.; Ting, C.; Yin, S.; Chen, Y.; Lin, S.; Liao, J.; Hsu, S. Berberine suppresses MEK/ERK-dependent Egr-1 signaling pathway and inhibits vascular smooth muscle cell regrowth after in vitro mechanical injury. *Biochem. Pharmacol.* **2006**, *71*, 806–817. [CrossRef] [PubMed]

80. Afzal, M.; Al-Hadidi, D.; Menon, M.; Pesek, J.; Dhami, M. Ginger: An ethnomedical, chemical and pharmacological review. *Drug Metabol. Drug Interact.* **2001**, *18*, 159–190. [CrossRef] [PubMed]

81. Lakhan, S.; Ford, C.; Tepper, D. *Zingiberaceae* extracts for pain: A systematic review and meta-analysis. *Nutr. J.* **2015**, *14*, 50. [CrossRef] [PubMed]

82. Thomson, M.; Al-Qattan, K.; Al-Sawan, S.; Alnaqeeb, M.; Khan, I.; Ali, M. The use of ginger (*Zingiber officinale* Rosc.) as a potential anti-inflammatory and antithrombotic agent. *Prostaglandins Leukot Essent Fatty Acids* **2002**, *67*, 475–478. [CrossRef] [PubMed]

83. Aimbire, F.; Penna, S.; Rodrigues, M.; Rodrigues, K.; Lopes-Martins, R.; Sertié, J. Effect of hydroalcoholic extract of *Zingiber officinalis* rhizomes on LPS-induced rat airway hyperreactivity and lung inflammation. *Prostaglandins Leukot Essent Fatty Acids* **2007**, *77*, 129–138. [CrossRef] [PubMed]

84. El-Abhar, H.; Hammad, L.; Gawad, H. Modulating effect of ginger extract on rats with ulcerative colitis. *J. Ethnopharmacol.* **2008**, *118*, 367–372. [CrossRef] [PubMed]

85. Podlogar, J.; Verspohl, E. Antiinflammatory effects of ginger and some of its components in human bronchial epithelial (BEAS-2B) cells. *Phytother. Res.* **2012**, *26*, 333–336. [CrossRef] [PubMed]

86. Shim, S.; Kim, S.; Choi, D.; Kwon, Y.; Kwon, J. Anti-inflammatory effects of [6]-shogaol: Potential roles of HDAC inhibition and HSP70 induction. *Food Chem. Toxicol.* **2011**, *49*, 2734–2740. [CrossRef] [PubMed]

87. Shibata, S. A drug over the millennia: Pharmacognosy, chemistry, and pharmacology of licorice. *Yakugaku Zasshi* **2000**, *120*, 849–862. [CrossRef] [PubMed]

88. Farese, R., Jr.; Biglieri, E.; Shackleton, C.; Irony, I.; Gomez-Fontes, R. Licorice-induced hypermineralocorticoidism. *N. Engl. J. Med.* **1991**, *325*, 1223–1227. [CrossRef] [PubMed]

89. Mumoli, N.; Cei, M. Licorice-induced hypokalemia. *Int. J. Cardiol.* **2008**, *124*, e42–44. [CrossRef] [PubMed]

90. Van Uum, S. Liquorice and hypertension. *Neth. J. Med.* **2005**, *63*, 119–120. [PubMed]

91. Palermo, M.; Quinkler, M.; Stewart, P. Apparent mineralocorticoid excess syndrome: An overview. *Arq. Bras. Endocrinol. Metabol.* **2004**, *48*, 687–696. [CrossRef] [PubMed]

92. van Uum, S.; Lenders, J.; Hermus, A. Cortisol, 11β-hydroxysteroid dehydrogenases, and hypertension. *Semin. Vasc. Med.* **2004**, *4*, 121–128. [CrossRef] [PubMed]

93. Walker, B.; Edwards, C. Licorice-induced hypertension and syndromes of apparent mineralocorticoid excess. *Endocrinol. Metab. Clin. N. Am.* **1994**, *23*, 359–377. [CrossRef]

94. Kaneko, T.; Chiba, H.; Horie, N.; Kato, T.; Kobayashi, M.; Hashimoto, K.; Kusama, K.; Sakagami, H. Effect of Scutellariae radix ingredients on prostaglandin E$_2$ production and COX-2 expression by LPS-activated macrophage. *In Vivo* **2009**, *23*, 577–582. [PubMed]

95. Kuo, C.; Chi, C.; Liu, T. The anti-inflammatory potential of berberine in vitro and in vivo. *Cancer Lett.* **2004**, *203*, 127–137. [CrossRef] [PubMed]

96. Kuo, C.; Chi, C.; Liu, T. Modulation of apoptosis by berberine through inhibition of cyclooxygenase-2 and Mcl-1 expression in oral cancer cells. *In Vivo* **2005**, *19*, 247–252. [PubMed]

97. Liang, Y.; Huang, B.; Song, E.; Bai, B.; Wang, Y. Constitutive activation of AMPK α1 in vascular endothelium promotes high-fat diet-induced fatty liver injury: Role of COX-2 induction. *Br. J. Pharmacol.* **2014**, *171*, 498–508. [CrossRef] [PubMed]

98. Leech, M.; Bartold, P. The association between rheumatoid arthritis and periodontitis. *Best Pract. Res. Clin. Rheumatol.* **2015**, *29*, 189–201. [CrossRef] [PubMed]

99. De Pablo, P.; Dietrich, T.; McAlindon, T. Association of periodontal disease and tooth loss with rheumatoid arthritis in the US population. *J. Rheumatol.* **2008**, *35*, 70–76. [PubMed]

100. Zhao, X.; Liu, Z.; Shu, D.; Xiong, Y.; He, M.; Xu, S.; Si, S.; Guo, B. Association of periodontitis with rheumatoid arthritis and the effect of non-surgical periodontal treatment on disease activity in patients with rheumatoid arthritis. *Med. Sci. Monit.* **2018**, *24*, 5802–5810. [CrossRef] [PubMed]

101. Araújo, V.; Melo, I.; Lima, V. Relationship between periodontitis and rheumatoid arthritis: Review of the literature. *Mediators Inflamm.* **2015**, *2015*, 259074. [CrossRef] [PubMed]

102. Kaur, S.; Bright, R.; Proudman, S.; Bartold, P. Does periodontal treatment influence clinical and biochemical measures for rheumatoid arthritis? A systematic review and meta-analysis. *Semin. Arthritis Rheum.* **2014**, *44*, 113–122. [CrossRef] [PubMed]

103. Javed, F.; Ahmed, H.; Mikami, T.; Almas, K.; Romanos, G.; Al-Hezaimi, K. Cytokine profile in the gingival crevicular fluid of rheumatoid arthritis patients with chronic periodontitis. *J. Investig. Clin. Dent.* **2014**, *5*, 1–8. [CrossRef] [PubMed]

104. Erciyas, K.; Sezer, U.; Ustün, K.; Pehlivan, Y.; Kisacik, B.; Senyurt, S.; Tarakçioğlu, M.; Onat, A. Effects of periodontal therapy on disease activity and systemic inflammation in rheumatoid arthritis patients. *Oral Dis.* **2013**, *19*, 394–400. [CrossRef] [PubMed]

105. Gümüş, P.; Buduneli, E.; Bıyıkoğlu, B.; Aksu, K.; Saraç, F.; Nile, C.; Lappin, D.; Buduneli, N. Gingival crevicular fluid, serum levels of receptor activator of nuclear factor-κB ligand, osteoprotegerin, and interleukin-17 in patients with rheumatoid arthritis and osteoporosis and with periodontal disease. *J. Periodontol.* **2013**, *84*, 1627–1637. [PubMed]

106. Silosi, I.; Cojocaru, M.; Foia, L.; Boldeanu, M.; Petrescu, F.; Surlin, P.; Biciusca, V. Significance of circulating and crevicular matrix metalloproteinase-9 in rheumatoid arthritis-chronic periodontitis association. *J. Immunol. Res.* **2015**, *2015*, 218060. [CrossRef] [PubMed]

107. Li, J.; Huang, Z.; Wang, R.; Ma, X.; Zhang, Z.; Liu, Z.; Chen, Y.; Su, Y. Fruit and vegetable intake and bone mass in Chinese adolescents, young and postmenopausal women. *Public Health Nutr.* **2013**, *16*, 78–86. [CrossRef] [PubMed]

108. Hardcastle, A.; Aucott, L.; Fraser, W.; Reid, D.; Macdonald, H. Dietary patterns, bone resorption and bone mineral density in early post-menopausal Scottish women. *Eur. J. Clin. Nutr.* **2011**, *65*, 378–385. [CrossRef] [PubMed]

109. Uchiyama, S.; Yamaguchi, M. Inhibitory effect of beta-cryptoxanthin on osteoclast-like cell formation in mouse marrow cultures. *Biochem. Pharmacol.* **2004**, *67*, 1297–1305. [CrossRef] [PubMed]

110. Matsumoto, C.; Ashida, N.; Yokoyama, S.; Tominari, T.; Hirata, M.; Ogawa, K.; Sugiura, M.; Yano, M.; Inada, M.; Miyaura, C. The protective effects of β-cryptoxanthin on inflammatory bone resorption in a mouse experimental model of periodontitis. *Mol. Med. Rep.* **2013**, *77*, 860–862. [CrossRef] [PubMed]

111. Zeng, W.; Jin, L.; Zhang, F.; Zhang, C.; Liang, W. Naringenin as a potential immunomodulator in therapeutics. *Pharmacol. Res.* **2018**, *135*, 122–126. [CrossRef] [PubMed]

112. Li, Y.; Chen, D.; Chu, C.; Li, S.; Chen, Y.; Wu, C.; Lin, C. Naringenin inhibits dendritic cell maturation and has therapeutic effects in a murine model of collagen-induced arthritis. *J. Nutr. Biochem.* **2015**, *26*, 1467–1478. [CrossRef] [PubMed]

113. La, V.; Tanabe, S.; Grenier, D. Naringenin inhibits human osteoclastogenesis and osteoclastic bone resorption. *J. Periodontal. Res.* **2009**, *44*, 193–198. [CrossRef] [PubMed]

114. Kimira, Y.; Taniuchi, Y.; Nakatani, S.; Sekiguchi, Y.; Kim, H.; Shimizu, J.; Ebata, M.; Wada, M.; Matsumoto, A.; Mano, H. Citrus limonoid nomilin inhibits osteoclastogenesis in vitro by suppression of NFATc1 and MAPK signaling pathways. *Phytomedicine* **2015**, *22*, 1120–1124. [CrossRef] [PubMed]

115. Gu, L.; Deng, W.; Liu, Y.; Jiang, C.; Sun, L.; Sun, X.; Xu, Q.; Zhou, H. Ellagic acid protects Lipopolysaccharide/ D-galactosamine-induced acute hepatic injury in mice. *Int. Immunopharmacol.* **2014**, *22*, 341–345. [CrossRef] [PubMed]

116. Beserra, A.; Calegari, P.; Souza Mdo, C.; Dos Santos, R.; Lima, J.; Silva, R.; Balogun, S.; Martins, D. Gastroprotective and ulcer-healing mechanisms of ellagic acid in experimental rats. *J. Agric. Food Chem.* **2011**, *59*, 6957–6965. [CrossRef] [PubMed]

117. Marín, M.; María Giner, R.; Ríos, J.; Recio, M. Intestinal anti-inflammatory activity of ellagic acid in the acute and chronic dextran sulfate sodium models of mice colitis. *J. Ethnopharmacol.* **2013**, *150*, 925–934. [CrossRef] [PubMed]

118. Mo, J.; Panichayupakaranant, P.; Kaewnopparat, N.; Songkro, S.; Reanmongkol, W. Topical anti-inflammatory potential of standardized pomegranate rind extract and ellagic acid in contact dermatitis. *Phytother. Res.* **2014**, *28*, 629–632. [CrossRef] [PubMed]

119. Allam, G.; Mahdi, E.; Alzahrani, A.; Abuelsaad, A. Ellagic acid alleviates adjuvant induced arthritis by modulation of pro- and anti-inflammatory cytokines. *Cent. Eur. J. Immunol.* **2016**, *41*, 339–349. [CrossRef] [PubMed]

120. Granica, S.; Kłębowska, A.; Kosiński, M.; Piwowarski, J.; Dudek, M.; Kaźmierski, S.; Kiss, A. Effects of *Geum urbanum* L. root extracts and its constituents on polymorphonuclear leucocytes functions. Significance in periodontal diseases. *J. Ethnopharmacol.* **2016**, *188*, 1–12. [CrossRef] [PubMed]

121. Ahmed, S.; Pakozdi, A.; Koch, A. Regulation of interleukin-1β-induced chemokine production and matrix metalloproteinase 2 activation by epigallocatechin-3-gallate in rheumatoid arthritis synovial fibroblasts. *Arthritis Rheum.* **2006**, *54*, 2393–3401. [CrossRef] [PubMed]

122. Yun, H.; Yoo, W.; Han, M.; Lee, Y.; Kim, J.; Lee, S. Epigallocatechin-3-gallate suppresses TNF-α-induced production of MMP-1 and -3 in rheumatoid arthritis synovial fibroblasts. *Rheumatol. Int.* **2008**, *29*, 23–29. [CrossRef] [PubMed]

123. Ahmed, S.; Marotte, H.; Kwan, K.; Ruth, J.; Campbell, P.; Rabquer, B.; Pakozdi, A.; Koch, A. Epigallocatechin-3-gallate inhibits IL-6 synthesis and suppresses transsignaling by enhancing soluble gp130 production. *Proc. Natl. Acad. Sci. USA* **2008**, *105*, 14692–14697. [CrossRef] [PubMed]

124. Gadagi, J.; Chava, V.; Reddy, V. Green tea extract as a local drug therapy on periodontitis patients with diabetes mellitus: A randomized case-control study. *J. Indian Soc. Periodontol.* **2013**, *17*, 198–203. [PubMed]

125. Sekiguchi, Y.; Mano, H.; Nakatani, S.; Shimizu, J.; Wada, M. Effects of the Sri Lankan medicinal plant, *Salacia reticulata*, in rheumatoid arthritis. *Genes Nutr.* **2010**, *5*, 89–96. [CrossRef] [PubMed]

126. Sekiguchi, Y.; Mano, H.; Nakatani, S.; Shimizu, J.; Kataoka, A.; Ogura, K.; Kimira, Y.; Ebata, M.; Wada, M. Mangiferin positively regulates osteoblast differentiation and suppresses osteoclast differentiation. *Mol. Med. Rep.* **2017**, *16*, 1328–1332. [CrossRef] [PubMed]

Permissions

All chapters in this book were first published by MDPI; hereby published with permission under the Creative Commons Attribution License or equivalent. Every chapter published in this book has been scrutinized by our experts. Their significance has been extensively debated. The topics covered herein carry significant findings which will fuel the growth of the discipline. They may even be implemented as practical applications or may be referred to as a beginning point for another development.

The contributors of this book come from diverse backgrounds, making this book a truly international effort. This book will bring forth new frontiers with its revolutionizing research information and detailed analysis of the nascent developments around the world.

We would like to thank all the contributing authors for lending their expertise to make the book truly unique. They have played a crucial role in the development of this book. Without their invaluable contributions this book wouldn't have been possible. They have made vital efforts to compile up to date information on the varied aspects of this subject to make this book a valuable addition to the collection of many professionals and students.

This book was conceptualized with the vision of imparting up-to-date information and advanced data in this field. To ensure the same, a matchless editorial board was set up. Every individual on the board went through rigorous rounds of assessment to prove their worth. After which they invested a large part of their time researching and compiling the most relevant data for our readers.

The editorial board has been involved in producing this book since its inception. They have spent rigorous hours researching and exploring the diverse topics which have resulted in the successful publishing of this book. They have passed on their knowledge of decades through this book. To expedite this challenging task, the publisher supported the team at every step. A small team of assistant editors was also appointed to further simplify the editing procedure and attain best results for the readers.

Apart from the editorial board, the designing team has also invested a significant amount of their time in understanding the subject and creating the most relevant covers. They scrutinized every image to scout for the most suitable representation of the subject and create an appropriate cover for the book.

The publishing team has been an ardent support to the editorial, designing and production team. Their endless efforts to recruit the best for this project, has resulted in the accomplishment of this book. They are a veteran in the field of academics and their pool of knowledge is as vast as their experience in printing. Their expertise and guidance has proved useful at every step. Their uncompromising quality standards have made this book an exceptional effort. Their encouragement from time to time has been an inspiration for everyone.

The publisher and the editorial board hope that this book will prove to be a valuable piece of knowledge for researchers, students, practitioners and scholars across the globe.

List of Contributors

Xiuqin Chen, Eric Banan-Mwine Daliri, Ramachandran Chelliah and Deog-Hwan Oh
Department of Food Science and Biotechnology, College of Agriculture and Life Sciences, Kangwon National University, Chuncheon 200-701, Korea

Elliot Mathieu, Véronique Robert, Vinciane Saint-Criq, Philippe Langella and Muriel Thomas
Micalis Institute, AgroParisTech, INRAE, Université Paris-Saclay, 78350 Jouy-en-Josas, France

Chad W. MacPherson, Jocelyn Belvis, Olivier Mathieu and Thomas A. Tompkins
Rosell Institute for Microbiome and Probiotics, Lallemand Health Solutions Inc., Montreal, QC H4P 2R2, Canada

Izabela Zieniewska
Doctoral Studies, Medical University of Bialystok, 24a M. Sklodowskiej-Curie Street, 15-274 Bialystok, Poland

Mateusz Maciejczyk
Department of Hygiene, Epidemiology and Ergonomics, Medical University of Bialystok, 15-022 Bialystok, Poland

Anna Zalewska
Experimental Dentistry Laboratory, Medical University of Bialystok, 24a M. Sklodowskiej-Curie Street, 15-274 Bialystok, Poland

Hessam Tabeian, Anouk V. ter Linde, Behrouz Zandieh-Doulabi, Vincent Everts and Astrid D. Bakker
Oral Cell Biology, Academic Centre for Dentistry Amsterdam, University of Amsterdam and Vrije Universiteit Amsterdam, 1081 LA Amsterdam, The Netherlands

Frank Lobbezoo
Oral Kinesiology, Academic Centre for Dentistry Amsterdam, University of Amsterdam and Vrije Universiteit Amsterdam, 1081 LA Amsterdam, The Netherlands

Beatriz F. Betti
Oral Cell Biology, Academic Centre for Dentistry Amsterdam, University of Amsterdam and Vrije Universiteit Amsterdam, 1081 LA Amsterdam, The Netherlands
Oral Kinesiology, Academic Centre for Dentistry Amsterdam, University of Amsterdam and Vrije Universiteit Amsterdam, 1081 LA Amsterdam, The Netherlands

Orthodontics, Academic Centre for Dentistry Amsterdam, University of Amsterdam and Vrije Universiteit Amsterdam, 1081 LA Amsterdam, The Netherlands

Cinthya dos Santos Cirqueira
Núcleo de Anatomia Patológica, Instituto Adolfo Lutz, São Paulo 01246-000, Brazil

Teun J. de Vries
Periodontology, Academic Centre for Dentistry Amsterdam, University of Amsterdam and Vrije Universiteit Amsterdam, 1081 LA Amsterdam, The Netherlands

Marije I. Koenders
Rheumatology, Radboud University Medical Center, 6525 GA Nijmegen, The Netherlands

Yukako Edo
Graduate School of Health Sciences, Showa University Graduate School, Yokohama 226-8555, Japan

Amane Otaki
Division of Nursing, Showa University School of Nursing and Rehabilitation Sciences, Yokohama 226-8555, Japan

Kazuhito Asano
Division of Physiology, Showa University School of Nursing and Rehabilitation Sciences, Yokohama 226-8555, Japan

Dorina Lauritano
Department of Medicine and Surgery, Centre of Neuroscience of Milan, University of Milano-Bicocca, 20126 Milan, Italy

Alberta Lucchese and Dario Di Stasio
Multidisciplinary Department of Medical and Dental Specialties, University of Campania- Luigi Vanvitelli, 80138 Naples, Italy

Fedora Della Vella
Interdisciplinary Department of Medicine, University of Bari, 70121 Bari, Italy

Francesca Cura and Annalisa Palmieri
Department of Experimental, Diagnostic and Specialty Medicine, University of Bologna, via Belmoro 8, 40126 Bologna, Italy

Francesco Carinci
Department of Morphology, Surgery and Experimental Medicine, University of Ferrara, 44121 Ferrara, Italy

Masataka Sunagawa, Kojiro Yamaguchi, Mana Tsukada, Nachi Ebihara, Hideshi Ikemoto and Tadashi Hisamitsu
Department of physiology, School of medicine, Showa University, Tokyo 142-8555, Japan

Daisuke Asai and Hideki Nakashima
Department of Microbiology, St. Marianna University School of Medicine, Kawasaki 216-8511, Japan

Taisei Kanamoto
Laboratory of Microbiology, Showa Pharmaceutical University, Machida, Tokyo 194-8543, Japan
Department of Microbiology, St. Marianna University School of Medicine, Kawasaki, Kanagawa 216-8511, Japan

Shigemi Terakubo and Hideki Nakashima
Department of Microbiology, St. Marianna University School of Medicine, Kawasaki, Kanagawa 216-8511, Japan

Yaeko Hara
Second Division of Oral and Maxillofacial Surgery, Department of Diagnostic and Therapeutic Sciences, Meikai University School of Dentistry, 1-1 Keyakidai, Sakado, Saitama 350-0283, Japan

Hiroshi Shiratuchi and Tadayoshi Kaneko
Department of Oral Maxillofacial Surgery, Nihon University School of Dentistry; 1-8-13 Kanda Surugadai, Chiyoda-ku, Tokyo 101-8310, Japan

Hiroshi Sakagami
Meikai University Research Institute of Odontology (M-RIO), 1-1 Keyakidai, Sakado, Saitama 350-0283, Japan

Christian-Alexander Behrendt and Eike Sebastian Debus
Department of Vascular Medicine, University Heart Center Hamburg, University Medical Center Hamburg-Eppendorf, 20251 Hamburg, Germany

Mark Kaschwich
Department of Vascular Medicine, University Heart Center Hamburg, University Medical Center Hamburg-Eppendorf, 20251 Hamburg, Germany
Department of Surgery, University Medical Centre Schleswig-Holstein, Campus Luebeck, Ratzeburger Allee 160, 23538 Luebeck, Germany

Andreas Bayer
Department of Surgery, University Medical Centre Schleswig-Holstein, Campus Luebeck, Ratzeburger Allee 160, 23538 Luebeck, Germany

Guido Heydecke, Udo Seedorf and Ghazal Aarabi
Department of Prosthetic Dentistry, Center for Dental and Oral Medicine, University Medical Center Hamburg-Eppendorf, 20246 Hamburg, Germany

Toshizo Toyama, Takenori Sato and Nobushiro Hamada
Division of Microbiology, Department of Oral Science, Kanagawa Dental University, 82 Inaoka-cho, Yokosuka 238-8580, Japan

Shuji Watanabe
Division of Microbiology, Department of Oral Science, Kanagawa Dental University, 82 Inaoka-cho, Yokosuka 238-8580, Japan
Odoriba Medical Center, Totsuka Green Dental Clinic, 1-10-46 Gumizawa, Totsuka-ku, Yokohama 245-0061, Japan

Mitsuo Suzuki
Division of Microbiology, Department of Oral Science, Kanagawa Dental University, 82 Inaoka-cho, Yokosuka 238-8580, Japan
Dental Design Clinic, 3-7-10 Kita-aoyama, Minato-ku, Tokyo 107-0061, Japan

Akira Morozumi
Morozumi Dental Clinic, 1-3-1 Miyamaedaira, Miyamae-ku, Kawasaki 216-0006, Japan

Hiromichi Yumoto and Masami Ninomiya
Department of Periodontology and Endodontology, Institute of Biomedical Sciences, Tokushima University Graduate School, Tokushima 770-8504, Japan

Katsuhiko Hirota
Department of Medical Hygiene, Dental Hygiene Course, Kochi Gakuen College, Kochi 780-0955, Japan

Kouji Hirao
Department of Conservative Dentistry, Institute of Biomedical Sciences, Tokushima University Graduate School, Tokushima 770-8504, Japan

Keiji Murakami and Hideki Fujii
Department of Oral Microbiology, Institute of Biomedical Sciences, Tokushima University Graduate School, Tokushima 770-8504, Japan

Yoichiro Miyake
Department of Oral Health Sciences, Faculty of Health and Welfare, Tokushima Bunri University, Tokushima, Tokushima 770-8514, Japan

Toshiaki Ara and Norio Sogawa
Department of Dental Pharmacology, Matsumoto Dental University, 1780 Gobara Hirooka, Shiojiri 399-0781, Japan

Sachie Nakatani and Kenji Kobata
Faculty of Pharmacy and Pharmaceutical Sciences, Josai University, 1-1 Keyakidai, Sakado, Saitama 350-0295, Japan

Chiharu Sogawa
Department of Dental Pharmacology, Okayama University Graduate School of Medicine, Dentistry and Pharmaceutical Sciences, 2-5-1 Shikata-cho, Okayama 700-8525, Japan

Index

www.ingramcontent.com/pod-product-compliance
Lightning Source LLC
Chambersburg PA
CBHW080522200326
41458CB00012B/4298

9 781639 276394